American Public Health Association
VITAL AND HEALTH STATISTICS MONOGRAPHS

Infant, Perinatal, Maternal, and Childhood Mortality in the United States

Infant, Perinatal, Maternal, and Childhood Mortality in the United States

SAM SHAPIRO / EDWARD R. SCHLESINGER /
ROBERT E. L. NESBITT, JR.

1968 / HARVARD UNIVERSITY PRESS

Cambridge, Massachusetts

Library of Congress Catalog Card Number 68-29183
Printed in the United States of America

PREFACE

Infant, maternal, and childhood mortality rates were sharply reduced during the first half of the twentieth century: by 1950 the infant mortality rate was one-fourth its level in the early 1900's, and maternal and childhood mortality rates were one-tenth of their earlier levels. Advances in medicine, the expansion and improvement of health facilities, the greater availability of medical and other health personnel, and aggressive action by public and private health and welfare agencies contributed to these declines in mortality. At midcentury there was little reason to expect a major change in the downward trend in mortality, and additional impressive gains might have been expected.

Events have not confirmed this expectation. By 1965 it was possible to look back over a 15-year period in which there had been no sizable decrease in the infant mortality rate. During the 1950's there were years in which the rate increased–a most unusual occurrence in half a century of vital statistics reporting in the United States. This situation has not gone unnoticed. The subject has been examined in the context of international, national, and local area changes in pregnancy loss rates (1-12),[1] and public health agencies have initiated determined measures to accelerate the decline in infant mortality. As this monograph approached publication, provisional infant mortality data appeared that show decreases in the rate for 1966 and 1967 (13, 14). The change is impressive, but it is too soon to judge whether it is the start of a major downward movement in the rate or only a temporary break from the relatively static picture of the 1950's and early 1960's.

While the slowdown in the decline in the infant mortality rate attracted most attention, lack of significant change in maternal and childhood mortality since the middle or late 1950's has also been a cause for concern. Even though maternal mortality risks during pregnancy and in childhood for the country as a whole are very low by any standard, there are still segments of the population having

---

[1]Numbers in parentheses refer to references for each chapter, to be found in the References section following the Appendix.

v

excessively high losses and there is room for improvement in reducing deaths from specific causes.

This monograph consists of four major sections. The first three
deal with infant and perinatal mortality (Part I), maternal mortality
(Part II), and childhood mortality (Part III). The pattern of presentation is the same in each section. Attention is first focused on the
circumstances leading to the current situation and the extent to
which some of the parameters of infant, maternal, and childhood
mortality have altered over the years. Long- and short-term trends,
as well as the basic variables of cause of death, sex of child, color,
and geography, are discussed. In the case of infant mortality, consideration is given to additional risk factors, such as age of mother,
birth order, and prior pregnancy history of the mother. Other components of pregnancy loss and damage among the offspring are also
discussed, since it has been apparent for some time that the attack
on infant and perinatal mortality must concern itself with these
types of loss and damage.

Most of the information presented in this monograph has been
derived from national vital statistics. Where national data were unavailable for examining infant and perinatal mortality, it proved
feasible in several instances to search for important relationships
among the vital statistics for upstate New York.[2] In addition, special studies conducted over the past two decades provide insights
into the epidemiology of pregnancy loss not obtainable from national statistics. Selected data derived from the special investigations have been used in the monograph in an effort to extend
information about variables found in vital statistics. Valuable as
these sources are they leave many questions unanswered and it is
clear that new series of data are urgently needed (15, 16).

While the analysis of mortality data is concerned with conditions
in the United States, comparisons with the situation in selected
countries that have long had comparatively low mortality are included. The final chapter in each of Parts I, II, and III provides a
perspective on the possible future course of mortality in this country. Part IV is devoted to a review of health services, medical and
paramedical manpower, facilities, and medical-care costs in the
United States, with particular emphasis on their relation to obstetrical and pediatric services.

---

[2]"Upstate New York" refers to New York State, excluding New York City.

The authors gratefully acknowledge the important advice received from Dr. I. M. Moriyama, National Center for Health Statistics, at critical junctures in the planning and preparation of the report, and wish to thank Mr. Mortimer Spiegelman, American Public Health Association, whose suggestions strengthened the monograph. Credit is due Mrs. Nancy Ampel for her highly competent preparation of tables and charts from material in a great variety of sources and for her assistance in editing the text.

Except where noted, all the vital statistics for the United States and its various subdivisions were obtained from the annual volumes on vital statistics published by the National Center for Health Statistics, Public Health Service, Department of Health, Education, and Welfare, and from special tabulations prepared by this office as requested for the monograph. Major additions to these data were made possible through the kind permission of the New York State Department of Health to obtain new tabulations of vital statistics for upstate New York. Vital statistics for foreign countries were obtained from the Demographic Yearbook (Thirteenth Issue), 1961, Statistical Office of the United Nations, and from the files of the Statistical Office except where otherwise noted. The authors wish to express their deep appreciation for the efforts made by the staffs of these organizations to facilitate the availability of the data needed. Thanks are also due to other individuals who made data available for the monograph. The specific individuals and their contributions are indicated in the relevant references.

April 1968

Sam Shapiro
Edward R. Schlesinger, M.D.
Robert E. L. Nesbitt, Jr., M.D.

CONTENTS

TABLES

FIGURES

FOREWORD

Rapid advances in medical and allied sciences, changing patterns in medical care and public health programs, an increasingly health-conscious public, and the rising concern of voluntary agencies and government at all levels in meeting the health needs of the people necessitate constant evaluation of the country's health status. Such an evaluation, which is required not only for an appraisal of the current situation, but also to refine present goals and to gauge our progress toward them, depends largely upon a study of vital and health statistics records.

Opportunity to study mortality in depth emerges when a national census furnishes the requisite population data for the computation of death rates in demographic and geographic detail. Prior to the 1960 census of population there had been no comprehensive analysis of this kind. It seemed appropriate, therefore, to develop for intensive study a substantial body of death statistics for a three-year period centered around that census year.

A detailed examination of the country's health status must go beyond an examination of mortality statistics. Many conditions such as arthritis, rheumatism, and mental diseases are much more important as causes of morbidity than of mortality. Also, an examination of health status should not be based solely upon current findings, but should take into account trends and whatever pertinent evidence has been assembled through local surveys and from clinical experience.

The proposal for such an evaluation, to consist of a series of monographs, was made to the Statistics Section of the American Public Health Association in October 1958, and a Committee on Vital and Health Statistics Monographs was authorized. The members of this Committee and of the Editorial Advisory Subcommittee created later are:

Committee on Vital and Health Statistics Monographs

Mortimer Spiegelman, Chairman
Paul M. Densen, D. Sc.
Robert D. Grove, Ph.D.
Clyde V. Kiser, Ph.D.
Felix Moore
George Rosen, M.D., Ph.D.

William H. Stewart, M.D. (withdrew June 1964)
Conrad Taeuber, Ph.D.
Paul Webbink
Donald Young, Ph.D.

Editorial Advisory Subcommittee

Mortimer Spiegelman, Chairman Eliot Freidson, Ph.D. (withdrew
Duncan Clark, M.D.   February 1964)
E. Gurney Clark, M.D.   Brian MacMahon, M.D., Ph.D.
Jack Elinson, Ph.D.   Colin White, Ph.D.

The early history of this undertaking is described in a paper that was presented at the 1962 Annual Conference of the Milbank Memorial Fund.[1] The Committee on Vital and Health Statistics Monographs selected the topics to be included in the series and also suggested candidates for authorship. The frame of reference was extended by the Committee to include other topics in vital and health statistics than mortality and morbidity, namely fertility, marriage, and divorce. Conferences were held with authors to establish general guidelines for the preparation of the manuscripts.

Support for this undertaking in its preliminary stages was received from the Rockefeller Foundation, the Milbank Memorial Fund, and the Health Information Foundation. Major support for the required tabulations, for writing and editorial work, and for the related research of the monograph authors was provided by the United States Public Health Service (Research Grant CH 00075, formerly GM 08262). Acknowledgment should also be made to the Metropolitan Life Insurance Company for the facilities and time that were made available to Mr. Spiegelman, now retired from its service, who proposed and administered the undertaking and served as general editor. The National Center for Health Statistics, under the supervision of Dr. Grove and Miss Alice M. Hetzel, undertook the sizable tasks of planning and carrying out the extensive mortality tabulations for the period 1959–1961. Dr. Taeuber arranged for the cooperation of the Bureau of the Census at all stages of the project in many ways, principally by furnishing the required population data used in computing death rates and by undertaking a large number of varied special tabulations. As the sponsor of the project, the American Public Health Association

[1] Mortimer Spiegelman, "The Organization of the Vital and Health Statistics Monograph Program," *Emerging Techniques in Population Research*, Proceedings of the 1962 Annual Conference of the Milbank Memorial Fund (New York: Milbank Memorial Fund, 1963), p. 230. See also Mortimer Spiegelman, "The Demographic Viewpoint in the Vital and Health Statistics Monographs Project of the American Public Health Association," *Demography*, vol. 3, No. 2 (1966), p. 574.

furnished assistance through Dr. Thomas R. Hood, its Deputy Executive Director.

Because of the great variety of topics selected for monograph treatment, authors were given an essentially free hand to develop their manuscripts as they desired. Accordingly, the authors of the individual monographs bear full responsibility for their manuscripts, and their opinions and statements do not necessarily represent the viewpoints of the American Public Health Association or of the agencies with which they are affiliated.

Berwyn F. Mattison, M.D.
Executive Director
American Public Health Association

NOTES ON TABLES

1. Symbols used in tables of data:
    - --- Data not available;
    - ... Category not applicable;
    - - Quantity zero;
    - 0.0 Quantity more than zero but less than 0.05.
2. Geographic classification.[1]
    a. Standard Metropolitan Statistical Areas (SMSA's): except in the New England States, "an SMSA is a county or a group of contiguous counties which contains at least one city of 50,000 inhabitants or more or 'twin cities' with a combined population of at least 50,000 in the 1960 census. In addition, contiguous counties are included in an SMSA if, according to specified criteria, they are (a) essentially metropolitan in character and (b) socially and economically integrated with the central city or cities." In New England, the Division of Vital Statistics of the National Center for Health Statistics uses, instead of the definition just cited, Metropolitan State Economic Areas (MSEA's) established by the Bureau of the Census, which are made up of county units.
    b. Metropolitan and nonmetropolitan: "Counties which are included in SMSA's or, in New England, MSEA's are called metropolitan counties; all other counties are classified as nonmetropolitan."
    c. Metropolitan counties may be separated into those containing at least one central city of 50,000 inhabitants or more or twin cities as specified previously, and into metropolitan counties without a central city.

[1] *Vital Statistics of the United States*, 1960 (Washington, D. C.: National Center for Health Statistics, 1963), Vol. 2 (*Mortality*), Part A, Section 7, p. 8.

Part I
Infant and Perinatal Mortality

1 / TRENDS AND RECENT STATUS

Trends in Infant Mortality

General Trends

Mortality in the first year of life was a fairly common experience at the beginning of the twentieth century. Although precise data are not available, it seems certain that at least 10 percent of the newborn died in infancy (Fig. 1.1). This was viewed as an intolerable situation that called for determined remedial action. By 1935 the infant death rate was about half that of the early 1900's. Between the mid-1930's and 1950 the rate was again greatly reduced (Appendix Table I.1a). The annual rate of decline was 4.7 percent, but year-to-year changes were very uneven: a few years would go by with comparatively minor changes, and then there would be a marked drop.[1] An extreme example of this is found in the World War II period, when the infant mortality rate decreased only about 5 percent from 1942 to 1945. In the immediate postwar years the drop was three times as great.

After 1950 the infant mortality rate began to level off. At first it might have been assumed that this was another temporary situation, but in time, it became clear that a fundamental change had occurred in the course of the infant mortality rate. Over the entire period 1951–64 the rate of decline was 0.9 percent per year, or a small fraction of the annual rate of change in the preceding period. Furthermore, some of the year-to-year fluctuations involved important increases in the infant mortality rate. It is only in the very recent period of 1966 and 1967 that there has been a significant decrease in infant mortality. The change was from 24.8 per 1,000 in 1965 to 22.1 per 1,000 in 1967 (provisional), the largest 2-year decline in almost 20 years.

Detailed consideration of changes in trend in infant mortality is restricted in this chapter to the period from the mid-1930's to the early 1960's. Data for the United States as a whole have been available only since 1933, when all states were included in the birth and death registration areas (1).[2] The birth registration area was

---

[1] Annual rates of decline were obtained by fitting straight lines by the method of least squares to the logarithms of the death rates. From the slopes of these fitted lines the annual rates of decline or increase (in percents) are derived. All rates of change are given in Fig. 1.5.

[2] Numbers in parentheses refer to references for each chapter, to be found in the References section following the Appendix.

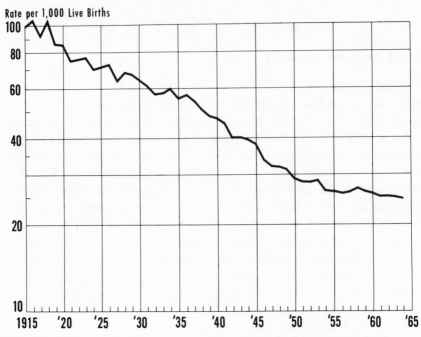

Fig. 1.1. Infant mortality rates, unadjusted: United States, 1915–64.

Source: National Center for Health Statistics, *Vital Statistics of the United States*, annual volumes.

Notes: Alaska included from 1959 and Hawaii from 1960. Unadjusted rates are infant deaths during the year per 1,000 live births occurring in the same year.

established by the Bureau of the Census in 1915, comprising ten states and the District of Columbia in which the registration of live births was relatively complete.[3] Periodically other states were added to the area as they met the minimum requirement of 90 percent completeness of birth registration. Generally the states that entered the area late have had comparatively high infant mortality rates.

Incompleteness of birth registration persisted as a serious problem in large sections of the country long after 1933, and it was not until the birth registration test of 1950 showed that 98 percent of the live births were being registered that the issue could be dismissed as inconsequential for the United States as a whole (2). There is no direct evidence about the relation between the completeness of live birth and of infant death registrations. The assumption often made

[3] The death registration area was established in 1900 for the annual collection of mortality statistics.

is that they are of the same order of magnitude and therefore that the errors cancel each other when rates are computed. However, this may be less true for very early infant deaths than for deaths later in infancy. Notwithstanding changes in registration completeness, inferences about the course of the infant mortality rate since the mid-1930's can be drawn with a fairly high degree of accuracy from data based on reported events.

Another point to bear in mind is that the discussion of trend in this chapter is in terms of conventional infant mortality rates, that is, the number of deaths under 1 year of age in a particular year related to the number of live births in that year. During a period of stability in annual number of live births, the rate closely approximates the risk of mortality in each of the years. A sharp increase in live births during a given year would result in a corresponding artificial decrease in the infant mortality rate during the subsequent year. Under such circumstances, as occurred in the immediate post-World War II period, a decrease in mortality would be overstated by conventional rates. The reverse would occur in the presence of a sharp decrease in number of live births (3).

Various approaches have been taken to remove the artificial effect of changing numbers of births and thereby to obtain a more accurate measure of the risk of death under 1 year of age in a calendar year. One commonly used method allocates deaths in a particular year to related live births in that year and the previous year to derive an adjusted infant mortality rate. Another method utilizes a cohort approach in which live births during a particular time period are followed to the end of the first year of life (4). The infant mortality rate is calculated by dividing the cumulated number of deaths by the number of live births in the cohort. It differs conceptually from other rates in that the rate for a year reflects mortality conditions over the 2-year period the cohort has to be followed to identify all infant deaths.

Table 1.1 shows the three types of rates, the unadjusted, the adjusted, and the cohort, for the time period 1935–63 (and the unadjusted rate for 1964). Conclusions about general changes in the direction of the infant mortality rate are the same regardless of the set of rates used. A closer view of the World War II period reveals some differences worth mentioning. Decreases between 1940 and 1945 appear more regular in the adjusted rate than in the

Table 1.1   Infant mortality rates, unadjusted, adjusted and cohort: United States, 1935-64.

Year	Unadjusted rate	Adjusted rate	Cohort rate	Year	Unadjusted rate	Adjusted rate	Cohort rate
1964	24.8			1949	31.3	31.4	30.8
1963	25.2	25.2	25.0	1948	32.0	31.8	31.9
1962	25.3	25.2	25.3	1947	32.2	32.8	32.0
1961	25.3	25.3	25.2	1946	33.8	34.6	34.6
1960	26.0	26.0	25.9	1945	38.3	38.1	37.0
1959	26.4	26.4	26.3	1944	39.8	39.4	39.0
1958	27.1	27.0	27.0	1943	40.4	40.7	39.7
1957	26.3	26.4	26.5	1942	40.4	41.2	41.3
1956	26.0	26.1	26.2	1941	45.3	45.9	44.5
1955	26.4	26.4	26.4	1940	47.0	47.4	47.7
1954	26.6	26.7	26.5	1939	48.0	48.0	47.3
1953	27.8	27.8	27.5	1938	51.0	51.4	50.5
1952	28.4	28.5	28.4	1937	54.4	54.7	53.3
1951	28.4	28.6	28.5	1936	57.1	57.1	57.7
1950	29.2	29.2	29.3	1935	55.7	55.7	54.9

Sources: Guralnick, L. and Winter, E. A note on cohort infant mortality rates. Public Health Reports, Vol. 80, No. 8, August, 1965; unpublished data, Division of Vital Statistics, National Center for Health Statistics; Annual volumes Vital Statistics of the United States, National Center for Health Statistics, Public Health Service, Washington.

Note: Alaska included beginning 1959, and Hawaii, 1960. Unadjusted rates are infant deaths during the year per 1,000 live births occurring in the same year; adjusted rates allocate deaths in a particular year to related live births in that year and the previous year; cohort rates are computed by observing a cohort of live births until all members are 1 year of age and dividing the number of deaths occurring in this cohort by the number of live births.

unadjusted, and the large decrease during 1946 already noted is dampened in the adjusted rate series. After 1948 both sets of rates are very similar. The cohort rates have an individuality of their own. In 1940 they show an increase instead of a decrease; the following year the drop is twice as great as in the other series of rates; and, in the immediate postwar period, the decreases in 1946 and 1947 are very similar. Afterwards, the cohort rates are almost identical with the unadjusted and the adjusted rates.

Age at Death
The trend in the infant mortality rate is the resultant of widely different trends in mortality at various ages during infancy. Selected for analysis are three age groupings in the neonatal period (under 1 day, 1–6 days, and 7–27 days) and two age groupings in the post-neonatal period (1–5 months and 6–11 months). These

provide a fairly complete basis for understanding changes in mortality that have taken place throughout infancy (Fig. 1.2).[4]

Mortality in the first day of life decreased between 1935 and 1951 rather steadily but at a substantially slower rate (2.9 percent per annum) than for the entire first year.[5] Then it leveled off, and from 1955 it began to increase slightly. By 1964 there was still no indication that the rate of loss in the first day after birth had resumed its former downward trend. In the balance of the first week of life (1–6 days) the mortality rate followed a course similar to that of the rate for under 1 day until the early 1950's, when, instead of increasing, it continued its slow downward movement (2.0 percent). After the first week the trend in the mortality rate showed great variability. At ages 7–27 days there were three different patterns. Between 1935 and 1945 the mortality rate declined at a fairly rapid rate (4.5 percent). This was followed by even larger reductions in the immediate postwar period. After 1950 the rate of decrease slowed down and was not much greater than at ages 1–6 days (2.8 percent).

The rate of decline in the mortality rate from 1935 to 1945 was larger in the post-neonatal period than at earlier ages. At ages 1–5 months the annual rate of decline was 5.4 percent. Following a sharp decrease in mortality immediately after World War II, the mortality rate at ages 1–5 months followed an erratic downward course until the mid-1950's. The precise year when the downward trend ended cannot be determined, but for purposes of the current discussion 1956 has been selected. In the next 2 years the mortality rate increased. Small decreases in 1959–61 brought the rate back to the 1955–56 figures, where it remained almost stationary from 1961 to 1964. The course of the mortality rate at ages 6–11 months resembles that at ages 1–5 months except that the decrease in each period has been greater.

Another way of examining changes in the mortality rate over time is to compare aggregate increases and decreases that occurred in successive periods. For this purpose two ten-year intervals are

[4] All rates in this section are obtained by relating deaths in a year to births in the same year. The previously discussed effect of changes in the number of births between adjacent years varies with age at death; it is negligible during the first month following birth, but it becomes appreciable in the post-neonatal period. The 1945–47 period is most affected by this situation, and the sharp drop in the single year from 1945 to 1946 at ages 1–5 months and 6–11 months would be dampened in a series of rates adjusted for changing numbers of births.

[5] All percentage changes in this section are per annum.

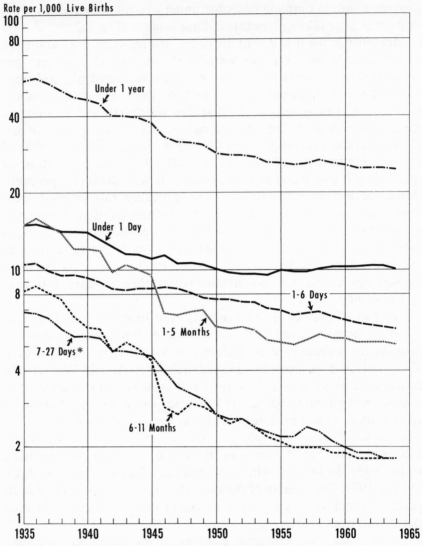

Fig. 1.2. Infant mortality rates by age: United States, 1935–64.

Source: National Center for Health Statistics, *Vital Statistics of the United States*, annual volumes.

Note: Alaska and Hawaii included from 1959.

*Rates for ages 7–29 days for the period 1935–48.

considered, the 1940 and 1950 decades, and changes for age at death are presented in greater detail than previously. It will be noted in Table 1.2 that during the 1940 decade, mortality in the first day after birth decreased by 26 percent; for the next 2 days the

Table 1.2   Percent changes in infant mortality rates by age and color:
United States, selected decennium periods

Age	Total		White		Nonwhite	
	Percent Decrease		Percent Decrease		Percent Decrease	
	1939-41 to 1949-51	1949-51 to 1959-61	1939-41 to 1949-51	1949-51 to 1959-61	1939-41 to 1949-51	1949-51 to 1959-61
Under 1 year	36.6	12.6	36.7	15.8	38.7	6.6
Under 1 day	26.4	+ 1.7	27.8	1.4	19.8	+ 11.6
1 - 2 days	10.7	13.2	8.8	15.0	21.8	7.0
3 - 6 days	27.5	26.1	26.7	27.3	33.3	25.5
7 - 13 days	43.3	29.1	43.3	32.1	45.7	25.2
14 - 27 days	53.7	25.7	55.0	31.4	51.8	15.8
28 - 59 days[1]	45.5	10.9	48.1	16.3	40.2	4.8
2 months	48.2	8.7	50.6	15.3	42.8	+ 0.7
3 months	48.4	16.3	49.6	23.3	47.4	5.0
4 months	49.2	23.0	50.2	31.1	49.2	9.9
5 months	50.8	25.9	52.5	32.9	48.7	16.0
6 - 8 months	54.0	31.4	54.5	36.5	55.3	24.2
9 - 11 months	58.5	31.5	58.6	35.2	60.3	26.6

Source: Annual volumes Vital Statistics of the United States, National Center
for Health Statistics, Public Health Service, Washington.

[1]In 1939-41, this category refers to deaths at age "one month."

decrease was much smaller, only 11 percent; and in the balance of
the first week of life the decline was 28 percent.   Thereafter the
percent decrease rose rapidly, and from the second week of life to
the end of the first year the rate was cut in half.   In the 1950 decade
the increase in mortality for under 1 day was followed by decreases
at 1 and 2 days of life which were similar to the changes in the
1940's; the relative size of the decrease in the balance of the first
week also paralleled those a decade earlier.   Immediately after the
first week and at every age to the end of the first year of life, the
decreases in the mortality rate during the 1950 decade lagged behind those in the 1940's.

Sex and Color
The trend in the infant mortality rate has been very similar for male
and female births (Fig. 1.3).   It is clear that the circumstances that
led to reductions in infant mortality did not favor one sex group
over the other in either the neonatal or post-neonatal period.
    The rates for white and nonwhite groups present a far different
situation.   Mortality trends for white infants closely parallel the

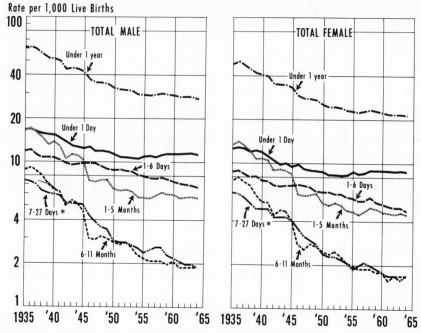

Fig. 1.3. Infant mortality rates by age and sex: United States, 1935–64.

Source: National Center for Health Statistics, *Vital Statistics of the United States*, annual volumes.

Note: Alaska and Hawaii included from 1959.

*Rates for ages 7–29 for the period 1935–48.

trends previously presented for all groups combined (Figs. 1.4 and 1.5). The only difference of any consequence is a slightly greater decrease in the death rate since 1950 for the white group than for the total population.

Until 1950 the rate of decrease in the loss during the first year of life was at least as great among the nonwhite births as the white. Since then the slowdown in the rate of decline has been more severe in the mortality rate for the nonwhite group. Larger differences than those suggested by the total infant mortality rate are found in the trends by age at death. Between 1935 and 1951 substantial decreases in mortality in the first day of life were scored by the white group; among nonwhite infants the decrease in the rate of loss under 1 day stopped in 1943. More recently—since 1952—the rate of increase in mortality at this age has been greater for the nonwhite than the white infants.

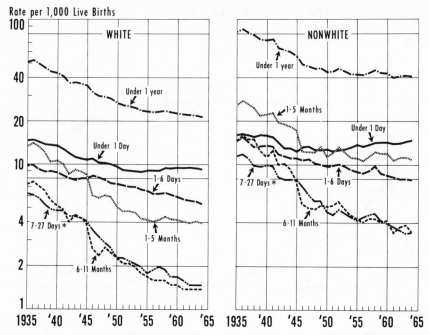

Fig. 1.4. Infant mortality rates by age, separately for white and nonwhite: United States, 1935–64.

Source: National Center for Health Statistics, *Vital Statistics of the United States*, annual volumes.

Notes: Alaska and Hawaii included from 1959. New Jersey excluded from data by color for 1962–63.

*Rates for ages 7–29 days for the period 1935–48.

A question might be raised about the comparative accuracy of the mortality trends for under 1 day among white and nonwhite children. Improvement in reporting of live births, accompanied by relatively more complete registration of deaths in early infancy, could artificially increase the mortality rate. It might be argued that this would be more significant for the rates among nonwhite babies in view of the reduction in the lag between nonwhite and white persons in the use of hospitals and in the completeness of registration of live births. These considerations are important, but it is unlikely that they completely explain events in the more recent period. The same situation is found in many areas of the country where the problems of under-registration and accuracy of reporting have been inconsequential for a long time. Another possibility is

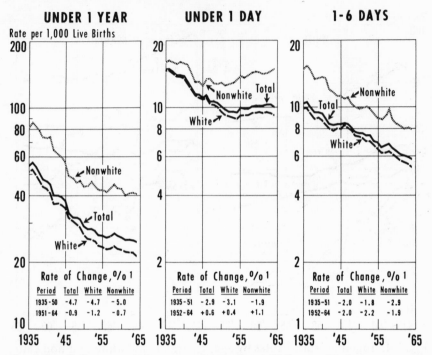

Fig. 1.5a. Infant mortality rates by color within specified age groups: United States, 1935–64.

Source: National Center for Health Statistics, *Vital Statistics of the United States*, annual volumes.

Notes: Alaska and Hawaii included from 1959. New Jersey excluded from data by color for 1962–63.

[1] Annual rate of change obtained by fitting least-square lines to logarithms of rates for specified time period and taking anti-log of slope of fitted line.

that with improvement in medical care there has been a shift in the timing of the death of some infants from the prenatal to the immediate postnatal period and that this has been more common among the nonwhite than the white births. This, too, is highly speculative, and it might be more fruitful to seek other explanations for the difference in trends between the rates for white and nonwhite infants.

Following the first day of birth and continuing until the end of the neonatal period, comparisons of mortality trends between the two color groups show a somewhat different set of relationships from those observed in under 1 day. There is some indication that the rate of decline in the 1–6 day age period was, at one time,

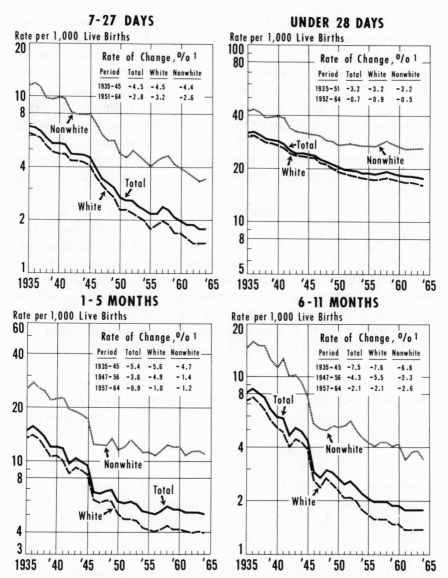

Fig. 1.5b. Infant mortality rates by color within specified age groups: United States, 1935–64.

Source: National Center for Health Statistics, *Vital Statistics of the United States*, annual volumes.

Notes: Alaska and Hawaii included from 1959. New Jersey excluded from data by color for 1962–63.

[1] Annual rate of change obtained by fitting least-square lines to logarithms of rates for specified time period and taking anti-log of slope of fitted line. For the period 1935–48 the ages at death were "7–29 days" and "under 1 month," respectively.

greater for the nonwhite than for white infants and that in more recent years the change in the loss rate has been similar in both groups. At 7–27 days the decline in losses was almost identical for white and nonwhite infants from 1935 through 1945. Since 1947 the rate of decline has been moderately greater among white births.

Taking the neonatal period as a whole, the reduction in death rates among the nonwhite births kept pace with the rate of decline among the white births until about 1951. Subsequently mortality in both groups decreased only slightly, with the rate of decline slowing down somewhat more among nonwhite infants than among the white.

Both groups made substantial gains in lowering post-neonatal mortality until the mid-1940's. The sharp drop in the death rate immediately after the war was shared by white and nonwhite infants. Since then the trends in the mortality rates for white and nonwhite births have differed. For almost a decade the rates among the white infants at ages 1–5 months and 6–11 months continued to decline briskly. The tendency of the rates to level off started about 1954 or 1955. In contrast, among the nonwhite infants the rate at 1–5 months flattened out shortly after the war ended, and this situation has persisted through 1964. Mortality rates at 6–11 months followed an erratic course among the nonwhite births after 1946. Increases in the rate were experienced for several years, but there have also been decreases and the trend has been generally downward.

Measures of aggregate change in the 1940 decade illustrate the high degree of consistency between the white and nonwhite groups in the large reductions in loss during the 1940's throughout most of infancy (Table 1.2). The only departures are in the first 3 days of life; under 1 day white infants experienced somewhat more of a reduction in mortality, but at ages 1–2 days the decrease was greater among the nonwhite. Data on overall changes by detailed age further emphasize that, except for a short period during the first week following birth, reductions in the 1950's lagged considerably behind those in the 1940's for both white and nonwhite infants. One additional point becomes clear: among nonwhite infants the only ages at which there were impressive gains in reducing mortality during the 1950's were 3–6 days, 7–13 days, and 6–11 months.

Cause of Death[6]

The decline in the overall infant mortality rate during the period prior to 1950 is generally accepted as reflecting the combined effect of advances in medicine, better maternal and child care, and improvement in medical facilities and economic and environmental conditions in the United States. About half of the decrease between 1939 and 1950 resulted from the lowering of mortality from infective and parasitic diseases, influenza and pneumonia, and infections of the digestive system (Fig. 1.6 and Appendix Table I.2a). The large decrease in the rate soon after World War II is due mainly to the reduction in mortality from these causes, a circumstance which is attributed largely to the increased availability of antibiotics in the postwar period.

This is one of the few instances in which a decrease in the infant mortality rate can be associated with a specific factor. Even here there is reason to moderate the conclusion. In the case of the rates for infective and parasitic diseases and for influenza and pneumonia the sharp drop after the war accentuated a decline that was already in progress. In the case of infections of the digestive system the large size of the reduction in the rate that followed the end of the war could be traced in part to the elimination of the increase in mortality from these conditions that occurred during the war.

Comparatively small but significant reductions in the mortality rate for "certain other diseases of early infancy" also occurred prior to 1950. These are the causes of death that are heavily weighted with conditions related to the development of the child in utero and conditions affecting the delivery. Difficult as it is to identify the contributions toward the decrease in mortality from infectious diseases made by specific medical and economic circumstances, the problem becomes even more complex in dealing with this class of

[6] Trends of cause-of-death rates start with the year 1939 rather than 1935 to reduce the effect of changes in rules for classification of causes of death that occurred during the 1930's. Since then there has been one fundamental change in classification rules that affects grouping of causes of death, that requiring mention of "immaturity" or "prematurity." In the Fifth Revision of the International Statistical Classification, 1938, prematurity was given priority over other diseases of early infancy, except injury at birth (5, 6). In the Sixth (1948) and Seventh (1955) Revisions, prematurity or immaturity was made a secondary axis of classification. The effect of this change is to understate rates for the following categories of disease in the period 1939–48 as compared with rates for succeeding years: 762, 763, 764, 768–774 (Seventh Revision, see Appendix Table I.2a). Similarly, 1939–48 rates for "immaturity, unqualified" are about 80 percent above the rates that would have been obtained under the classification rules of the Sixth and Seventh Revisions.

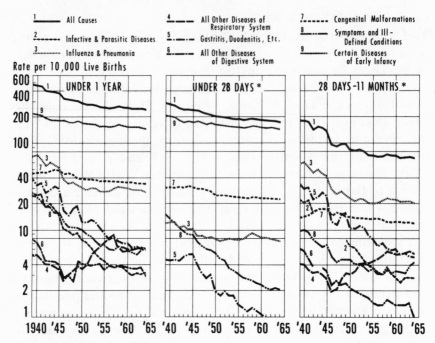

Fig. 1.6. Infant mortality rates for selected causes of death by age: United States, 1939–64.

Source: National Center for Health Statistics, Vital Statistics of the United States, annual volumes.

Notes: Data not available by age at death for 1943–48 for "infective and parasitic diseases" and for 1943 for "all other diseases of digestive system." "Pneumonia of the newborn" included with "influenza and pneumonia"; "diarrhea of the newborn" included with "gastritis, duodenitis, etc." Alaska included from 1959 and Hawaii from 1960.

*Prior to 1949 these categories refer to deaths at ages "under 1 month" and "1–11 months," respectively.

causes of death. Public health programs pertaining to the prenatal and postnatal periods appear to be central factors, although quantitative confirmation of the effectiveness of specific measures is not available.

Since 1950 the infant mortality rates for the infective diseases and infections of the digestive system have declined still further, but the rates for respiratory diseases have not. Actually the combined rate for acute upper respiratory infections, bronchitis, and other diseases of the respiratory system (excluding influenza and pneumonia) has increased. To a large extent this rise reflects interest stimulated in the late 1940's and in the 1950's in hyaline membrane and abnormal pulmonary ventilation as stated causes of death. In 1958 classification changes transferred hyaline membrane from the category of other respiratory diseases to ill-defined diseases peculiar to early infancy. The rate for "other respiratory diseases" was thereby appreciably reduced but even so it has remained at a higher level than in the 1940's.

The increased attention given to "other respiratory diseases" in no way diminishes the importance of the rate for influenza and pneumonia, which still account for more infant deaths than all other infectious diseases combined. The lack of significant decreases in this rate over the past 10–15 years has been one of the major reasons for the comparative stability in the post-neonatal mortality rate.

The infant mortality rate for the category "certain diseases of early infancy" decreased slowly and irregularly for several years after 1950 and then flattened out. This is, of course, indicative of the general lack of progress in reducing mortality in early infancy.

An important feature of the cause-of-death trends is that the rate for congenital anomalies has changed little in almost a quarter of a century. The rate of decline in this cause of death has consistently lagged behind the decline in the total infant mortality rate both during the period when the infant mortality rate fell rapidly and for the past decade, when it decreased only moderately.

Examination of the causes that comprise "certain diseases of early infancy" indicates that the overall picture shown by this category is a composite of divergent trends. The rates for birth injuries, hemolytic diseases, and immaturity unqualified decreased by about 30 percent during the 1950's. There was an increase in the rates for postnatal asphyxia and atelectasis and ill-defined peculiar to early infancy. In view of the suspected changes in styles of reporting, it is not known to what extent the trend in the rate for most of these rates is real. An exception is hemolytic disease of the newborn, which is specific and which is known to have benefited from the increased use of exchange blood transfusions in the early neonatal period.

There is a remarkable similarity in the trends of specific causes of death for male and female infants. This parallelism holds for almost all cause groups, both those related to prenatal conditions and those having their etiology in postnatal environmental circumstances. The consistency of the trends could result from innate constitutional qualities of males and females, which are not affected by improvements in general or by specific health measures.

Trends in cause-of-death rates for white and nonwhite infants also have some elements in common (Fig. 1.7). In both color groups the loss rates from infective and parasitic diseases have dropped to a tenth of what they were 20–25 years ago. The long-term decline in mortality from pneumonia and influenza and infectious diseases of the digestive system has also been impressive for both white and nonwhite infants. However, the magnitude of the decline in the rates for these diseases has not been the same in the two color groups. During the period of rapid reduction in mortality from pneumonia and influenza (from 1939 until shortly after World War II) the relative gain was greater among white infants. Subsequently the differences in rates of decline increased. The

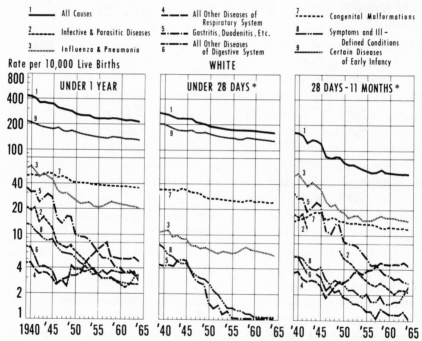

Fig. 1.7a. Infant mortality rates for selected causes of death by age and color: United States, 1939–64.

Source: National Center for Health Statistics, *Vital Statistics of the United States*, annual volumes.

Notes: Data not available by age at death for 1943–48 for "infective and parasitic diseases" and for 1943 for "all other diseases of digestive system." "Pneumonia of the newborn" included with "influenza and pneumonia"; "diarrhea of the newborn" included with "gastritis, duodenitis, etc." Alaska included from 1959 and Hawaii from 1960. New Jersey excluded from data by color for 1962–63.

*Prior to 1949 these categories refer to deaths at ages "under 1 month" and "1–11 months," respectively.

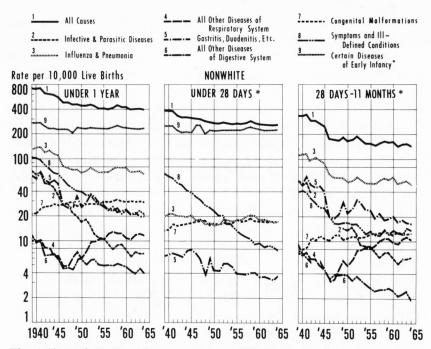

1 ——— All Causes	4 —··— All Other Diseases of Respiratory System	7 ------ Congenital Malformations
2 ------ Infective & Parasitic Diseases	5 —·—·— Gastritis, Duodenitis, Etc.	8 —···— Symptoms and Ill-Defined Conditions
3 ·········· Influenza & Pneumonia	6 —·—·— All Other Diseases of Digestive System	9 ·········· Certain Diseases of Early Infancy*

Rate per 10,000 Live Births   NONWHITE

UNDER 1 YEAR   UNDER 28 DAYS *   28 DAYS–11 MONTHS *

1940 '45 '50 '55 '60 '65   '40 '45 '50 '55 '60 '65   '40 '45 '50 '55 '60 '65

Fig. 1.7b. Infant mortality rates for selected causes of death by age and color: United States, 1939–64.

Source: National Center for Health Statistics, *Vital Statistics of the United States*, annual volumes.

Notes: Data not available by age at death for 1943–48 for "infective and parasitic diseases" and for 1943 for "all other diseases of digestive system." "Pneumonia of the newborn" included with "influenza and pneumonia"; "diarrhea of the newborn" included with "gastritis, duodenitis, etc." Alaska included from 1959 and Hawaii from 1960. New Jersey excluded from data by color for 1962–63.

*Prior to 1949 these categories refer to deaths at ages "under 1 month" and "1–11 months," respectively.

death rate due to pneumonia and influenza among nonwhite children leveled off several years before the rate among the white. As for the loss from infectious diseases of the digestive system, major decreases were scored during the 1950's in the rate for the white infants. Among the nonwhite, there were also important decreases in the rate for these diseases, but the decline was interrupted by periodic large-scale increases.

It is apparent that the rates for the more important causes of death reflecting the influence of postnatal environmental conditions are substantially lower in both color groups than in the early 1940's. However, except for the infective and parasitic diseases the gap between the rates for white and nonwhite infants has widened. In 1964 mortality from pneumonia and influenza was higher among the nonwhite births than the corresponding rate of loss among the white births 25 years earlier; mortality from infectious diseases of the digestive system showed almost a 20-year lag for the nonwhite infants. These observations must be qualified because of the changes in the proportion of the deaths in the nonwhite group that were attributed to ill-defined diseases. In 1939–41 about 14 percent were so classified; in 1959–61 only 5 percent. The proportions of deaths so classified in the white group have consistently been very low: 1 percent in 1959–61 and 3 percent 20 years earlier.

Congenital malformation mortality rates for white and nonwhite infants have undergone only slight changes over the years. The rates have been lower among the nonwhite group, although color differences in these rates are now much smaller than years ago. While the rate among nonwhite infants has slowly increased, the rate among white has slowly decreased. The classification issue relating to ill-defined diseases that was previously discussed may also apply to the long-term comparison of congenital malformation rates, but the more recent courses of these rates could hardly be affected.

Generally, trends in mortality rates among white children from "certain diseases of early infancy" followed the same pattern as all deaths in the first few weeks of infancy. This does not hold for the long-term trend among nonwhite infants. For example, between the early 1940's and the early 1960's there was no change in the mortality rate attributed to certain diseases of early infancy among nonwhite children, but their total neonatal mortality rate decreased by about one-fourth. This apparently anomalous situation resulted from the shift of large numbers of deaths among nonwhite infants from the category of ill-defined causes of death to categories included under certain diseases of early infancy.

Recent Status of Infant Mortality

Age, Sex, and Color
In 1964 the infant mortality rate in the United States was 24.8 per 1,000 live births. About two-fifths (41 percent) of the deaths were concentrated in the first 24 hours after birth (Appendix Table

I.3). Another 24 percent of the deaths occurred during the balance of the first week, and 7 percent in the second through the fourth week of life. The risk of dying decreased with each succeeding month and the loss in the last month of infancy was only a fraction of 1 percent of the total deaths.

Close examination of the changes in the mortality rates as age progresses during infancy reveals a number of interesting turning points in the rates of decrease. The decrease in the mortality rate immediately after the first day of life is extraordinarily large (Fig. 1.8). Throughout the balance of the first week of life each succes-

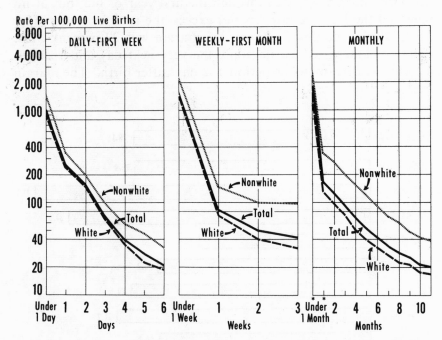

Fig. 1.8. Infant mortality rates by color and detailed age: United States, 1964.

Source: National Center for Health Statistics, *Vital Statistics of the United States, 1964.*
*These categories refer to deaths at ages "under 28 days" and "28-59 days," respectively.

sive day shows a marked decrease in the risk of mortality, although there seems to be a definite slowing down in the rate of decline starting with age 4 days. Decreases in the mortality rate continue as the child advances in age after the first week. After 7 months of age, the monthly rate of decrease in the rate is comparatively small and only a fraction of the declines earlier in the post-neonatal period. Characterizing the changes at the end of the first year as "small" should not obscure the fact that they are highly significant. The point is that the decreases are between short age intervals, that is, one month of age to the next month, and even the 6 percent decrease that occurs between 10 and 11 months of age, if continued for a full year, would represent a major decline.

Chances of dying during infancy were 29 percent greater among males than females during 1959–61. The margin between the mortality rates for males and females varied appreciably as the newborn infant progressed through the first year of life, but at no point did the loss rate for females exceed the rate for males (Fig. 1.9). During the first 24 hours, the margin was 29 percent. The differential increased substantially the very next day and reached its peak, 41 percent, in the period 1–2 days after birth. The margin

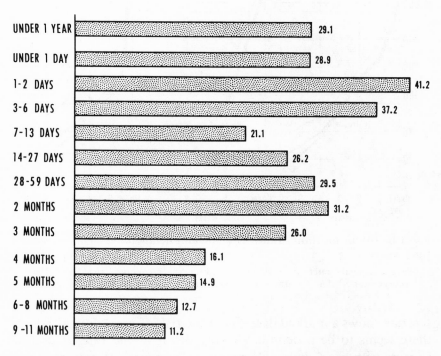

Fig. 1.9. Percent excess of male over female infant mortality rates by age: United States, 1959–61.

Source: National Center for Health Statistics, special tabulations.

remained comparatively high until 3 months of age and then dropped to only 11 percent at 9–11 months of age.

The infant mortality rate for nonwhite children was 86 percent above the rate for white children during 1959–61. In the first 24 hours following birth the differential was 50 percent (Fig. 1.10).

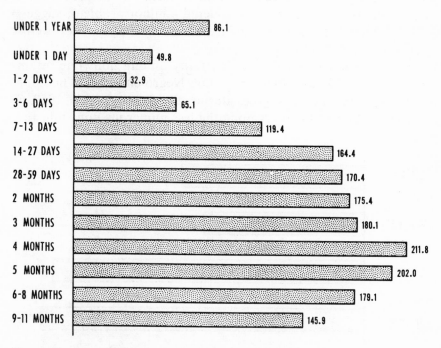

UNDER 1 YEAR	86.1
UNDER 1 DAY	49.8
1-2 DAYS	32.9
3-6 DAYS	65.1
7-13 DAYS	119.4
14-27 DAYS	164.4
28-59 DAYS	170.4
2 MONTHS	175.4
3 MONTHS	180.1
4 MONTHS	211.8
5 MONTHS	202.0
6-8 MONTHS	179.1
9-11 MONTHS	145.9

Fig. 1.10. Percent excess of nonwhite over white infant mortality rates by age: United States, 1959–61.

Source: National Center for Health Statistics, special tabulations.

It dropped to 33 percent at ages 1–2 days. But with each successive day to the end of the first week of life the differential increased sharply, and at the ages of 7–13 days the mortality rate among the nonwhite infants was more than twice the rate among the white. The differential continued to widen and at ages 4 and 5 months the rate for the former group was about three times that for the latter. The margin narrowed only moderately in the balance of the first year.

It is unlikely that the progression from comparatively small differentials soon after birth to sizable differentials thereafter merely reflects the effect of reporting problems. Nationally, it may well be that the early infant deaths are less completely reported for the nonwhite births than for the white. Nevertheless, the existence of a smaller color differential during the neonatal period than later on in every part of the country and in large urban areas, where under-reporting of deaths is considered a minor problem, suggests that the general picture obtained from official vital statistics is close to the true state of affairs.

For the country as a whole, mortality among nonwhite infants reflects essentially the situation among Negro children. The infant mortality rate among Negroes during the 2-year period 1959–60 averaged 44.6 per 1,000. Among the less numerous nonwhite race

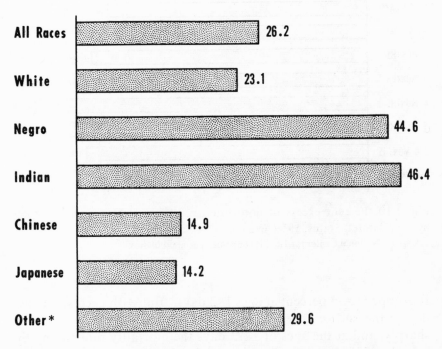

Fig. 1.11. Infant mortality rates per 1,000 live births by race: United States, 1959–60.

Source: National Center for Health Statistics, *Vital Statistics of the United States*, annual volumes.

Note: Includes Alaska in 1959 and 1960; Hawaii in 1960.

*Includes Aleutian, Eskimo, Hawaiian, Part Hawaiian, and Filipino.

groups, the rate varied widely. The rate for Indian children based on registered births and deaths was very close to the rate for Negroes. Infant mortality among those of Chinese and Japanese stock was exceptionally low (14–15 per 1,000) even when compared with the loss among the white infants (23 percent) (Fig. 1.11). The fact that an ethnic group has been identified as having a loss rate well below 20 per 1,000 suggests that there is a potential for a major reduction in infant mortality from the general level of 25 per 1,000 in 1964. Unfortunately, no national data are available on cause of death or age at death for detailed races to provide a basis for closely examining the low rates among infants of Chinese and Japanese stock.

Cause of Death

Restrictions

Because of the concentration of infant mortality in the first few days of birth, a large proportion of the deaths are not clearly the culmination of a known, specific disease process. About two-fifths of the deaths are ascribed to a generalized state such as immaturity unqualified and postnatal asphyxia and atelectasis or to ill-defined diseases peculiar to early infancy. In almost another 10 percent of the cases the cause of death is birth injury, a category which combines many different circumstances and often does not reflect the underlying cause of death as much as the known, immediate mechanism which caused the death. Actually, almost the entire set of conditions included under the general heading "certain diseases of early infancy" is vague and probably subject to considerable variation from place to place, from one population group to another, and in what the physician records as the particular cause of death. This restriction is of lesser importance for the other causes of death, although here, too, uncertainty as to the cause of death does occur.

Autopsy studies of neonatal deaths by Potter (7) throw light on the nature of some of the difficulties in obtaining consistent reports of causes of death in early infancy. In one of these investigations it was found that "most of the infants designated (by the pathologist) as dying of prematurity showed widespread atelectasis and many of those designated as dying of atelectasis were premature. It was largely a matter of terminology that was responsible for differentiating atelectasis, prematurity, and unknown." These three categories were then grouped together under the heading "abnormal pulmonary ventilation," with the statement that they "showed no specific pathological lesions outside the lungs—and [death] could be accounted for only on the basis of inadequate functioning of the lungs." Postmortem examinations indicated further that some deaths ascribed to atelectasis by the attending physician were actually caused by pneumonia.

The other condition most often missed without autopsy was intracranial hemorrhage. It was determined that congenital debility (classified under ill-defined diseases peculiar to early infancy) often applied to a death caused by intracranial hemorrhage. However, the effect of this situation does not appear to be great for birth injuries as a whole.

Starting about 15 years ago, hyaline membrane and abnormal pulmonary ventilation began to appear with increasing frequency as causes of death shortly after birth. Previously most of these deaths would undoubtedly have been ascribed to postnatal asphyxia and atelectasis or to immaturity. As noted in the earlier discussion of trends, hyaline membrane was for several years classified as a respiratory disease, but since 1958 it has been included in the general category of ill-defined diseases peculiar to early infancy. Abnormal pulmonary ventilation has always been included with other respiratory diseases.[7]

Despite severe limitations imposed by imprecision of many of the clinical diagnoses and lack of knowledge about the role of maternal conditions, cause-of-death data for the neonatal period have served a useful function. They define the relative order of importance of the various causes of death, and vague as some are, they do have meaning to the clinician and those concerned with public health programs. Even such indefinite entries as "immaturity" on the death record have served a positive function. They have directed attention to the critical role of immaturity in infant mortality and aided in the development of programs designed to cope with the problem. Furthermore, difficulties with cause-of-death statistics become less serious as one moves further away from the date of

[7] For a review of the difficulties and different points of view regarding the causes of the symptoms of respiratory difficulty among premature infants in the first few days of life, see reference 8. For an early discussion of pathologic findings that led to the use of the term hyaline membrane, see reference 9.

birth and as most of the mortality is related to postnatal environmental conditions.

Major Causes of Death

Congenital malformations and influenza and pneumonia (including pneumonia of newborn) predominate among the more specific causes of infant deaths. Approximately 14 percent of the deaths under 1 year in 1959–61 were accounted for by each of these groups of causes of death (Table 1.3 and Appendix Table I.4a). All of the diseases of the digestive system (including diarrhea of newborn) accounted for only 4 percent of the infant deaths, and the infective and parasitic disease category was responsible for an even smaller proportion of the mortality (1 percent). Hemolytic diseases and accidents were also responsible for small fractions of the infant deaths (2 and 3 percent, respectively, for the two causes). Outweighing the more specific causes are those subject to the restrictions discussed above. Postnatal asphyxia and atelectasis and immaturity unqualified accounted for about one-third of the infant deaths (35 percent), birth injuries for 9 percent, and ill-defined diseases peculiar to early infancy for 7 percent.

The relative importance of the various causes of death shifts radically as the infant advances in age. In a matter of a few days the overwhelming concentration among causes that reflect the influence of conditions present before the birth or that occur during the birth is attenuated. At ages 7–27 days certain diseases of early infancy account for only about half of the deaths; in the post-neonatal period this category is of negligible significance. In the post-neonatal period, the infectious diseases, particularly pneumonia and influenza, dominate as causes of death. Also, accidents begin to assume a major role in mortality. There is, however, evidence that some of these presumably accidental deaths are sudden deaths of varied and, to a large extent, unknown origin(10). Mortality attributed to congenital malformations is an important factor both early and late in infancy. The rate for this cause varies less from one age group to the next than the rate for any other condition. Accordingly, in the first day of life, when mortality is very high, congenital malformations account for only 9 percent of the loss; later the proportion is substantially higher.

Cause-of-death data give the strong impression that no special group of conditions is responsible for the excess mortality among

Table 1.3   Infant mortality from 5 leading causes of death by age at death and color:
United States, 1959-61.

(Ranked on the basis of the average annual rates for all races.
Numbers after causes of death are category numbers
of the Seventh Revision of the International Lists, 1955)

Rank Order	Cause of Death	Rates per 10,000 live births			Percent of total deaths		
		Total	White	Non-white	Total	White	Non-white
	Under 1 Year						
	All causes	259.0	228.5	425.3	100.0	100.0	100.0
1	Postnatal asphyxia and atelectasis (762)	45.7	42.2	64.8	17.6	18.5	15.2
2	Immaturity unqualified (776)	45.4	39.4	77.8	17.5	17.2	18.3
3	Congenital malformations (750-759)	36.4	37.5	30.4	14.1	16.4	7.1
4	Influenza and pneumonia, including pneumonia of newborn (480-493,763)	31.0	22.9	75.2	12.0	10.0	17.7
5	Birth injuries (760,761)	23.9	23.4	26.9	9.2	10.2	6.3
	Under 1 Day						
	All causes	103.1	95.6	143.3	100.0	100.0	100.0
1	Immaturity unqualified (776)	31.3	27.5	51.6	30.4	28.8	36.0
2	Postnatal asphyxia and atelectasis (762)	27.4	24.9	41.2	26.6	26.0	28.8
3	Birth injuries (760,761)	15.9	15.7	16.9	15.4	16.4	11.8
4	Congenital malformations (750-759)	9.5	10.1	6.4	9.2	10.6	4.5
5	Ill-defined diseases peculiar to early infancy, including nutritional maladjustment (772,773)	8.6	7.7	13.3	8.3	8.1	9.3
	1 - 6 Days						
	All causes	63.9	60.0	85.3	100.0	100.0	100.0
1	Postnatal asphyxia and atelectasis (762)	16.4	15.8	20.0	25.7	26.3	23.4
2	Immaturity unqualified (776)	12.2	10.6	21.0	19.1	17.7	24.6
3	Congenital malformations (750-759)	8.9	9.3	6.8	13.9	15.5	8.0
4	Ill-defined diseases peculiar to early infancy, including nutritional maladjustment (772,773)	7.6	7.4	8.6	11.9	12.3	10.1
5	Birth injuries (760,761)	7.4	7.1	8.9	11.6	11.8	10.4
	7 - 27 Days						
	All causes	20.2	16.6	40.1	100.0	100.0	100.0
1	Congenital malformations (750-759)	5.5	5.6	4.6	27.2	33.7	11.5
2	Influenza and pneumonia, including pneumonia of newborn (480-493,763)	4.2	3.0	10.4	20.8	18.1	25.9
3	Immaturity unqualified (776)	1.6	1.1	4.3	7.9	6.6	10.7
4	Postnatal asphyxia and atelectasis (762)	1.2	1.0	2.3	5.9	6.0	5.7
5	Gastritis, duodenitis, enteritis and colitis, including diarrhea of newborn (543,571,572,764)	1.0	0.5	3.6	5.0	3.0	9.0
	28 Days - 11 Months						
	All causes	71.9	56.3	156.7	100.0	100.0	100.0
1	Influenza and pneumonia, including pneumonia of newborn (480-493,763)	22.4	16.3	56.1	31.2	29.0	35.8
2	Congenital malformations (750-759)	12.5	12.5	12.6	17.4	22.2	8.0
3	Accidents (E800-E962)	7.4	6.2	14.0	10.3	11.0	8.9
4	Gastritis, duodenitis, enteritis and colitis, including diarrhea of newborn (543,571,572,764)	5.8	3.4	19.1	8.1	6.0	12.2
5	Other diseases of respiratory system[1] (470-475,500-527)	5.5	4.6	10.1	7.6	8.2	6.4

Source: Special tabulations of the Division of Vital Statistics, National Center for Health Statistics, Public Health Service, Washington.

[1]Includes acute upper respiratory infections, bronchitis and all other diseases of respiratory system except influenza and pneumonia.

males during infancy (Appendix Tables I.4b and c). The rate for every major cause of death is substantially higher among males than females. To be sure, the relative margin fluctuates from one cause group to another. For example, the difference between rates for congenital malformations is about 17 percent, while the difference between rates for birth injuries is especially large (43 percent). But the basic observation remains: male infants have higher rates than females in all important cause-of-death categories. Among the comparatively low frequency causes, hemolytic disease of the newborn stands out as an exception to the rule. Here the difference between the rates for males and females is negligible. Another exception occurs in the subgroup, congenital malformations of the central nervous system and sense organs. Mortality attributed to these causes is relatively more frequent for girls than boys.

Throughout infancy, as the male-female differential in overall mortality varies, the margin in most of the causes of death keeps pace. For example, at ages 1–6 days, when excess mortality among males reaches a peak of 40 percent, almost all causes of death showed at least a 40-percent male-female differential. Comparable situations are found at the other ages. An interesting departure occurs in the rate for congenital malformations. Both very early in infancy (under 1 day) and in the post-neonatal period, the male-female gap in mortality is very low, under 10 percent. At ages 1–6 days and 7–27 days the differential is greater but not as large as for most other causes. When congenital malformations of the central nervous system and sense organs are excluded, the relative differential between male and female rates for other anomalies becomes comparable at most ages in infancy to the situation for all causes combined.

Little consistency is found when cause-of-death rates are compared for white and nonwhite infants. Although styles of reporting causes of death may differ for these two population groups, it is clear that infectious diseases of all types are more common causes of death both early in infancy and later on among the nonwhite births than the white (Appendix Tables I.4d and e). Compared to the margins for these causes, the rates for other digestive diseases and birth injuries are very similar for the two color groups. In two cause groups, congenital anomalies and hemolytic diseases, the rates are higher among white than nonwhite infants. Many of these relationships change rapidly as age increases. For example, the similarity in the birth injury death rates for white and nonwhite children is confined to the first day of life. After this, the rates diverge. Nonwhite children have lower congenital malformation death rates in the neonatal period; later the rates for white and nonwhite infants are the same. More generally, the essential point is that mortality rates for most causes become increasingly disadvantageous for the nonwhite children as age progresses.

Infant Mortality in Geographic Areas

Trends

The major changes in the infant mortality rate during the 1930's and 1940's already considered for the country as a whole were shared by almost all geographic areas in the United States. Whether one looks at the situation from the standpoint of large aggregates of areas, such as urban and rural and geographic regions, or in terms of political entities, such as individual states or cities, the reduction in the rate was little short of phenomenal, and by 1940 the infant mortality rate had fallen below 40 per 1,000 in many areas. Nevertheless, for a broad expanse of the country, cutting across the entire southern area from the Atlantic to the Rockies, the rate in 1939–41 was close to 60 per 1,000 (Appendix Table I.5). In these areas the rates for the white population varied between 50 and 60 per 1,000; rates for the nonwhite population in the South were 70–80 per 1,000, and in the Mountain division, where Indians predominate among the nonwhite races, the rate for all the nonwhite combined was 160 per 1,000.

Large-scale reductions in infant mortality continued well into the 1940's in most parts of the country. Areas with high rates and those with low rates experienced major decreases in the post-World War II period. By and large, these decreases were proportionately of about the same magnitude and there was only a modest reduction in the gap between the rates of high and low areas.

The leveling off in the infant mortality rate that is usually viewed as starting in 1950 for the country as a whole spread at an uneven pace. It began immediately after the postwar drop in a number of areas, and by the mid-1950's almost every part of the country had been affected. Infant mortality rates among white children in areas with relatively high rates continued to show decreases longer than the others, thereby reducing the range between the extremes (Appendix Table I.5). In fact, the 1950 decade witnessed a major reduction in the variation of both neonatal and post-neonatal rates among the white infants throughout the country. Among nonwhite children, if the Mountain area (with its progress in reducing mortality among the Indians) is excluded, there was no comparable reduction in the spread between high and low areas.

General observations on infant mortality trends in urban-rural areas[8] bear a great resemblance to those derived from data on aggregates of states, despite the entirely different character of the geographic unit. The details of what happened in these areas, however, are important in understanding events since 1940.

During the 1940's both urban and rural areas experienced major decreases in infant mortality (Fig. 1.12 and Appendix Table I.6). Among white infants the reduction in the rural rate was somewhat greater than in the urban rate, so that the excess mortality in rural areas was almost eliminated by the end of the decade. After 1950 the urban rate for white children leveled off a little earlier than the rural, and for the first time in many years the urban rate began to exceed the rural. The margin was small but it has persisted to the early 1960's (Table 1.4).

Among nonwhite infants urban rates dropped sharply between 1945 and 1950; this was followed by minor year-to-year fluctuations in the rate. The level of the rate in 1963 was slightly below what it had been in 1950. The last time infant mortality decreased significantly among nonwhite children in rural areas was immediately after the war. Since then, there has been no persistent decrease in the infant mortality rate among nonwhite rural residents, and their rate has been well above the urban rate for a number of years.

An interesting feature of these trends is that they have left unchanged the direction of urban-rural differentials in neonatal mortality and in post-neonatal mortality. The neonatal rate has remained lower among rural births; the post-neonatal rate has stayed higher among rural births. This situation holds for both white and nonwhite children. Among the white births the elimination of the disadvantage in infant loss that was prevalent in rural

[8] In general, urban areas include incorporated places with 2,500 or more inhabitants; all remaining places are classified as rural. Difficulties in classifying usual residence for vital events such as birth and death may result in an overstatement of mortality rates for urban areas and an understatement of the rates for rural areas (11).

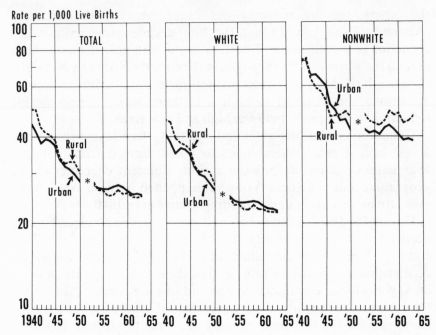

Fig. 1.12. Infant mortality rates by color for urban and rural areas: United States, 1940–63.

Source: National Center for Health Statistics, Vital Statistics of the United States, annual volumes.

Notes: Alaska included from 1959 and Hawaii from 1960. New Jersey excluded from data by color for 1962–63. In general, urban includes incorporated places with 2,500 inhabitants or more; all remaining places are classified as rural.

*Data not available for 1951–52.

areas until the 1950's was brought about by a particularly large reduction in post-neonatal mortality. Nonwhite infants in rural areas, on the other hand, experienced an increase in the post-neonatal mortality rate, a circumstance which contributed substantially to the widened difference between urban and rural infant mortality in this color group.

The category "urban" is a composite of communities that range from large, densely populated cities such as New York and Chicago to small cities of 2,500–10,000 persons. Although these different size places vary in economic and medical resources, all of them showed major decreases in infant mortality during the 1940's (Appendix Table I.6). One might have assumed a highly uneven dissemination of the benefits of medical advances, but it is apparent

Table 1.4   Ratio of rural to urban area infant mortality rates
             per 1,000 live births by age at death and color:
             United States, selected years.

Age and Color	1963[1]	1960[1]	1950	1940[2]
Total				
Under 1 year	0.99	0.98	1.07	1.13
Under 28 days	0.90	0.89	0.92	0.99[2]
28 days - 11 months	1.27	1.24	1.53	1.39[2]
White				
Under 1 year	0.98	0.97	1.05	1.12
Under 28 days	0.93	0.91	0.92	0.99[2]
28 days - 11 months	1.17	1.13	1.46	1.38[2]
Nonwhite				
Under 1 year	1.21	1.19	1.10	0.99
Under 28 days	0.92	0.91	0.88	0.88[2]
28 days - 11 months	1.85	1.75	1.58	1.14[2]

Source: Annual volumes Vital Statistics of the United States,
National Center for Health Statistics, Public Health Service, Washington.

[1]Includes Alaska and Hawaii in 1960 and 1963; New Jersey excluded
from data by color for 1963; color not reported on vital record.

[2]In 1940, these categories refer to deaths "under 1 month" and
"1 to 11 months" respectively.

that circumstances were ripe everywhere in the postwar period for
changes in the infant mortality rate. After the downward plunge in
the infant mortality rate, the situation changed. Decreases in the
larger cities soon slowed down and many experienced increases,
mainly in the post-neonatal period. Much of the increase reflects
changes in the color composition of the major cities, but this should
not obscure the fact that the later improvement in the infant mortality rate among white children in these cities was often negligible.
In smaller cities infant mortality continued to decrease well into the
1950's. Reductions in these areas occurred in the rates for white and
nonwhite children during both the neonatal and post-neonatal
periods.

The category "rural" is also a composite of very diverse areas. It
consists of suburbs, which are heavily influenced economically,

socially, and medically by nearby large urban centers, as well as of wide expanses of farm land remote from a major city. To a limited extent these differences are taken into account by separating the rural in metropolitan counties from rural in nonmetropolitan counties.[9] Despite the different nature of the two "rurals," the white infant mortality rate decreased during the 1950's to approximately the same extent in both areas. Among nonwhite infants, the rate in rural nonmetropolitan counties increased, while in rural metropolitan counties it went down slightly (Appendix Table I.7).

Neonatal and post-neonatal mortality decreased less in metropolitan counties than in nonmetropolitan counties during the 1950's. This reflects the failure of the rate to decrease in very large cities. Almost all of the decreases in these two aggregates of areas were concentrated among white children; the decreases in rates among the nonwhite were inconsequential. Actually, changes in rates among the nonwhite were so small that in 1960–61, in all city size places and in rural areas, they were far above the corresponding white rates ten years earlier (1950).

Recent Status

The uneven changes in infant mortality rates during the 1950's brought the rates in various parts of the country closer together than at any other time since national statistics have been available. This does not mean that differences among all geographic areas have disappeared. In 1959–61 the margin between geographic divisions with the low and high infant mortality rates was about 40 percent (New England—22.5 per 1,000, and East South Central —31.7 per 1,000).

When rates are examined separately for the white population, the range is quite small (Appendix Table I.5). Despite the variation in economic composition, in degree of urbanization, and in medical resources, only 19 percent separates the geographic division

[9] The division between metropolitan and nonmetropolitan counties is based on the Standard Metropolitan Area definition established by the Federal Committee on Standard Metropolitan Areas (SMA). In 1950, except in New England, an SMA was a county or group of counties which contained at least one city of 50,000 inhabitants or more. In 1960 the definition changed mainly in that under certain circumstances an area containing two contiguous cities with a combined population of at least 50,000 qualified the area as a Standard Metropolitan Statistical Area. The category "nonmetropolitan" contains not only rural areas of the type mentioned but small cities remote from large cities. Metropolitan is associated with heavy concentrations of urban population, although it does contain some smaller cities and rural areas.

(Mountain) with the highest rate (25.7 per 1,000) from the division (West North Central) with the lowest rate (21.6 per 1,000). The neonatal mortality rate for white infants in the high area is 15 percent above the rate in the low area. During the post-neonatal period the rates diverge, and the margin between low and high areas increases to almost 40 percent.

The situation is quite different among nonwhite births. The nonwhite infant mortality rate ranges from 30.4 per 1,000 in the Pacific division to 48.7 per 1,000 in the Mountain division. The composition of the nonwhite population is, however, different in these two areas. Over a third of the nonwhite persons in the Pacific area are of Oriental stock, and three-fourths in the Mountain division are American Indian. In the other divisions all but a small proportion are Negro. When the comparison is confined to Negroes, the gap between low and high is still substantially larger than that among the white infants. This is due to major geographic differentials in the post-neonatal rates for Negro infants. Post-neonatal rates in the South Atlantic and East South Central parts of the country (19.3 per 1,000 and 19.9 per 1,000, respectively, in 1959–61) are almost twice the rates in the New England, Middle Atlantic, East North Central, and Pacific Areas. The variation among the neonatal rates is negligible by comparison (Appendix Table I.8).

Geographic variations in the infant mortality rates for other nonwhite groups are even greater than for Negroes. To a large extent this reflects the heterogeneity of the category. Other nonwhite groups in the Pacific Division, where the rate was 24.6 per 1,000, are heavily weighted by persons of Oriental stock in California and Hawaii; in the Mountain Division, with its rate of 50.0 per 1,000, other nonwhites are mainly Indian.

Generally a geographic area with a comparatively low rate among white infants has a comparatively low rate among the nonwhite; this is also true for high rates. A more important observation is that infant mortality is far greater everywhere among the nonwhite children. In most areas the white-nonwhite margin indicates the high mortality among Negro children. The only other nonwhite groups with rates comparable to the Negroes are located in the Mountain and West North Central Regions. The interesting feature of the rates for other nonwhite groups (mainly Indian) in these areas is that they are exceptionally low in the first week after birth. There is some question about the reliability of rates of loss in early infancy among the Indians, although it has been argued that registration has improved sufficiently among them to allow acceptance of the recorded rates of early infancy loss as approximately correct (12). Following the first week the mortality rate is relatively high among the other nonwhite groups in these divisions, and in the post-neonatal period they exceed the corresponding rates for Negroes anywhere in the country.

Pursuing the issue of geographic variability in infant mortality rate on the basis of smaller aggregates of population than geographic division leads to a number of inferences that are highly relevant to the present discussion. Taking the state as the unit, it is clear that with only a few exceptions the state rates for white births cluster closely around the national average; for nonwhite births the spread is substantial (Appendix Table I.9 and Fig. 1.13). In every state with sufficient numbers of births to make the comparison (except Hawaii), infant mortality in the nonwhite group is considerably above the rate in the white. These findings are consistent with what has already been pointed out for the geographic divisions. They support the fact that geography does not alter certain fundamental properties of the infant mortality rate at the present time, that is, an underlying similarity in the level of the rate for the white population when large areas are the unit of analysis and a wide gap between the loss rates for white and nonwhite children almost everywhere.

This is also confirmed when other geographic aggregates are examined. Comparison of mortality rates for metropolitan counties with those for nonmetropolitan counties leads to the same conclusion (Appendix Tables I.7 and I.10). Among white children the favorable edge that metropolitan areas have in the mortality rate is consistently small throughout the country. Among nonwhite children the variability is greater, with nonmetropolitan areas having the higher rates due to a wide gap in the post-neonatal rates. Area for area in all regions infant mortality in the nonwhite group is substantially above the loss rate in the white group.

As a further test of the thesis advanced, infant mortality rates in the 51 cities with a population of 250,000 or more in the 1960 census have been compared. For white infants the lowest rate was 20.3 per 1,000 in 1960–61; the highest, 29.6. A majority of the cities fell in the narrow range of 20.3–25.5 (Appendix Table I.11). In about half of the cities the rate among the nonwhite infants was at least 50 percent above the figure for the white. It should be noted that the

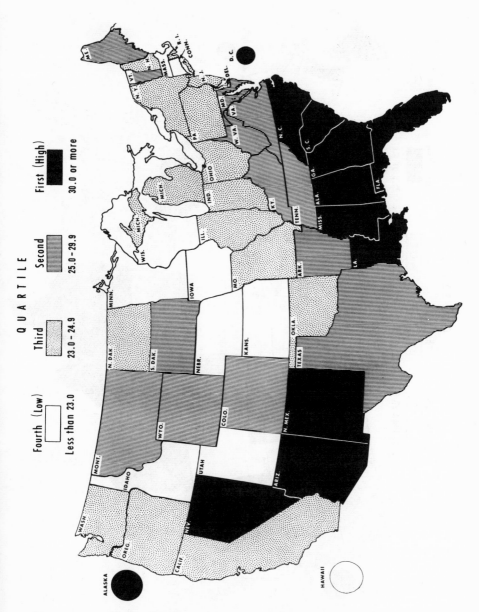

Fig. 1.13a. Infant mortality rates per 1,000 live births: Each state, 1959–61.

Source: National Center for Health Statistics, special tabulations and *Vital Statistics of the United States*, annual volumes.

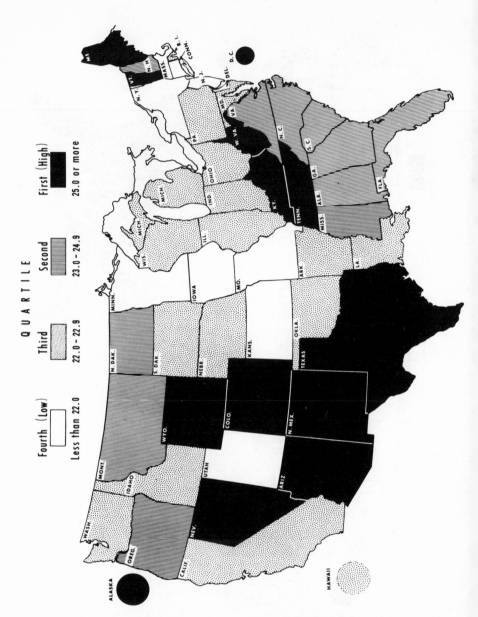

Fig. 1.13b. Infant mortality rates per 1,000 live births for white population: Each state, 1959–61.

Source: National Center for Health Statistics, special tabulations and Vital Statistics of the United States, annual volumes.

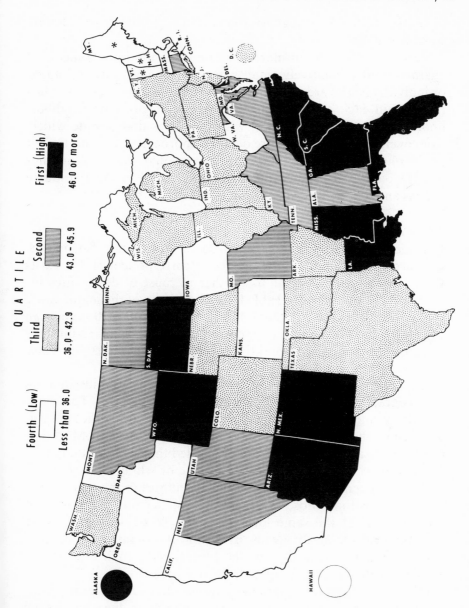

Fig. 1.13c. Infant mortality rates per 1,000 live births for nonwhite population: Each state, 1959–61.

Source: National Center for Health Statistics, special tabulations and *Vital Statistics of the United States*, annual volumes.

*Rates not computed, based on fewer than 20 deaths, for Maine, New Hampshire, and Vermont.

cities are scattered throughout the country—in the North, South, East, and West.

Variation in the infant mortality rate for white infants has been characterized as relatively small when states, aggregates of states, or individual cities are considered. This should not obscure the fact that within each of the areas there are subregions or neighborhoods (as in the case of cities) with loss rates that deviate widely from overall averages. A more detailed approach to the question of geographic variability in infant mortality would lead to groupings of area based on demographic, economic, and medical resource indices and to a clear identification of special problem areas.

Cause of Death

Considering the nature of cause-of-death information for infants, it is surprising to find the high degree of correspondence that exists from one geographic region to another in cause-of-death rates for white children (Appendix Table I.10). For many of the major cause groupings, the range from high to low was less than 20 percent in 1959–61. The West had the highest mortality rates for respiratory diseases and shared comparatively high accident mortality rates with the South.

Among nonwhite infants there was far greater variability among the geographic regions in their cause-of-death rates. The comparatively high infant mortality rate in the South is heavily influenced by the rates for all types of infectious diseases. Mortality attributed to accidents in this area exceeded the corresponding rate in other areas even more than in the case of white children. The rates for congenital anomalies and birth injuries in the South were slightly lower than those in other regions; the rate for postnatal asphyxia was at the same level as in the West, where nonwhite infants had a comparatively low overall mortality rate. It is hard to say what this means in view of the exceptionally high rates in the South for categories containing ill-defined conditions.

Metropolitan-nonmetropolitan contrasts in cause of death rates for white children show quite different patterns in the early weeks after birth and later in infancy (Appendix Table I.10). In the neonatal period, during which mortality rates in metropolitan and nonmetropolitan areas were close in each geographic region, differences by cause were generally marginal and showed no special pattern. Later, when environmental factors become more important and the margin between metropolitan and nonmetropolitan rates increased somewhat, greater losses from infectious diseases and accidents accounted for the higher nonmetropolitan loss.

If residents of metropolitan and nonmetropolitan areas in every geographic region had the same cause-of-death rates and these were the lowest attained in 1959–61 in any of these regions, the post-neonatal mortality rate for white children in the United States would be 4.3 per 1,000 instead of 5.6. Applying the same approach in the case of neonatal mortality the reduction would be from 17.2 per 1,000 to 14.6. Combining the neonatal and post-neonatal rates would result in a mortality rate for white children in the first year of life of 18.9 per 1,000 or 17 percent below the 1959–61 rate of 22.9.

Among nonwhite children, although neonatal rates are very similar for metropolitan-nonmetropolitan residents, there are major differences in the stated causes of death. Nonmetropolitan areas have higher rates for infectious diseases and for the conglomeration of causes contained in the residual category. This situation is counterbalanced principally by a far lower rate for postnatal asphyxia and atelectasis in nonmetropolitan areas. Rates for immaturity unqualified and ill-defined diseases of early infancy are also slightly lower in nonmetropolitan areas. In the post-neonatal period almost every cause of death contributes to the major differential in mortality between metropolitan and nonmetropolitan residents, the most important exceptions being respiratory diseases (other than influenza and pneumonia) and congenital malformations. Half of the margin is accounted for by deaths from influenza and pneumonia and from infectious diseases of the digestive system.

The assumptions used in arriving at the "low" rate of 18.9 per 1,000 for white children have also been applied in the case of non-white infants. This time, however, because of differences in composition of the nonwhite group, the calculation has been made excluding the West. The projected infant mortality rate for the nonwhite population in the rest of the country becomes 30.2 per 1,000 as compared with an actual figure for the United States, excluding the West, of 43.6 per 1,000.

Fetal and Perinatal Mortality

Trends
Much of the public concern about reproductive loss has been concentrated on the mortality among the live-born infants. How-

ever, the heavy concentration of infant deaths in the period immediately following birth has for a long time indicated the desirability of simultaneously examining the problem of fetal mortality. The circumstances responsible for the overwhelming majority of the deaths in early infancy arise from conditions established before the delivery or from stresses during the birth process itself. Although national data are not available on causes of fetal death, these same circumstances must, of course, also be responsible for the loss of viable fetuses. The various conditions may differ in their relative importance for neonatal and fetal deaths, but they are present in both mortality categories. This has led to the introduction of the concept of perinatal mortality, which provides for combining fetal deaths with loss in early infancy.

Another reason advanced for the use of the perinatal mortality measure is that it overcomes artifacts due to differences among physicians and hospitals in how they report a death that occurs immediately after birth. There is evidence that some of these births are reported as fetal deaths, but it is not at all certain how much this problem affects each of the components of the perinatal mortality rate. Also, as previously mentioned, there is the possibility that some of the pregnancies now terminating in live-born children who die soon after birth would formerly have terminated in fetal deaths.

It should be realized that a penalty of unknown dimensions is incurred when the perinatal mortality rate is used. This arises from the underreporting of fetal deaths, which may vary in magnitude with time, place, and population subgroup. Fragmentary data available on the issue of under-reporting indicate that it is heavily influenced by an area's reporting requirements and its special efforts to improve registration completeness. The problem of under-reporting of fetal deaths is generally assessed as being a serious matter in most places even today(13).

Turning first to fetal mortality, trends can be examined from 1942 onward for fetal deaths of 20 weeks or more gestation and for those of 28 weeks or more gestation (Appendix Table I.12a and Fig. 1.14). Very much the same impression is obtained from the two sets of loss ratios. Between 1942 and the mid-1950's large decreases occurred in fetal mortality; after that the trend lines leveled off. Compared with the neonatal mortality rates, the decline in fetal loss after 1942 extended into a later period and was steeper.

Fetal loss trend data by sex and race are available only since 1945

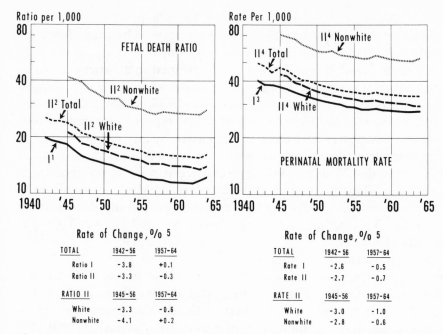

Fig. 1.14. Fetal death ratios and perinatal mortality rates by color: United States, 1942–64.

Source: National Center for Health Statistics, special tabulations and *Vital Statistics of the United States*, annual volumes.

Notes: Alaska included from 1959 and Hawaii from 1960. Data by color not available for 1942–44. New Jersey excluded from data by color for 1962–63.

[1] Includes fetal deaths of 28 weeks' or more gestation and a proportionate number of fetal deaths of unknown gestation per 1,000 live births.

[2] Includes fetal deaths of 20 weeks' or more gestation plus all not stated gestation age per 1,000 live births.

[3] Infant deaths under 1 week plus fetal deaths of 28 weeks' or more gestation and a proportionate number of fetal deaths of unknown gestation per 1,000 live births plus specified fetal deaths.

[4] Infant deaths under 28 days plus fetal deaths of 20 weeks' or more gestation plus all not stated gestation age per 1,000 live births plus specified fetal deaths.

[5] Annual rate of change obtained by fitting least-square lines to logarithms of rates for specified time period and taking anti-log of slope of fitted line.

and are limited to rates for all fetal deaths of 20 weeks or more gestation. With regard to male-female comparisons the observation made about infant mortality trends holds for fetal loss trends. In both cases there has been no narrowing of the gap between the mortality rates for the two sexes. Males have consistently had the higher fetal loss rates, although the margin has been far less than in the total infant mortality or neonatal mortality rates.

Trends in the fetal mortality rates among the white and nonwhite populations were strikingly similar for the period 1945 to the mid-1950's, when the rates declined sharply. The rate of decline since 1956 has been negligible for both groups.

The perinatal mortality rate can be defined in a variety of ways, but conclusions about the rate of decline or when the trend changed directions are not materially altered by the definition used. Rates based on two definitions are given in this report. One definition is the most inclusive that has been proposed by any group, that is, it includes fetal deaths of 20 weeks or more gestation and infant deaths under 28 days. For convenience it will be referred to as PMR II. The other definition, referred to as PMR I, is restricted to fetal deaths of 28 weeks or more gestation plus infant deaths under 7 days. This definition has been recommended by the American Medical Association as coming closer than PMR II to the theoretical purpose of a perinatal mortality rate (14).

Ideally, the perinatal mortality rate should be confined to fetal and infant deaths influenced by prenatal conditions and circumstances surrounding the delivery. Given the present stage of knowledge and the limited information of the vital records, the criteria for defining perinatal mortality rest on less certain grounds than is implied by this concept. In all statistical series derived from official records, the definition relies entirely on a time-of-death criterion. PMR I does have the advantage of limiting the infant death group to an age range (under 1 week) which is less affected than the balance of the neonatal period by postnatal environmental factors. Also, fetal deaths of gestation ages 28 weeks or more are believed to be better reported than earlier fetal deaths. In favor of the PMR II is the fact that a longer time series of data is available for such variables as color, sex, and geographic area. This circumstance has led to the more frequent use of PMR II in this report.

In any event, wherever it is possible to examine trends by means of both PMR I and PMR II, the same conclusions are reached. The decreases in these rates paralleled each other between 1942 and 1964. Both rates declined rapidly until 1956, when they leveled off (Appendix Table I.12b and Fig. 1.14). The decline continued until 1956 in the face of a leveling off in the early infant mortality rates that started several years earlier. Fetal mortality decreased enough during this period to overcome the tendency of the mortality rate in early infancy to flatten out.

No new insights are obtained about trends from the perinatal mortality rates by sex or race. There has been no reduction in the sex or racial differences in PMR II between 1945 and 1964. Male births have been subject to a 20–23 percent higher risk of perinatal death than female throughout this period. Nonwhite births have had a 70–80 percent higher risk than white.

Recent Status

As discussed above, national data on fetal mortality are most extensive for fetal deaths of 20 weeks or more gestation. About 85 percent of the population in the United States lives in areas covered by laws that limit fetal death reporting to this gestational age. In most of the other areas reporting is required for all products of conception without regard to gestational age. Unless otherwise stated, measures of fetal loss discussed below refer to fetal deaths of 20 weeks or more gestation (plus fetal deaths of unknown gestation age).

The fetal death ratio in 1964 was 16.4 per 1,000 live births (Appendix Table I.12a). This almost equals the neonatal death rate (17.9). The male-female differential in fetal loss was 11 percent; this is considerably less than the differential found in the neonatal mortality rate (32 percent). On the other hand, the margin between the white and nonwhite color groups is much greater for fetal loss (100 percent) than for neonatal deaths (64 percent).

Fetal death ratios for geographic divisions have a wider dispersion around their national average than is the case for neonatal death rates (Appendix Table I.13). Even so, the range from high to low is not extraordinary in the white population; in the nonwhite the range is 57 percent among the divisions whose nonwhite populations are almost exclusively Negro.

This assessment of the variation among geographic divisions is based on an adjustment of the ratios for the Middle Atlantic division of states. The white and nonwhite ratios are higher in this area than anywhere else because of an artifact of reporting. Because of special promotional campaigns to obtain reports of all fetal deaths, New York City, which is contained in the Middle Atlantic division, has an especially high ratio for fetal deaths in the category 20 weeks or more gestation and gestation not stated (28.0 per 1,000 live births in 1959–61). Excluding the New York City experience from the Middle Atlantic division lowers the 1959–61 ratios to 15.8 for the geographic area. With these adjustments the areas that emerge as having the highest fetal death ratios are the South Atlantic and East South Central. These are the two divisions that also had the highest neonatal death rates.

The perinatal mortality rates do not alter materially relationships indicated by the neonatal mortality rates. This, of course, results from the similarity in the direction of differences in fetal and early infant loss rates for the variables sex, race, and geographic area. Compared with mortality rates for early infancy, the perinatal mortality rates show a narrower male-female margin, a larger white-nonwhite differential, and greater geographic variation (Appendix Tables I.12–I.15).

2 / OTHER PARAMETERS OF PREGNANCY LOSS

It is recognized that the racial, sex, and geographic variations considered in Chapter 1 represent only a starting point in determining the circumstances that influence pregnancy loss. In the present chapter other factors that have long been implicated in pregnancy loss are considered. These include birth weight, gestation age, age of mother, birth order, prior pregnancy outcome, socioeconomic status, and seasonality. The data greatly broaden our understanding of the role of a host of parameters in infant and perinatal mortality, thereby helping to identify high-risk groups for program purposes; the data also provide leads for intensive studies into the etiology of pregnancy loss.

Birth Weight

Distributions

One of the most important themes that runs through any consideration of infant mortality is the critical role of the maturity of the infant at birth. For years the primary measure used in statistical studies to classify the newborn infant by developmental maturity has been weight at birth. From the beginning the imperfections of this measure have been recognized. A major source of dissatisfaction arose from the clinical observation that a particular birth weight reflects different levels of maturity in various population subgroups. In favor of relying on birth weight has been the comparative ease of collecting on a mass scale reasonably uniform data subject to less error than such other measures of maturity as gestation age and heel-to-crown length. The live birth and fetal death certificates have contained an item on "length of gestation" for many years, but gross errors in the data have prevented its extensive use. New measures to improve gestation age information center on revision of the item on the certificates to call for the reporting of date of last menses.

Widespread improvement in gestation age reporting will help overcome the problems inherent in dealing with birth weight alone and will strengthen investigations of pregnancy loss (1). Although the main brunt of the analysis that follows is borne by the birth-weight item, some indication of what may be learned through the joint use of birth weight and gestation age data is also provided.

One out of 12 children born in 1964 (8.2 percent) weighed 2,500 grams or less (Appendix Table I.16 and Fig. 2.1). Very small babies

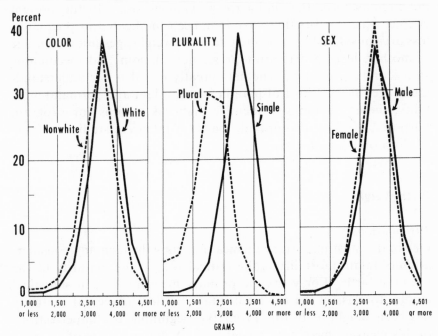

Fig. 2.1. Percent distribution of live births by birth weight and selected characteristics: United States, 1964.

Source: National Center for Health Statistics, *Vital Statistics of the United States, 1964.*

(1,500 grams or less) accounted for 1.3 percent of all live births. A somewhat higher proportion weighed 1,501–2,000 grams (1.5 percent). With increasing weight the proportion rose sharply, and 5.4 percent, or two-thirds of all those weighing 2,500 grams or less, were in the category 2,001–2,500 grams. The modal weight group 3,001–3,500 grams contained 38 percent of the live-born infants. Above this weight the decrease was rapid, and only 1.4 percent were born at the very high weights 4,501 grams or more.

Members of plural sets represented 2.0 percent of all live births, but they accounted for 14 percent of the children weighing 2,500 grams or less at birth. Over half of the children in multiple deliveries (56 percent) as compared with 7.2 percent among single births, were at these low weights. Fully 11 percent of the live births in plural sets weighed 1,500 grams or less at birth. A somewhat higher proportion (15 percent) had birth weights of 1,501–2,000 grams and about 30 percent were found in each of the weight groups 2,001–2,500 and 2,501–3,000 grams. Only 16 percent of the children born in plural sets weighed more than 3,000 grams as compared with 74 percent among single births.

Birth-weight differentials which are of a considerable smaller magnitude but which are nevertheless highly important exist between males and females and between whites and nonwhite infants. Female babies are more likely than male infants to have low birth weights. An interesting feature of this relationship is that almost the entire excess in low birth weights is concentrated in the 2,001–2,500-gram weight group. Under 2,001 grams the proportions are similar for males and females in each weight group.

The modal weight in both sexes in 1964 was 3,001–3,500 grams. However, the distributions in the immediate vicinity of this weight interval differed considerably, with a much higher proportion of births in the male group falling to the right of the interval than was the case for female births.

Color differences in birth weight are marked. The likelihood of a nonwhite infant being born at a low birth weight is almost twice as great as for a white infant. The excess is not concentrated in any particular weight subgroup but is found at every low birth weight, starting with 1,000 grams or less and ending at 2,001–2,500 grams. Peak percentages are in the same weight group, 3,001–3,500 grams, among white and nonwhite infants. As weight increases, the distribution falls off more sharply for nonwhite children.

Birth-weight distributions have been more stable over time for white children than for nonwhite (Appendix Table I.16). During the 1950's there were slight decreases in the proportion of white children born weighing 2,500 grams or less, but in 1964 (7.1 percent) this proportion was at about the same point as in 1950 (7.2 percent). Among nonwhite children, changes of far greater significance occurred. Since 1950 there has been a steady increase in the proportion of children at low birth weights (2,500 grams or less), and the figure in 1964 is one-third higher than in 1950 (13.9 percent and 10.4 percent for the 2 years, respectively). An increased proportion of births is found at every weight level below 2,501 grams. This situation might conceivably result from a shift from fetal loss to neonatal loss among the low birth-weight groups. The possibility that improvement in registration was also a factor cannot be dismissed, but the increase was too general, occurring in almost every type of geographic area, to be primarily accounted for in this way.

This discussion of low birth weight has focused on the national scene, but several observations of interest can be made from the limited information available on low birth weights in various geographic areas. An important qualification is that the accuracy of reported birth weight may vary from one area to another. Although the overwhelming majority of the births take place in hospitals, practices in weighing the newborn may differ depending on size or type of institution.

Among the geographic regions, there is moderate variation among the white babies in the proportion of children under 2,501 grams at birth, the North Central area having the lowest figure (Table 2.1). The spread among the nonwhite babies is considerably greater, with the West having a much smaller proportion in the low birth-weight group than any other section of the country. In interpreting the relatively more favorable birth weights in the West,

Table 2.1   Percent of live births with birth weights of 2,500 grams or less by color: United States and each geographic region, 1964.

Region	Total	White	Nonwhite
United States	8.2	7.1	13.9
Northeast	8.3	7.3	15.7
North Central	7.4	6.6	14.5
South	9.1	7.4	13.7
West	7.7	7.2	11.2

Source: Vital Statistics of the United States, 1964, National Center for Health Statistics, Public Health Service, Washington.

it should be borne in mind that in this part of the country a significant segment of the nonwhite group consists of persons of Oriental stock and Indians, whereas elsewhere Negroes represent almost the total nonwhite population. Among both white and nonwhite children low birth weight was most common in the larger cities; generally the proportion weighing 2,500 grams or less at birth decreased with decreasing size of the urban place and was lowest in rural areas. Again, variability was much larger for the nonwhite group.

Mortality

The only set of national data available on the relation of birth weight to mortality was compiled by the National Vital Statistics Division from a special study of the experience in January–March 1950 (2). There is no reason to believe that the associations have changed materially since this study. As previously stated, in making comparisons between subgroups of the population, similar birth weights may often involve children with quite dissimilar physical development.

Among infants weighing 2,500 grams or less at birth, 174 in 1,000 died within 4 weeks after birth (Appendix Table I.17 and Fig. 2.2). This rate is extremely high in comparison with the rate for all other infants, 7.8 per 1,000. In fact, although children with low birth weights represented only 7.4 percent of all the live-born, deaths among these children accounted for two-thirds of all neonatal deaths.

An extremely high proportion of the children under 1,001 grams died during the first 28 days (872 per 1,000). Chances of survival improved considerably with a moderate increase in weight, but a little over half (551 per 1,000) of those weighing 1,001–1,500 grams also died. Mortality continued to decline steeply with each added 500 grams of weight, and neonatal deaths at 2,001–2,500 grams amounted to 50.4 per 1,000 infants. Substantial decreases were recorded well into the higher weight groups; the optimum birth weight for the survival of infants was 3,501–4,000 grams (5.6 deaths per 1,000 live births). Additional weight, particularly when it brought the weight above 4,500 grams, was, on the average, decidedly disadvantageous.

Primarily because of the heavy preponderance of plural births at the low weights, the neonatal mortality rate for babies born in mul-

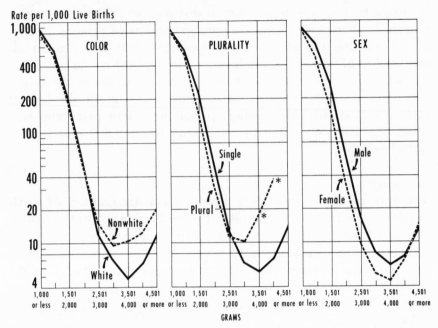

Fig. 2.2. Neonatal mortality by birth weight and selected characteristics: United States, January–March, 1950.

Source: Chap. 2, Ref. 2.

Note: Massachusetts excluded from data.

*Based on fewer than 20 deaths.

tiple sets was five to six times the rate for single births. On a weight-specific basis the mortality risk among plural births was actually lower than among the single births between 1,001 and 3,000 grams. Above this point multiple births were at a major disadvantage.

During the neonatal period the mortality risk for males and females differed greatly at almost every weight level. The prognosis was considerably better for girls than for boys at most birth weights. Neonatal mortality rates for females at weights between 1,001 and 4,000 grams were one-half to three-fourths of those for the males. Only in the highest weight group (4,501 grams or more) was the rate lower for males. Thus, despite a less favorable weight distribution, girls had a lower total neonatal mortality rate than did boys.

Below 2,001 grams the nonwhite infants had a better chance of survival than did the white. The mortality rates for the two groups differed only slightly at 2,001–2,500 grams. At all higher weights the mortality risk among nonwhite births was the greater, with the gap between the rates for the two color groups becoming relatively wider at each successive level through 3,501–4,000 grams and then narrowing slightly.

The most favorable birth-weight group was 3,001–3,500 grams for the nonwhite, and 3,501–4,000 grams for the white. Mortality rates at these two low points differed considerably, with the nonwhite rate being double the white rate.

These mortality data and the figures on distribution of live births by weight indicate that the large excess in overall neonatal mortality among nonwhite children results from the combination of greater mortality rates at birth weights over 2,500 grams and higher proportions of births at the poor-risk birth weights. In 1950 each of these factors was responsible for about half the differential in mortality. Increases since then in the proportion of nonwhite children with low birth weights have contributed significantly to the widening of the differential between white and nonwhite children in their neonatal mortality during the 1950's and early 1960's.

Gestation Age
The need for introducing gestation age data when examining pregnancy loss by birth weight is so compelling that despite serious reporting errors there is value in the cautious use of the gestation item on the birth certificate (3). In the national study of neonatal mortality among January–March 1950 live births, it was found that the heavier babies at each gestation age level fared better than the lighter ones (Table 2.2) (4). Similarly, among children falling in the same weight group, those at gestations at or near term had the best chance of survival. This set of relationships was examined more closely for single births in upstate New York in 1949–51 with substantially the same results (5). Of considerable interest is the additional finding that birth weight and gestation age have a joint influence on mortality throughout the neonatal period. The effect is most pronounced in the first day after birth but subsequently it is also of major importance.

Gestation age information might be expected to clarify some of the neonatal mortality differences between white and nonwhite births, single and plural births, and male and female births taken up in the previous section. This is true even when rather crude gestation age data must be used. In each instance, the group of

Table 2.2   Neonatal mortality rates per 1,000 live births by birth weight, weeks of gestation, and color: United States, January-March 1950.

Color and birth weight (in grams)	Under 28 weeks	28-31 weeks	32-35 weeks	36 weeks	37 weeks and over
White					
1,000 or less	914.7	828.8	787.0	*	485.3
1,001-1,500	762.2	560.0	416.6	377.5	351.1
1,501-2,000	593.9	345.8	204.8	142.6	119.5
2,001-2,500	400.0	187.6	92.7	49.9	33.5
2,501-3,000	*	108.4	51.3	18.1	10.1
3,001-3,500	*	*	23.8	8.3	5.9
3,501-4,000	*	*	*	6.1	4.8
4,001-4,500	*	*	190.5	9.6	5.9
4,501 or more	*	*	*	13.9	11.5
Nonwhite					
1,000 or less	865.9	800.0	766.7	*	419.4
1,001-1,500	743.3	467.8	383.7	383.0	347.5
1,501-2,000	566.7	284.9	155.7	141.4	134.9
2,001-2,500	*	190.6	86.1	54.9	32.9
2,501-3,000	*	151.9	44.9	13.3	14.4
3,001-3,500	*	*	*	11.3	9.2
3,501-4,000	*	*	*	9.4	10.4
4,001-4,500	*	*	*	10.7	11.9
4,501 or more	*	*	*	16.3	20.7

Source: National Office of Vital Statistics: Weight at birth and its effect on survival of newborn in the United States, early 1950, by S. Shapiro and J. Unger. Vital Statistics-Special Reports, Selected Studies, Vol. 39, No. 1, Public Health Service, Washington.

Note: Based on deaths under 28 days among children born January 1 to March 31, 1950. Excludes data for Massachusetts. Births and deaths with birth weight or gestation age not stated are distributed.

*Rates not computed, less than 10 deaths.

infants that had the more favorable neonatal mortality rates at low birth weights had smaller proportions born under 36 weeks' gestation. Use of such differences in gestation age to explain the observed differentials in mortality at low birth weights between the white and nonwhite, single and plural, male and female births is, however, not a simple, straightforward affair. For example, by means of more refined data in New York City, evidence has been offered that the better survival of nonwhite children at low weights is not a function of their more advanced maturity, at least insofar as maturity is measured by duration of gestation (6). In the case of male-female mortality differentials, the rate is substantially lower among females not only at low birth weights but at the favorable weights 3,001–4,000 grams, in which gestation age distributions might be expected to be similar for the two sex groups.

The point is that the preceding observations related to gestation age require critical re-examination with more accurate and detailed information. One would like to determine with greater confidence, for example, what the optimum birth weight is for survival at each gestation age. Also, what is the nature and magnitude of pregnancy loss and damage when only the birth-weight or only the gestation age criterion is satisfied, or when both criteria are met; and how the causes of low birth weight differ from the causes of early termination of pregnancy.

Several studies are beginning to probe into this area with some interesting results. In a recent report from the Cooperative Study of Child Development, Oakland, California, a five-point classification of gestation age and birth weight is provided (7). This separates births of $3\frac{1}{2}$ pounds or less, regardless of gestation age, into a very high risk category. The remaining births are placed in one of four categories through the joint use of two classes of birth weight (3 pounds 9 ounces to 5 pounds 8 ounces, and 5 pounds 9 ounces or more) and two classes of gestation age (less than 37 weeks, and 37 weeks or more). The effect on neonatal mortality rates of the particular combination used is striking (Table 2.3). As compared with the neonatal mortality rate for mature newborn, there is a threefold increase in the loss among those satisfying only the gestation age criterion for immaturity[1]; the rate is at least doubled again for infants meeting only the birth-weight criterion; and there is a further threefold increase for infants meeting both criteria, even when excluding the very small babies of $3\frac{1}{2}$ pounds or less. After the neonatal period the gradient diminishes, but large differences in mortality risk among the various classes persist throughout the first year of life. There is, in addition, a suggestion in the data that small infants of gestation 37 weeks or more "have relatively many more

[1] The term immaturity is applied to births of 5 pounds 8 ounces or less and to those of less than 37 weeks' gestation.

Table 2.3   Neonatal and postneonatal mortality rates according to birth weight and
length of gestation for white single live births: New York City, 1957-59.

Birth weight, grams (lb., oz.)	Gestation (weeks)	Neonatal deaths per 1,000 live births	Postneonatal deaths per 1,000 survivors of neonatal period
Total number of deaths		4,922	1,706
Group I 1,588 (3,8) or less	All gestations	656.2	44.4
Group II 1,617 to 2,500 (3,9 to 5,8)	< 37	93.7	16.8
Group III 1,617 to 2,500 (3,9 to 5,8)	37 or more	30.3	11.3
Group IV 2,524 (5,9) or more	< 37	13.7	7.7
Group V 2,524 (5,9) or more	37 or more	4.7	4.1
Total		14.1	4.9
Total immature; I-IV	...	79.9	11.4
By gestation; I, II, IV	...	100.4	11.4
By birth weight; I-III	...	135.9	14.9
By birth weight and gestation; I, II	...	260.2	20.6

Source: Yerushalmy, J., van den Berg, B. J., Erhardt, C. L., and Jacobziner, H.:
Birth weight and gestation as indices of "immaturity" — neonatal mortality and
congenital anomalies of the "immature." A. M. A. J. Dis. Child. 109:51, Jan. 1965.

severe anomalies than the small infants of short gestation. The latter, however, have higher neonatal mortality rates."

Prior Pregnancy Experience and Age of Mother

No parameters of pregnancy loss have been as completely or as frequently explored as parity and age of mother. The reason is quite simple. These are items that appear on vital records, and therefore tabulations based on large numbers of births can be obtained to satisfy many of the interests of epidemiologists, clinicians, and program agencies. In the current period of intensive study of pregnancy loss new sources of data are being developed through research projects conducted outside the orbit of official vital statistics. Despite the diversity in methodology, time, and place of these studies, there is considerable consistency in findings related to variables they have in common with vital statistics.

The national study of live births early in 1950 probed into the association between birth order, age of mother, and prior fetal loss, and the incidence of low birth weight and neonatal mortality (8). It was found that the rate of low birth weight varied only moderately by birth order (Appendix Table I.18). The rate was highest among first births and births of fifth and higher order (7.7 per 100). This was not much greater than the low figure found among second-order births (6.9). Excluding births to mothers at ages 15-19 years, where the risk was particularly high (9.0 per 100), the variation by age of mother was also modest. The rate was at a minimum at ages 25–29 years (6.7) and then increased moderately to a high of 7.7 after age 35 years.

Interaction of birth order and age of mother results in a far greater variation in the rates of low birth weight than is indicated when each of these parameters is considered separately (Fig. 2.3).

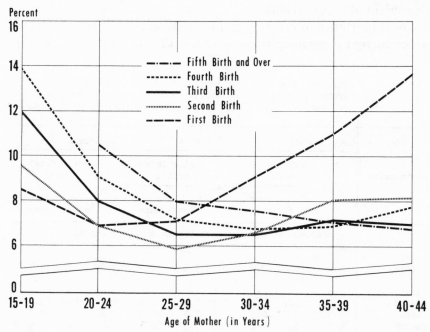

Fig. 2.3. Percent of live births by birth weights of 2,500 grams or less, by age of mother and total-birth order: United States, January-March 1950.
Source: Chap. 2, Ref. 8.
Notes: Total-birth order refers to number of children ever born to mother, including fetal deaths. Massachusetts excluded from data.

The rate among first births was at its lowest point among women 20–24 years of age. From age 30–34 on the risk increased sharply and about 1 of 8 of the firstborn infants to women 40–44 years old weighed 2,500 grams or less. Rates for the other birth orders followed, in general, an inverted J-shaped curve, with the highest rates usually found at the very young ages 15–19 years.

Intervening variables unquestionably exert an important influ-

ence on the relationships discussed. Illegitimacy is particularly high
under 20 years of age when the relative frequency of children with
low birth weights is also very high (9). The explanation for the
sizable increase under age 30 in the risk of low birth weight that
accompanies increasing birth order (except for first births) is not
known. On the surface, the demographic parameters that are implicated include socioeconomic status, child spacing, and prior fetal
loss. However, parity and age may have biological significance independent of these variables.

The importance of prior pregnancy outcome in assessing the risk
in the current pregnancy is unequivocal (Table 2.4). The propor-

Table 2.4   Percent of single live births at birth weights of 2,500
              grams or less, by total-birth order, outcome of previous
              deliveries, and color: United States, January-March 1950.

Birth order	Total			White			Nonwhite		
	Total	Prior fetal deaths		Total	Prior fetal deaths		Total	Prior fetal deaths	
		None	1 or more		None	1 or more		None	1 or more
	Percent of current live births at birth weights 2,500 grams or less								
Total	6.4	6.2	10.0	6.0	5.9	10.0	8.6	8.4	10.1
First	7.3	-	-	6.8	-	-	11.4	-	-
Second	6.0	5.9	10.5	5.6	5.5	9.9	9.1	8.9	13.8
Third	5.9	5.7	10.5	5.6	5.4	10.4	7.8	7.5	10.7
Fourth	6.1	5.7	10.2	5.9	5.5	10.1	7.0	6.5	10.8
Fifth & over	5.9	5.4	9.5	5.7	5.1	9.7	6.6	6.0	9.1

Source: National Office of Vital Statistics: Weight at birth and
survival of new-born, by age of mother and total-birth order, by J. Loeb.
Vital Statistics-Special Reports, Vol. 47, No. 2. Public Health Service.
Washington, 1958.

Notes: Total-birth order refers to number of children ever born to
mother, including fetal deaths. Excludes data for Massachusetts. Figures
for birth weight and birth order not stated are distributed.

tion of children weighing 2,500 grams or less at birth was more than
one and a half times as high among births of women who had reported at least one prior fetal death as among other births (10.0 and
6.2 per 100 single live births, respectively). Birth-order differentials

do not explain these relationships. On the contrary, the increase in the risk of low birth weight among births preceded by a fetal death is more marked when comparisons are made by birth order than when birth order is ignored.

As might be expected, the associations between low birth weight and birth order and age of mother are generally paralleled by the neonatal mortality rates (Appendix Table I.19 and Fig. 2.4). The

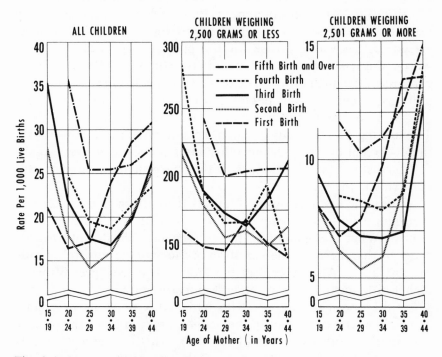

Fig. 2.4. Neonatal mortality rates by birth weight, age of mother, and total-birth order: United States, January–March 1950.

Source: Chap. 2, Ref. 8.

Notes: Based on deaths under 28 days among children born January 1–March 31, 1950. Total-birth order refers to number of children ever born to mother, including fetal deaths. Massachusetts excluded from data.

loss rate among first births was moderately high among women 15–19 years of age. It dropped sharply to a low point at ages 20–24 and climbed rapidly as age increased beyond 30 years. Second-order births among women aged 25–29 had a particularly low loss rate. In fact, the lowest neonatal mortality rate for any age-birth-order group was in this category (14.3 per 1,000 live births as compared with the rate of 20.0 for all birth orders and ages combined).

Although the patterns of neonatal mortality rates have some similarity to those of the incidence of low birth weight, there are notable differences. Between ages 20 and 34 the relative margins among the neonatal death rates by birth order are greater than those among the low birth-weight rates. Fifth and higher order births with their high mortality at these ages contribute greatly to this situation. Another difference is that the shape of the curves for neonatal death rates more nearly approximate a "U" than a reversed "J," as was the case for the prematurity rates. In other words, the risk for mortality definitely swings up after age 30 regardless of the birth order. The reason for this is found in the mortality experience among babies born weighing more than 2,500 grams. Here the mortality curve is J-shaped for every birth order. The turning points occur at different ages, but the picture is the same—exceptionally high mortality after 35 years of age. Again, first births are an exception, with the sharp increase in mortality occurring in the early 30's.

Among the low birth-weight infants the pattern is not nearly as clear and definite as among children with birth weights over 2,500 grams. What is apparent is that for second-, third-, and fourth-order births, there is little variation in the neonatal mortality rates at most ages. Also, except at the more advanced ages, fifth and higher order births have the highest mortality rate.

Children born to mothers who had had a previous pregnancy ending in a fetal death had in the neonatal period twice the mortality rate of the other children (Table 2.5). This increased mortality risk was present at all birth orders. Only part of the increased risks were due to a higher rate of births at low weights. In general, neonatal mortality was greater among children born to mothers who had had a previous fetal loss, whether or not the infant had a birth weight of 2,500 grams or less.

As in the case of neonatal deaths, fetal mortality (at 20 weeks' gestation or later) is strongly related to age of mother and birth order (Appendix Table I.20 and Fig. 2.5). The most favorable loss rates are found among gravida 2 and 3 women in their 20's, who accounted for 30 percent of all pregnancies of 20 weeks' or more gestation. More generally, the low fetal mortality rate for women

Table 2.5   Neonatal mortality rates per 1,000 single live births, by birth weight, color, total-birth order, and outcome of previous deliveries: United States, January-March 1950.

Color and birth order	Birth weight of current live birth								
	All birth weights			2,500 grams or less			2,501 grams or more		
	Total	Prior fetal deaths		Total	Prior fetal deaths		Total	Prior fetal deaths	
		None	1 or more		None	1 or more		None	1 or more
Total									
Total	18.3	17.6	35.8	173.4	168.8	237.6	7.7	7.5	13.3
First	18.4	-	-	17.2	-	-	27.6	-	-
Second	16.2	15.8	34.6	173.4	171.3	223.3	6.3	6.1	12.4
Third	17.8	16.9	33.0	185.9	180.6	233.0	7.2	7.1	9.6
Fourth	19.1	17.2	38.9	183.6	170.9	259.4	8.4	8.0	13.8
Fifth & over	23.4	21.3	36.5	212.6	205.5	236.9	11.4	10.8	15.5
White									
Total	17.3	16.6	36.1	176.7	172.0	250.1	7.1	6.9	12.4
First	17.2	-	-	156.1	-	-	7.0	-	-
Second	15.4	15.0	32.0	175.6	173.6	228.1	5.9	5.8	10.5
Third	17.4	16.6	32.6	192.1	186.5	242.3	7.0	6.9	8.3
Fourth	18.1	16.3	39.5	182.6	168.6	270.4	7.9	7.4	13.7
Fifth & over	22.7	20.4	38.9	226.2	217.9	256.9	10.5	9.8	15.6
Nonwhite									
Total	24.4	23.5	34.9	159.5	154.9	204.0	11.7	11.3	15.9
First	27.6	-	-	136.6	-	-	13.6	-	-
Second	23.3	22.3	47.5	161.6	159.0	206.1	9.4	9.0	22.0
Third	20.4	19.2	34.7	157.6	153.8	190.8	8.8	8.3	15.8
Fourth	23.4	21.8	36.8	187.3	179.8	224.5	11.1	10.7	14.0
Fifth & over	25.1	23.4	32.4	184.1	178.2	201.6	13.8	13.5	15.3

Source: National Office of Vital Statistics: Weight at birth and survival of newborn, by age of mother, and total-birth order, by J. Loeb. Vital Statistics-Special Reports, Vol. 47, No. 2. Public Health Service. Washington, 1958.

Notes: Based on deaths under 28 days among children born January 1-March 31, 1950. Total-birth order refers to number of children ever born to mother, including fetal deaths. Excludes data for Massachusetts. Figures for birth weight and birth order not stated are distributed.

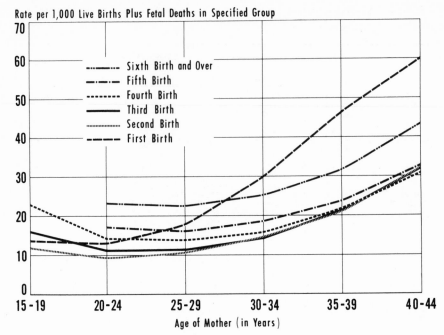

Fig. 2.5. Average fetal death rates by age of mother and total-birth order: United States, 1960–61.

Source: National Center for Health Statistics, *Vital Statistics of the United States,* annual volumes.

Notes: Birth order and age of mother not stated distributed. Includes only fetal deaths for which period of gestation was 20 weeks (or 5 months) or more or was not stated. Total-birth order refers to number of children ever born to mother including fetal deaths. Massachusetts excluded from data.

of a specified gravidity was at about the same age as occurred in the case of neonatal mortality.

The extent to which the number of prior fetal deaths is a factor in subsequent reproductive loss has been explored on the basis of vital statistics for white single births in upstate New York during 1959 and 1960 (Table 2.6) (10). Both neonatal and fetal mortality (20 weeks' or more gestation) rose steeply as the number of prior fetal deaths increased. The neonatal mortality rate went from 14.4 per 1,000 live births where there was no prior fetal death to 129.3 per 1,000 live births where three or more fetal deaths had preceded the current pregnancies. The corresponding fetal death rates showed a much bigger spread: 11.8 to 221.4.

Perinatal mortality rates provide even clearer evidence of the high risk associated with prior fetal loss. Almost one-third of the

Table 2.6   Neonatal, fetal, and perinatal mortality rates for white single births, by
total-birth order and prior fetal deaths: Upstate New York, 1950-52 and
1959-60.

Period and birth order[1]	Prior fetal deaths					
	Total	None	1 or more	1	2	3 or more
1959-60						
Deaths under 28 days[2]						
Total	15.1	14.4	36.8	33.1	49.0	129.3
First	14.5	14.5	-	-	-	-
Second	14.4	14.1	38.0	38.0	-	-
Third	14.3	13.7	36.4	32.8	132.3*	-
Fourth and over	16.8	15.3	37.1	32.4	42.0	129.3
Fetal deaths, 20 weeks or more[3]						
Total	13.4	11.8	61.9	48.2	141.0	221.4
First	12.9	12.9	-	-	-	-
Second	9.3	8.8	46.0	46.0	-	-
Third	11.6	10.5	51.0	48.3	116.8*	-
Fourth and over	18.6	14.8	67.1	48.6	143.0	221.4
Perinatal deaths[4]						
Total	28.3	26.1	96.4	79.8	183.1	322.1
First	27.2	27.2	-	-	-	-
Second	23.6	22.9	82.3	82.3	-	-
Third	25.8	24.2	85.5	79.6	233.7*	-
Fourth and over	35.0	29.8	101.3	79.4	179.0	322.1
1950-52						
Deaths under 28 days[2]						
Total	16.3	15.6	40.3	35.9	73.4	91.3
First	15.8	15.8	-	-	-	-
Second	15.0	14.7	34.0	34.0	-	-
Third	16.2	15.3	37.6	35.1	97.0*	-
Fourth and over	19.9	17.5	43.8	37.2	69.8	91.3
Fetal deaths, 20 weeks or more[3]						
Total	15.8	14.3	64.6	55.3	109.8	226.5
First	16.6	16.6	-	-	-	-
Second	11.3	10.4	64.8	64.8	-	-
Third	15.4	13.8	51.1	46.4	151.9	-
Fourth and over	23.0	18.1	71.2	56.5	103.0	226.5
Perinatal deaths[4]						
Total	31.8	29.7	102.3	89.3	175.1	297.0
First	32.1	32.1	-	-	-	-
Second	26.1	24.9	96.6	96.6	-	-
Third	31.3	28.9	86.8	79.9	234.2	-
Fourth and over	42.5	35.3	111.8	91.6	165.7	297.0

Source: Special tabulations, New York State Department of Health.

[1]Birth order refers to number of births the mother has had, including fetal deaths.

[2]Rates per 1,000 live births in specified group.

[3]Rates per 1,000 live births plus fetal deaths in specified group.

[4]Fetal deaths of 20 weeks or more gestation (and not stated) plus infant deaths under 28 days
per 1,000 fetal deaths plus live births in specified group.

*Rate based on less than 20 deaths.

women who had had three or more previous fetal deaths had their pregnancies terminate with a perinatal death. This is an extreme situation, but women with two prior fetal deaths also had an especially high risk, with one of six of their current pregnancies ending in a perinatal death.

Investigations of "familial susceptibility to perinatal loss" which utilized upstate New York data both preceded and followed the national study described above (11, 12). These studies combined prior fetal and child losses as reported on the vital records in determining the association between perinatal mortality in the current pregnancy and previous adverse outcome. While there are differences in detail between the relations shown by the national data and the mortality rates for upstate New York, the conclusion is the same: that is, a history of previous loss is a major factor in predicting future perinatal loss. Furthermore, judging from the upstate New York data, this relation is not greatly modified by general changes in economic or medical care conditions. (The New York studies covered 1936 and 1951, two years that spanned a period of major change in these conditions).

Socioeconomic Status
One of the major gaps in national data on factors influencing infant and perinatal mortality relates to socioeconomic status. From the earliest days of recording births and fetal deaths, the vital records have contained an item on occupation of child's father which could serve as a direct indicator of socioeconomic status. But, because of difficulties in reporting and coding, the item has never been used for national studies of infant mortality. Most of the information on the relation between socioeconomic status and infant loss comes from city and state studies. The most comprehensive of these covers the period 1950–52 for single white births from upstate New York (13). Because of the passage of time, it cannot be assumed that the gradients found in that study are applicable today, even in upstate New York. Nevertheless, the data are useful since they indicate what the situation was like in a populous state at the start of the slowdown in the decline in infant mortality.

In general, there was an inverse relation between neonatal, postneonatal, and fetal mortality and socioeconomic level as measured by father's occupation, that is, mortality increased as the socio-

Table 2.7   Infant mortality rates by age at death, fetal death ratios and perinatal mortality rates
by socio-economic class: Upstate New York, 1950-52.

(Deaths among single white live births, New York State exclusive of New York City)

Father's Occupation at Time of Infant's Birth	Infant Mortality Rates	Neonatal Mortality Rates	Post- neonatal Mortality Rates	Fetal Death Ratios	Perinatal Mortality Rates
Total	21.6	16.3	5.2	16.1	31.9
Non-Agricultural					
Professional and managerial	18.0	14.5	3.5	13.2	27.3
Sales and clerical workers	18.8	14.6	4.2	14.8	29.0
Craftsmen	21.0	16.0	5.0	15.8	31.3
Operatives	23.3	17.4	5.9	18.1	34.9
Service workers and non-farm laborers	26.9	18.7	8.3	18.2	36.2
Agricultural	23.0	16.5	6.6	18.1	33.9
Not classified	29.4	22.8	6.7	23.2	44.9

Source: Chase, H.: Father's occupation, parental age, and infant's birth rank. "The Relationship of
Certain Biologic and Socioeconomic Factors to Fetal, Infant, and Early Childhood Mortality", Part I.
Washington, D.C. Children's Bureau, 1964.

Note: Infant mortality rates are per 1,000 live births. Fetal death ratios are all reported fetal deaths of
20 weeks or more gestation (plus not stated) per 1,000 live births. Perinatal mortality rates are reported
fetal deaths (20 weeks or more gestation plus not stated) plus neonatal deaths per 1,000 live births plus fetal deaths.

economic level decreased (Table 2.7). Differences among the
various socioeconomic groups in the distributions of births by ages
of parents and birth order did not explain this association.

The gradient in neonatal mortality rates, which reflect mainly the
effect of circumstances present during the prenatal period and at
delivery, was moderate. Mortality in the group with the highest
rate, nonfarm laborers and service workers, was almost 30 percent
above that of the white-collar occupation groups. The margin between high and low fetal loss rates by occupation of father was also
relatively modest. In the post-neonatal period, when mortality is
largely influenced by environmental conditions, the difference between low and high rates increased sharply; the rate among children
of nonfarm laborers was more than double the rates among children of professional and managerial workers.

By far the highest neonatal and fetal loss rates were found in the
group "occupation not classified." In the main, this category consists of illegitimate births, and the rates indicate the extremely high
mortality risk associated with out-of-wedlock pregnancies. Elevated risk in this group extends into the post-neonatal period, although at these ages the increased risk does not represent a sharp
break from the experience in all other groups as in the case of neonatal and fetal loss.

More recent data for New York City (1961–63) indicate that in this area there is about a 50 percent gradient in neonatal mortality among major occupation of father groups for both white and Negro births[2] (Fig. 2.6) (14). Illegitimate births, as represented by the group with no information about the father on the birth record, have a higher loss rate than any of the other categories.

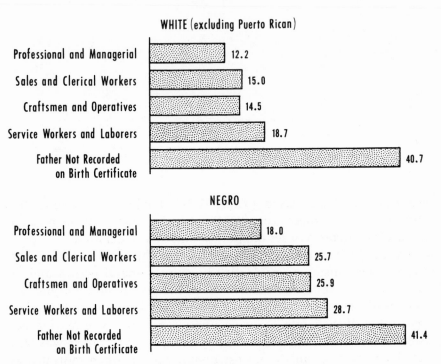

Fig. 2.6. Neonatal mortality rates per 1,000 live births by occupation of father and race: New York City, 1961–63.

Source: Chap. 2, Ref. 14.

Note: Rates are infant deaths under 28 days, 1961–63, per 1,000 live births, 1962, multiplied by 3.

The extent to which the neonatal mortality rates for Negroes exceed the rates for white persons varies from one occupation group to another, the range being from 48 percent to 79 percent.[3] These differentials are less than the observed difference between the

[2] Puerto Rican births are excluded from the rates.

[3] This excludes births with no information on the father and referred to in the discussion as illegitimate. Neonatal mortality rates for this group are very similar among white and Negro births.

loss among white and Negro births when all occupations are combined (84 percent).[4] Adjustment for the variations in occupational and age-of-mother distributions reduces the margin in mortality between the two color groups but a substantial difference remains (64 percent).

The complexity of interpreting the large residual difference between rates for white persons and Negroes is illustrated by one other observation that can be made from the data for New York City. It will be noted that the neonatal mortality rate among Negroes in the highest socioeconomic class is close to the rate in the laborer and service worker category among the whites. A related finding based on births several years earlier (1955) indicated that nonwhite patients of private physicians had a perinatal loss rate similar to that of white patients admitted to the general service wards of hospitals (15). These relationships emphasize the need for more intensive studies of economic, social, and medical forces that underly color differences in mortality than is possible through information on vital records. In this instance, the descriptive data derived from the vital records, limited as they are, could clarify the course to be taken in such investigations.

Less direct measures of the relation between socioeconomic factors and infant mortality are available for a number of other cities (16, 17). In these areas, neighborhoods (census tracts) are grouped by one or more of such indicators of socioeconomic status as family income, educational attainment, occupation, cost and quality of housing to form a gradient that reflects differences in levels of living. While there are difficulties in dealing with this type of data, they do support the premise that infant mortality varies inversely with socioeconomic status and that there is an important gap between the high and low mortality groups in the population.

Seasonality

Seasonality in infant mortality can be measured in several distinct ways, each of which is designed to answer a different set of questions. The most commonly used measure is based on the month of death and directs attention to conditions in particular months that are unfavorable for survival (Appendix Table I.21b). These death

---

[4] Including illegitimate births, the differential increases to 105 percent because of the higher proportion of illegitimate births among Negroes.

rates (adjusted for changing number of births) reach a peak each year in December or January and a low point in July, August, or September. The winter peak reflects a seasonal increase in respiratory diseases which are responsible for about one-third of the post-neonatal deaths. Departures from the regular pattern are of special importance for investigating epidemic conditions in the newborn's environment.

Another measure considers the changes in risk of dying during the first year of life among children born at different times of the year (Appendix Table I.21a) (18). Each month's births constitute a cohort, and deaths under 1 year are cumulated without regard to when they occurred. As expected, these cohort death rates show a very different type of seasonal variability than the more usual death rates. They are lowest in February or March and highest in May through August. Equally important is the appreciably smaller amplitude between the peak and low points in the cohort rates than in the month-of-death rates. This implies that month of birth is of lesser significance in determining infant mortality risks than is the seasonality in adverse environmental conditions.

The opportunity to examine seasonality in pregnancy loss from another standpoint is now opening up. Through the presence of the item "month of last menses" on the live birth and fetal death certificates it becomes possible to investigate the relation between month of conception and pregnancy loss and thereby clarify the influence that certain conditions may have on the development of the fetus in utero. Increasing numbers of registration areas now have this item on their birth certificates, and a start has been made by the New York City Department of Health in using it for seasonality studies (19). Preliminary data for New York City show that when month of conception is used there is a "clear downward trend in perinatal losses among pregnancies originating in February, with a rate of 35.7, to those of October, with a rate of 28.4; while the rate among November to January conceptions vary about the annual mean." More specific uses of month-of-conception data are anticipated. For example, it is expected that this type of information, when applied to the period covered by the rubella epidemic in 1963-64, will more clearly reveal the effects of the epidemic on perinatal mortality and congenital anomalies in New York City than month-of-birth statistics.

Suboptimal Pregnancy Outcome

Infant and perinatal mortality rates provide only a partial view of the total loss and disability associated with pregnancy. They are the best documented measures of loss and historically have attracted most attention. However, as the attack against mortality concentrates increasingly on conditions that affect the development of the fetus, the desirability of including the total spectrum of loss and congenital defects among children becomes apparent. It is this perspective that has led some investigators to postulate a continuum of pregnancy wastage involving different types of loss that have similar etiologies (20, 21).

Special studies now in progress are beginning to produce data designed to measure the components of this loss and disability and to uncover clues to their etiology. Selected for presentation here are several observations drawn from research with which one of the authors is associated. The data represent only a small proportion of the information that will eventually be derived from the intensive investigations of the National Institute of Neurological Diseases and Blindness, the Cooperative Study of Child Development of the University of California in Berkeley, the Kaiser Foundation Research Institute, the Fetal Life Study at Babies Hospital (New York City), the Pregnancy Outcome Study of the Health Insurance Plan of Greater New York (H.I.P.), and other research projects (22).

Fetal Loss

It is well known that fetal loss of 20 weeks' or more gestation is only a small fraction of the total volume of fetal deaths of all gestational ages. Precisely how many women become pregnant each year and how many of these pregnancies end with a dead conceptus is unknown. Even in an area such as New York City, where determined efforts have been made to obtain complete reporting, it is clear that many fetal deaths remain unreported. There are many reasons for this, including the possibilities that the woman herself may not have been aware that she was pregnant or that the pregnancy may have terminated so early and with so little discomfort that a physician was not seen.

By applying life-table techniques in local area studies, Erhardt (23) and French and Bierman (24) have independently estimated the magnitude of fetal loss as being considerably in excess of 20 percent of all pregnancies (30 percent in the case of Erhardt's estimate).[5] No study has produced so high a figure directly from reported events. However, in a recent investigation of a population insured for comprehensive medical care (H.I.P. in the New York City area), it was found that about 14 percent of the pregnancies known to the physicians terminated in a fetal death (25, 26). Because of the methodology it was concluded that this was close to the limit of reporting accuracy that might be reached in a large-scale study. A restriction on the generalization of rates obtained from this study is that it is known that women under the care of H.I.P. obstetricians have lower prematurity and perinatal mortality rates than do other patients of private physicians in New York City (15). Nevertheless, distributions and relationships coming from the study clarify a number of the issues in fetal and infant mortality which cannot readily be dealt with through official vital statistics.

Almost half of the fetal deaths in the H.I.P. study were at gestation ages under 12 weeks, 32 percent were at ages 12–19 weeks, and 12 percent were at 20 weeks' or more gestation. The proportion of "medically known" pregnancies that terminate in a fetal death at a particular gestation age appears to follow a bimodal distribution.[6] The first peak is at about 10 weeks; the other after 39 weeks (Fig. 2.7). There is probably little reason to question the general form of the curve except for the early gestation ages. The question remains, however, how best to measure the fetal mortality rates under 12 weeks' gestation. Pregnancy tests at short intervals would appear to be the only precise way to do so but no large-scale investigation using this technique has as yet been conducted.

The life-table approach mentioned earlier represents a statistical method for estimating fetal loss. The underlying assumption is that the probability of fetal death at a particular gestation age is independent of when the pregnancy comes to medical attention (or otherwise becomes known). This assumption may result in overstating fetal mortality at early gestation ages and the derived rates represent upper limits of the current estimates of the loss. Data in Table 2.8 indicate that in the H.I.P. study, the probabilities of fetal loss based on the above assumption are far greater than the rates

[5] Erhardt's study was based on a special inquiry among physicians and clinics in New York City; French and Bierman's investigation was located in Kauai, Hawaii.

[6] Percentages plotted refer to the proportion of all pregnancies that reached a specified gestation age that terminated in a fetal death during that gestation age.

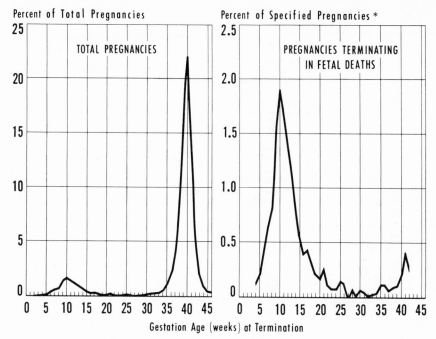

Fig. 2.7. Total pregnancies and fetal deaths by duration of gestation: Health Insurance Plan, 1958–59.

Source: Chap. 2, Ref. 25.

*Percent of pregnancies attaining specified gestation age terminating in fetal deaths.

plotted in Fig. 2.7 for gestation ages under 10 weeks.[7] Differences decrease with advancing gestation age and after about the 14th or 15th week they have little impact on the overall measure of fetal loss. The total fetal death rate derived from probabilities calculated as in Table 2.8 for all gestation ages, starting with 4 weeks, is 21 per 100 pregnancies in the H.I.P. study.

For most analytical purposes involving parameters of fetal loss, the life-table approach becomes cumbersome, and relations are usually explored by means of data classified by gestation age without regard to when the pregnancy became known. This type of information from the H.I.P. study provides new insights into the

[7] It should be noted that extraordinarily high fetal loss rates in the first 2 months following LMP are not universally accepted as a fact. Potter points out that the "embryonic sac develops normally only where it contains an embryo, but it may actually grow for about three months with a very abnormal embryo or none at all," and then concludes that "more abortions occur at 10 to 14 weeks than at any other time" (27). The last is, of course, a speculation since there are no data free of the problems discussed.

Table 2.8   Fetal loss rates at specified gestation ages, 4-19 weeks of gestation: Health Insurance Plan, 1958-60. (Single Deliveries).

Gestation Age	Percent of pregnancies attaining specified gestation age that terminate in a fetal death during week[1]	Probability (per 100) of fetal death among pregnancies under medical observation during the specified gestation age[2]
4 weeks	0.15	2.81
5 weeks	0.29	2.40
6 weeks	0.51	2.18
7 weeks	0.80	1.73
8 weeks	1.20	1.90
9 weeks	1.74	2.23
10 weeks	1.98	2.28
11 weeks	1.90	2.28
12 weeks	1.58	1.65
13 weeks	1.02	1.08
14 weeks	0.82	0.82
15 weeks	0.60	0.57
16 weeks	0.49	0.49
17 weeks	0.41	0.39
18 weeks	0.34	0.30
19 weeks	0.30	0.29

Source: Unpublished data from the HIP Pregnancy Study.

[1]Derived by dividing number of fetal deaths at specified gestation age by the total number of pregnancies known to have reached that gestation age without regard to when they came under medical observation. Data are based on experience of two years of pregnancies in the HIP study; data in Figure 2.7 are based on one year of pregnancies and differ slightly from those in the table.

[2]Probabilities are calculated as follows: $q_i = d_i/(p_i + \frac{1}{2}n_i)$
where d_i = number of fetal deaths during gestation week i;
   p_i = number of pregnancies known medically and not terminated at beginning of gestation week i; and
   n_i = number of pregnancies that first became known medically during the week of gestation i.
Excluded from these calculations are fetal deaths that terminated during the same gestation week as they came to medical attention. Almost all involve women who sought medical care when they experienced difficulties following a miscarriage.

Table 2.9   Fetal death rates per 1,000 pregnancies by period of gestation, age of mother, and gravidity: Health Insurance Plan, 1958-59.

(Single and plural deliveries included.)

Age of mother at LMP and gravidity	Total pregnancies[1]	Period of gestation			
		Total	Under 12 weeks	12-19 weeks	20 weeks or more
Age of mother					
Total[1]	6,844	141.7	67.9	48.9	19.4
Under 20	161	124.2	*	*	*
20-24	1,385	96.8	40.4	40.6	14.9
25-29	2,222	115.2	52.2	39.9	16.3
30-34	1,812	156.2	71.7	57.7	20.2
35 & over	1,190	219.3	120.2	64.9	29.6
Gravidity					
1	1,504	97.1	41.9	36.1	17.3
2	1,869	107.0	55.1	35.7	14.1
3	1,499	138.1	63.4	56.3	18.9
4 & over	1,898	186.5	93.3	62.8	27.3

Source: Shapiro, S., Jones, E. W., and Densen, P. M.: A life table of pregnancy terminations and correlates of fetal loss. Milbank Mem. Fund Quart. 40:7-45, Jan. 1962.

Note: Rates specific for gestation age are based on total number of pregnancies less the number terminating prior to specified age.

[1]Totals include pregnancies with age of mother, gravidity, and/or gestation age not stated.

*Rate not computed, less than 15 deaths.

relevance of age of mother and birth order to the risk of fetal loss at all gestational ages. Elevated risks at ages over 30 and at the higher birth orders were found among fetal deaths under 12 weeks and at 12–19 weeks' gestation as well as at 20 weeks or more (Table 2.9). The overall impression is that with only minor exceptions the pattern of risk shown by national vital statistics for occurrences at 20 weeks' gestation or later is a continuation of similar patterns of risk at earlier gestation ages. A possible exception concerns gravida 1 women who appear to have a lower risk than gravida 2 women early in pregnancy (under 12 weeks' gestation).

Congenital Anomalies

Until recently there was considerable underestimation of the magnitude of this problem. Vital statistics could not be expected to do anything more than provide information on those severe anomalies that were detectable at time of birth or reported on the death certificate. With the appearance of a report on congenital anomalies by McIntosh and associates in 1954 it became clear that the problem was of major proportions (28). In their study of a clinic population (Babies Hospital, Sloan Hospital in New York City) about 8 anomalies were diagnosed per 100 children. The H.I.P. study had a very similar finding, 7 anomalies per 100 children. Both of these figures refer to definite anomalies diagnosed by the time the child reached 2 years of age. They omit conditions, principally orthopedic defects, about which there might be some question as to whether they are malformations.

An Index of Suboptimal Pregnancy Terminations

A loss-disability index which covers the total range of mortality and defects related to prenatal circumstances has been derived from the experience in the H.I.P. investigation (29). (Also see Kauai pregnancy study) (30). Although it must be interpreted as an understatement of the situation in the general community, it is high indeed.[8] The index shows that about one-fourth (24 percent) of all pregnancies that come to medical attention end in either a fetal death (14 percent) or in a live-born child who dies during the neo-

[8] The understatement is due to the type of population studied and the fact that the measure refers to single births among women 19–40 years of age. Also, no adjustment is made for the understatement of very early fetal deaths.

natal period (0.8 percent); has a significant anomaly[9] that requires medical care or will interfere with normal functioning (4.5 percent); or has a low birth weight (4.0 percent). In the last three percentages shown, children are counted only once even if, for example, they died and had a congenital anomaly and a low birth weight.[10]

The magnitude of special risks of all types in the current pregnancy that might be associated with how the last prior pregnancy terminated is now becoming clearer. The H.I.P. study indicated

Table 2.10 Fetal death rates per 1,000 pregnancies by outcome of last prior pregnancy, age of mother, and gravidity: Health Insurance Plan, 1958-59.

(Multigravidae only. Single and plural deliveries included.)

Age of mother at LMP and gravidity	Outcome of last prior pregnancy		
	Total[1]	Live Birth	Fetal death
Age of mother			
Total	127.9	110.2	222.2
20-24	105.5	83.9	157.9
25-29	115.7	93.1	151.4
30-34	153.3	111.2	284.5
35 & over	199.3	155.0	257.6
Gravidity			
Total - 2 and 3	120.8	100.3	186.5
2	107.0	91.6	156.3
3	138.1	111.6	216.5
4 & over	186.5	131.2	255.4

Source: Shapiro, S., Jones, E. W., and Densen, P. M.: A life table of pregnancy terminations and correlates of fetal loss. Milbank Mem. Fund Quart. 40:7-45, Jan. 1962.

[1]"Not stated" are included in totals but are not shown separately.

[9] The study was restricted to conditions diagnosed in the normal course of providing medical care during the first 2 years of the child's life. Neurological damage that becomes manifest later is, therefore, not included.

[10] The priority sequence was death, then congenital anomaly, followed by low birth weight.

Table 2.11   Pregnancy loss disability for single deliveries, by outcome of last prior pregnancy: Health Insurance Plan, 1958-60.

Outcome of last prior pregnancy	Total pregnancies	Outcome of current pregnancy						Loss disability index[3]
		Fetal deaths		Live births				
		Rate per 100 pregnancies[1]		Total live births	Rate per 100 live births			
		Total	12 weeks or more gestation		Deaths under 4 weeks	2,500 grams or less	"S" anomaly[2]	
Total[4]	5,984	14.4	6.9	5,123	0.98	5.9	5.5	23.7
Gravida 1								
Total[4]	1,193	9.7	5.3	1,077	0.56	7.4	4.4	19.9
Gravida 2 and 3								
Total[4]	3,025	12.4	6.1	2,651	0.87	5.4	5.3	21.4
Live birth	2,671	11.3	5.5	2,368	0.93	4.9	5.2	20.0
Premature[5]	183	8.7	4.6	167	*	16.8	9.0	30.0
Mature	2,371	10.1	5.2	2,132	0.94	4.0	5.0	18.0
Fetal death	338	19.5	11.3	272	*	8.8	5.5	30.5
Gravida 4 or more								
Total[4]	1,700	18.5	8.9	1,386	1.52	5.7	6.7	28.2
Live birth	1,256	14.7	6.7	1,071	1.49	5.8	6.7	24.9
Premature[5]	68	14.7	9.4	58	*	24.1	*	41.2
Mature	1,108	12.4	5.7	970	1.34	4.9	6.8	22.2
Fetal death	388	26.6	15.5	285	*	5.6	5.6	34.8

Source: Shapiro, S. , Ross, L.J., and Levine, H. S.: Relationship of selected prenatal factors to pregnancy outcome and congenital anomalies. Am. J. Pub. Health 55:268-282, Feb. 1965.

[1]Rates relate to pregnancies at risk in specified gestation age range.

[2]Live-born children with one or more severe or significant congenital anomalies diagnosed before 2 years of age. Anomalies included are those that will probably make a difference in the child's life by affecting his survival or by necessitating parental, medical, surgical, educational, and/or public attention not required by a majority of the individuals at the same age.

[3]Loss-disability index is the total number of pregnancies that terminated in either a fetal death (of any gestational age), a low birth-weight child, a child who died in the neonatal period, or a child who has an "S" anomaly per 100 pregnancies.

[4]Not stated are included in totals but are not shown separately.

[5]Determined primarily from obstetrical notes recorded at first prenatal visit. Entries were, for the most part, in terms of birth weight.

*Rates not computed, 5 or fewer deaths.

that throughout the pregnancy, from the earliest weeks on, women whose previous pregnancy had ended in a fetal death were considerably more likely to have their current pregnancy end in a fetal death than other women. The influence of prior pregnancy experience was about the same regardless of the age of mother or birth order of child (Table 2.10).

One other observation from this study is of interest to the present discussion (Table 2.11). It was found that women whose last prior pregnancy ended in either a fetal death or low birth-weight infant had relatively high reproductive loss or damage in the current pregnancy (that is, fetal mortality plus neonatal death, low birth weight, and congenital anomalies). Furthermore, there was a tendency for successive pregnancies to repeat themselves with regard to the type of loss or disability incurred. If the last pregnancy ended in a low birth-weight infant, the excess in loss-disability in the current pregnancy was heavily weighted with low birth weights; if the prior outcome was a fetal death, the loss-disability excess was heavily weighted with fetal deaths. This finding is consistent with results from other investigations (31).

The high-risk group of women whose last pregnancy ended in fetal death or low birth-weight infant has an appreciable impact on the overall rate of pregnancy loss and disability. These women accounted for one in six pregnancies in the H.I.P. study. If their experience had paralleled that of other women, the total loss-disability rate would have been 19.4 percent instead of 23.7 percent.

3 / FACTORS INFLUENCING TREND

The evidence already presented points to the fact that every major segment of the population had by the early 1960's experienced a levelling off in the infant mortality rate. This generalization is important but there is a need to probe beyond it for relations that might be obscured by the apparent pervasiveness of the change in the trend. In particular, it is relevant to ask, To what extent does the slowdown in the rate of decline in infant mortality reflect changes in correlates of infant loss? Also, did any of the high-risk groups deviate from the general pattern of small decreases in the loss rate?

These questions are explored on the basis of events during the 1950 decade, the period of decisive change in the trend in the infant mortality rate. As a background, some of the demographic changes that took place in the 1950's are reviewed briefly.

Demographic Changes

Birth Rates

The crude birth rate increased during World War II and rose sharply in the early postwar years (1, 2). After several years of stability at the comparatively high level of the mid-1920's (25–26 live births per 1,000), the rate began a slow decline, and in 1960 it was 23.7 per 1,000, or slightly below the figure 10 years earlier (24.1 per 1,000). The general fertility rate (live births per 1,000 women aged 15–44 years) followed the same pattern as the crude birth rate, except that the rate in 1960 was still above the 1950 level. To a great extent, the maintenance of a high fertility rate was due to the rate at which families were increasing in size with the birth of a fourth, fifth, or higher birth-order child. Between 1950 and 1960 there were uninterrupted increases in the rates at these birth orders. In 1960, 30 percent of all the live births were at fourth or higher birth orders as compared with 21 percent in 1950. In view of the changes in birth-order specific rates it might have been expected that especially large increases in birth rates would have occurred among women over 30 years of age. Actually, it was at ages 20–29 years that the major increases took place between 1950 and 1960. Joint consideration of data on birth order and age of mother shows the effect of the postponement of births prior to and during the war and the influence of decreasing age at marriage following the war. In 1950 births among women over 30 were more heavily weighted with first, second, and third children than in 1960. Most of the children born to women aged 20–29 were at these birth orders in both years, but in 1960 fourth and fifth children became a more common occurrence among women in their 20's.

Since 1960 the crude birth rate has decreased rapidly, and by 1965 it was 19.4 per 1,000, which is the level of the rate in the period immediately prior to World War II (3). Women at all child-bearing ages have experienced decreases in their birth rates since 1960; also, there has been a decline in the rate at all birth orders, including those representing a fourth, fifth, or higher birth-order child.

Economic Status

Most indicators of socioeconomic status point toward a major improvement in the living standards of the population as a whole during the 1950's. The changes came on top of impressive gains in the 1940's. Educational attainment increased and family income rose (even after taking into the account the rise in the cost of living) (4). However, some groups lagged considerably behind others in the improvement they experienced (see section on differentials by color below). Also, an indicator of social difficulties, such as the illegitimacy rate, showed an upward trend in this period (5).

One might assume that the improvement in socioeconomic status in the population as a whole was paralleled by similar changes among families with children born during the 1950's. This may very well have been the case, but there are no national data bearing directly on the point. Some inferences may be drawn from fertility rates (children ever born per 1,000 women) obtained from the 1950 and 1960 censuses. These data suggest that fertility rates in families with higher educational attainment increased relatively more than the rates for other families (6). In a period such as the 1950's, when there was general improvement in educational attainment, this would mean that families with higher socioeconomic status (as measured by education) accounted for an increasing proportion of the total number of births. A restriction on this inference is that fertility rates based on the number of children ever born apply to the aggregate experience over a number of years and it is not certain that birth rates derived from vital statistics for specific years would show the same relationships.

Mobility

Another strong demographic force is represented by the large-scale shifts in the geographic distribution of the population during the 1950's which rivaled the massive movement in the previous decade. Half of the population in 1960 was living in a house different from the one occupied 5 years earlier (7). Nine percent moved to another county in the same state. The movement was out of rural areas and into urban centers in every section of the country. By 1960 about 70 percent of the population was living in a city or the urbanized area around a city. Increasing proportions of the population took up residence in the West, and in 1960 almost one in six persons lived in this region.

Differentials by Color

There are many broad similarities in the demographic changes experienced by the white and nonwhite groups during the 1950's. Fertility in the two color groups started to decline in 1957 or 1958, but at the end of the decade the rates were still above the 1950 figures. Also, white and nonwhite persons were highly mobile during the decade. Nevertheless, there were significant differences between the white and nonwhite groups in the nature of these changes. Mobility among the white population, for example, was strongly characterized by a movement into the urban fringes from both the core cities and the rural areas, whereas in the nonwhite population, the most important factor appeared to be the migration from the rural areas in the South into the core cities in all parts of the country. With regard to socioeconomic status, it has been found that "(a) increases in the level of living and educational status of nonwhites over the last decade or so have not been sufficient to eliminate—or in some instances, even to narrow—differences between whites and nonwhites; (b) greatest white-nonwhite differences are in the rural population and particularly within the farm population; and (c) in many respects—particularly the education associated with occupational placement—the position of Negroes in 1960 was about that of whites 20 years earlier" (8).

Changes in Correlates of Infant Loss and Their Effect on Trend

Limited information is available on the extent to which changes in several parameters of infant mortality may have slowed the rate of decline in the death rate during the 1950's. Other parameters, such as child-spacing and socioeconomic status, would unquestionably add greatly to the understanding of events in the 1950's, but there is no direct evidence on these variables through mortality rates that would be useful for this purpose.

The variables that can be studied include color, birth order, age of mother, geography, and birth weight. Nonwhite persons have consistently had higher birth rates than have white persons for as long as vital statistics have been available. Color differentials in the birth rate increased during the 1950's over the previous decade. But since white births still represented a large majority of all births, the effect of the increased birth rate differentials on changes in the infant mortality rate was negligible. If the color composition of the live births had not altered, the infant mortality rate would have decreased between 1949–51 and 1959–61 by about 14 percent, which is almost the same as the 13 percent decrease observed.

The influence of changes in the distributions for birth order and age of mother among live births has also been examined. Two circumstances of potential importance for the infant mortality rate were operating during the 1950's. As mentioned, age at marriage continued to go down and there was a persistent trend toward higher birth orders. The net result was that the age-of-mother and birth-order distributions of births were more unfavorable for survival of the newborn infant in 1960 than in 1950; a small part of the slowdown in the rate of decline of the neonatal death rate[1] is attributable to this factor. The basic data follow:

| | Neonatal mortality rates[2] per 1,000 live births | | |
	Total	White	Nonwhite
Adjusted 1950–51	19.9	18.8	26.4
Expected 1960–61	21.0	20.0	26.7
Observed 1950–51	20.3	19.2	27.4
Observed 1960–61	18.6	17.1	26.6

[1] This issue could be tested only in relation to the neonatal mortality rate, since mortality rates by age of mother and birth order were available on a national scale only for the neonatal period.

[2] "Expected" rates were obtained by applying the neonatal mortality rates by birth order and age of mother from the special study of January–March 1950 to the appropriate subgroups in 1960–61. "Adjusted" rates for 1950–51 were obtained in a similar manner. The adjustment was required since the birth-order and age-of-mother rates were for January–March 1950. Rates exclude Massachusetts, where birth-order data were not collected. "Observed" rates also exclude Massachusetts.

The above figures indicate that if only the distribution of births by birth order and age of mother had changed, the neonatal mortality rate for the United States would have increased by 6 percent between 1950–51 and 1960–61 instead of decreasing by the observed 8 percent. Thus, if age of mother and birth order had not changed, a decrease of about 13 percent in the neonatal rate might have been expected. This is still far below the 28 percent decrease that occurred during the 1940 decade.

This approach to evaluating the impact of changes in age-of-mother and birth-order distributions on the neonatal mortality rate for white infants shows that the overall decrease between 1950–51 and 1960–61 would have been 16 percent instead of the 11 percent actually observed if it had not been for the more adverse distributions. The observed decrease in the previous decade was 27 percent. Among nonwhite infants the changes in distribution of these two variables resulted in only a 1 percent reduction in the decline of the neonatal rate. In short, the shift toward a greater proportion of births in relatively poor-risk age-of-mother and birth-order categories exerted a small but noticeably deterrent effect on the downward trend in the neonatal mortality rate for the United States as a whole and for white births in particular.

Geographic changes in the distribution of the population might be expected to have an important effect on infant mortality rates, particularly since at the beginning of the 1950 decennium there was considerable variability in the rate among geographic areas and since a high degree of population mobility characterized the 1950's. Nevertheless, as shown below, when the average rates for 1949–51 are applied to the 1959–61 births classified by groupings of geographic areas, the resulting rates are in almost all cases below the observed rates for 1949–51.

	Infant mortality rates per 1,000 live births		
	Total	White	Nonwhite
Observed 1949–51	29.6	27.1	45.5
Observed 1959–61	25.9	22.8	42.5
Expected 1959–61			
(a) Based on nine major geographic divisions	29.4	27.1	44.6
(b) Based on metropolitan-nonmetropolitan groupings of counties	28.3	25.9	43.3

These data lead to the conclusion that without the geographic shifts the decline in the white and nonwhite rates might have been slightly less than did occur. It could be argued that for the non-white infants, in particular, the altered distribution of births by geographic area was accompanied by improvement in registration completeness and possibly by an increased likelihood that a death in early infancy would be reported as both a live birth and death instead of as a fetal death.

The issue of changes in registration can not be ignored, but other questions can be raised about the effect of mobility on mortality trends that are undoubtedly far more important. For example, what is the impact of the migrant group on available resources in the community and are there changes in these resources to respond to the needs of the new group? Also, is the migrant group sufficiently different economically and socially to modify the composition of the areas from which they come and the composition of the areas to which they migrate?

An examination of the change in infant mortality rates among nonwhite infants for cities of 500,000 or more in 1960 suggests that these questions are highly pertinent. The average rates for 1950 and 1960–61 were compared in each of the 19 cities which had more than a third increase in their nonwhite population during the 1950's. In 10 of these cities the rate increased. Rates for white infants do not lend themselves as easily to this type of analysis, but some cities have had an increase in the infant mortality rate among white children. The role of changing composition of both the white and nonwhite populations of the cities is certainly worthy of further study.

By far the strongest discriminating variable in neonatal mortality is weight at birth. Changes in birth-weight distributions which result in even moderate increases or decreases in low birth-weight groups could have an important effect on neonatal mortality. Between 1950 and 1960 there was no change in any respect in the birth-weight distribution for white and nonwhite births combined. When the two color groups are considered separately, changes in opposite directions are found. The distribution for white infants showed a small decrease in the proportion of low birth-weight babies, while the distribution for nonwhite infants showed a marked increase. Application of neonatal mortality rates for January–March 1950 to detailed distributions of live births by birth weight for 1950 and 1960 results in the following neonatal rates:

| | Neonatal mortality rates per 1,000 live births | | |
	Total	White	Nonwhite
Adjusted 1950	19.8	18.6	27.2
Expected 1960	20.9	18.6	32.8

From these figures it is clear that the changes in birth weight among white children were too small to have an effect on the trend in the neonatal mortality rates for white infants. The increasing proportion of low birth-weight infants among the nonwhite births, however, was a major factor during the 1950's in the lack of significant decrease in the neonatal mortality rate in this group.

Changes in High Mortality Risk Groups

The slower rate of decline in the nonwhite infant mortality rate has already been considered, but it is worth returning to this point and drawing it to a conclusion within the context of the current discussion by defining nonwhite infants in the aggregate as a high mortality risk group. Events during the 1950's widened the margin between the mortality rates for white and nonwhite children both early and later in infancy. This is clearly seen in the following figures:

| | Percent decrease in rates from 1949–51 to 1959–61 | |
	White	Nonwhite
Infant mortality	16	7
Neonatal mortality	12	3
Post-neonatal mortality	26	11

| | Percent excess of nonwhite over white rates | |
	1959–61	1949–51
Infant mortality	86	68
Neonatal mortality	56	43
Post-neonatal mortality	180	133

Geography has traditionally been a useful parameter in identifying population groups with particularly high mortality risks. Until more recent years even large aggregates of areas such as geographic divisions and metropolitan and nonmetropolitan areas served this function well. Events during the 1950 decade changed the situation for white infants. Actually, the most impressive departure from the general pattern of small decreases in infant mortality during the 1950 decade was the substantial decrease in mortality among white infants in areas that had comparatively high rates. At the end of this period the East and West South Central and Mountain geographic divisions were no longer outstandingly high risk areas in infant mortality for the white population, and the gap between the rates for nonmetropolitan and metropolitan counties was eliminated for all practical purposes. It seems clear that for geography to become once again a strong discriminating variable in infant mortality, it will be necessary to expand current series of data for local areas and subdivisions within these areas.

Among nonwhite infants it is still useful to think in terms of large aggregates of geographic areas in identifying relatively high risk groups. Omitting the Mountain division, the variation in infant mortality rates among geographic divisions was not reduced during the 1950's and high-risk areas still have infant mortality rates far in excess of the loss in other areas. Examination of mortality rates in small areas would, of course, sharpen the search for high-risk groups and thereby provide information needed for local community action programs.

Within each geographic area, large or small, nonwhite infants represented the high-risk segment of the population at the beginning of the 1950 decade. Ten years later in almost all areas there was either the same relative gap or a larger one.

One of the more critical variables to consider in a discussion of high-risk groups is birth weight. In the absence of national data on changes that have occurred during the 1950's in the mortality by birth weight, it is useful to examine the experience of upstate New York. This was a period of relatively small decreases in infant mortality for upstate New York, as it was for the country as a whole. Another point of interest is that this area experienced a decrease in mortality among low birth-weight infants before the 1950's; the neonatal mortality rate for this category was 228 per 1,000 live births in 1945 and 183 per 1,000 in 1950 (9, 10).

Table 3.1   Infant mortality rates for single births, by birth weight, color, and age at death: Upstate New York, 1950-52 and 1959-60.

Birth weight and color	1959-60[1]			1950-52		
	Total[2]	Under 28 days[2]	28 days- 11 months[3]	Total[2]	Under 28 days[2]	28 days- 11 months[3]
White						
Total[4]	19.0	15.1	4.0	21.6	16.3	5.4
1,000 grams or less	954.2	950.9	*	944.8	941.2	*
1,001-1,500 grams	565.4	549.3	35.8	566.5	544.2	48.8
1,501-2,000 grams	216.6	203.3	16.7	228.5	207.3	26.6
2,001-2,500 grams	54.1	43.4	11.2	55.0	43.0	12.6
2,501-3,000 grams	14.9	9.5	5.5	16.8	10.2	6.7
3,001-3,500 grams	7.0	3.7	3.3	9.6	4.9	4.7
3,501 grams or more	6.2	3.5	2.7	8.0	4.4	3.7
2,500 grams or less	183.7	172.7	13.4	178.0	164.2	16.5
2,501 grams or more	8.3	4.8	3.3	10.4	5.8	4.7
Nonwhite						
Total[4]	37.4	27.7	9.9	35.8	23.9	12.2
2,500 grams or less	194.6	173.4	25.7	179.7	150.7	34.2
2,501 grams or more	15.0	7.0	8.1	17.5	7.6	10.0

Source: Unpublished data for 1959-60 received from Dr. A. Gittlesohn, New York State Department of Health; unpublished data for 1950-52 received from Dr. J. Yerushalmy, University of California, School of Public Health.

[1]Mortality rates for 1959-60 adjusted to birth-weight distributions in 1950-52 follow (adjustment is made by applying mortality rates by 500-gram intervals for 1959-60 to the distributions in the earlier period):

		Total	Under 28 days	28 days- 11 months
White:	2,500 grams or less	175.8	164.7	13.3
	2,501 grams or more	8.3	4.8	3.5
Nonwhite:	2,500 grams or less	175.0	153.0	25.8
	2,501 grams or more	15.0	7.0	8.0

[2]Rates per 1,000 live births in specified group.

[3]Rates per 1,000 survivors of neonatal period.

[4]Not stated birth weights are included in totals but not distributed in 1950-52. Three percent of infant deaths had birth weight not stated; in 1959-60 the figure was 1 percent.

*Rates not computed, less than 20 deaths.

Assessment of changes in the 1950 decade is based on mortality rates in the two time periods 1950–52 and 1959–60 (Table 3.1) (11, 12). Mortality risks shortly after birth among low birth-weight infants were not lowered, in either the white or nonwhite groups. Among nonwhite infants the neonatal mortality rate for the birth-weight group 2,500 grams or less was appreciably higher in the more recent period than at the beginning of the 1950 decade. This excess is primarily due to an increase in the proportion of infants of very low birth weights, among whom mortality rates are extremely high. The same situation was found among white children, but to a lesser extent. Despite these circumstances the main conclusion holds: during the 1950's there was apparently no decrease in neonatal mortality among infants at low birth weights (see adjusted mortality rates in Table 3.1).

Once the neonatal period was passed, babies weighing under 2,501 grams at birth had a better chance of surviving to the end of the first year of life in the more recent period 1959–60 than previously. The reduction in mortality was substantial and was shared by white and nonwhite infants. Among children born weighing over 2,500 grams, decreases in mortality occurred during both the neonatal and post-neonatal periods. The gains were much greater in the white group than in the nonwhite. Among white infants the improvement was more marked above 3,000 grams than in the weight class 2,501–3,000 grams. This further supports the impression that the most impressive gains occurred in those weight groups that already had the most favorable chances of surviving.

Upstate New York data also provide an opportunity to look at "prior fetal loss," another variable that distinguishes between comparatively high-risk and low-risk pregnancies (Table 2.6). The time periods involved are the same as mentioned above. Whether one examines neonatal or fetal mortality in the current pregnancy, the gap between the poor-risk groups (that is, pregnancies preceded by at least one fetal death) and the others did not appear too close.

4 / PREGNANCY OUTCOME AND MATERNAL CONDITIONS AND COMPLICATIONS

Introduction

Despite vigorous efforts to identify clinical factors which are inimical to perinatal welfare, only modest progress has been made in determining the etiology and mechanism of pregnancy loss and infant damage. Most of the information currently available has come from experiences with groups of clinic and hospital patients. In many cases the data pose problems of interpretation because of the inability to define the nature of the selectivity associated with the patients studied and the difficulties in obtaining suitable comparison groups. In some instances, however, the evidence is either so overwhelming or has been reproduced in so many different settings that there is little reason to doubt the existence of an association, although its strength may not be precisely established.

The first section of this chapter presents some of the findings of studies based on selected groups of patients, usually obtained from clinics or hospitals. In a few instances, as in the discussion of low birth weight, the evidence is drawn from general population studies. No attempt has been made to be comprehensive in the coverage of available material; to do so would require a volume devoted entirely to the subject. Instead, consideration has been limited to some of the more prominent manifestations of insult to the fetus and what appears to be known about their etiology.[1] Also excluded are the clinical approaches to reduce the occurrence or effect of the great variety of maternal conditions adversely influencing the pregnancy outcome (1, 2).

The second section is devoted to a detailed examination of the role of several complications of pregnancy and operative procedures in determining pregnancy outcome, that is, fetal and neonatal mortality and low birth weight. Information for this section is drawn entirely from the birth and fetal death certificates in upstate New York.

---

[1] The reader is referred to the discussion of causes of infant deaths in Chapter 1, for which much of the material of this section is relevant.

Special Population Studies

Hypoxia

Clinical and pathological studies have indicated that hypoxia is a major cause of perinatal mortality and morbidity, accounting for perhaps one-quarter of all the deaths (3, 4). A number of complications of pregnancy which are recognized as potential causes of intrauterine hypoxia include (5): (a) reduced oxygen in the maternal circulation such as might occur in severe anemia, shock, hemorrhage, pulmonary disease, or improper anesthesia; (b) reduced oxygen in the fetal circulation due to faulty placental function, as in abruptio placenta (premature separation of the placenta), placenta previa, dysfunctional labor, or gross infarction and degeneration of the placenta, that is, toxemias of pregnancy; (c) reduced fetal oxygen resulting from abnormalities of circulation through the umbilical cord, as from prolapse, true knots or stretching, entanglement around the neck, or compression; and (d) reduced fetal oxygen due to fetal anemia, hemolytic disease, rupture of fetal vessels in placental separation, or vasa previa, accidental incision of the placenta in Caesarean section, fetal bleeding into the maternal circulation, and vascular anastomoses in monochorial placentas in twins.

It has also been observed that the most common cause of fetal anoxia due to interference with the passage of oxygen from mother to fetus is abruptio placenta (4). Fetal prognosis depends in large measure upon the severity of disruption, the presence of associated toxemia, the time needed to accomplish delivery, the degree of shock, and the stage of pregnancy at the time of the event. Recent studies have shown the nutritional status of both mother and fetus is often poor and that defective folate metabolism may be the underlying cause of placental abruption, while hypertensive toxemia is encountered in a relatively insignificant percentage of such cases (6).

Intracranial Hemorrhage

Although intracranial hemorrhage without obvious cause may follow normal birth, more often than not the fetus has been subjected to abnormalities of labor or other maternal complication. Any condition that interferes with transport of oxygen to the fetus may result in anoxic brain injury. These fetuses may exhibit extensive intracranial hemorrhages at different sites without evidence of mechanical trauma. Only about one-quarter of fetuses and infants dying of intracranial hemorrhage are delivered in the absence of some type of significant maternal complication (7). The more important complications noted were uterine inertia, prolonged labor, antepartal or intrapartal bleeding, intrapartal sepsis, and difficult delivery. About 40 percent of these fetuses were delivered normally, while 30 percent were delivered by breech extraction and 13 percent by mid-forceps operations.

Congenital Malformations
Important maternal factors which have been definitely implicated in anomalous fetal development are rubella infections during the early months of pregnancy (8,9), ingestion of certain teratogenic drugs, such as thalidomide taken during the first trimester of pregnancy (10), and toxoplasmosis (11). Some investigators have pointed to a wide variety of other maternal complications and chemical drugs and agents as possible etiological factors in the production of fetal anomalies, but for the most part these have not been proved for the human (12).

The teratogenic effects of rubella are particularly significant, since the incidence of embryopathy may be as high as 50 percent when the disease is acquired during the first 8 weeks of pregnancy, and comparatively large numbers of women are at risk for the disease. The classic defects include intrauterine growth retardation (9), congenital heart disease, ear and eye defects, hepatosplenomegaly, and to a lesser extent, thrombocytopenic purpura, bone lesions, adenopathy, hepatitis and anemia (13). The effectiveness of gamma globulin in preventing rubella infection in pregnant women exposed to the disease is still debatable since very mild infections with viremia may occur (14).

Respiratory Conditions
The respiratory distress syndrome, in which pulmonary hyaline membrane is often but not uniformly found in cases with a fatal outcome, occurs particularly in low birth-weight infants and in infants of diabetic mothers or those delivered by Caesarean section. There is good evidence that the pulmonary hyaline membrane may be the result of intrauterine asphyxia which in many instances is associated with maternal bleeding (15). Most affected infants ex-

hibit respiratory difficulties immediately after delivery and develop a characteristic pattern of obstructive breathing within 6 hours after birth (1).

Pneumonia in infancy includes infections originating in the antenatal, natal, and postnatal periods (16). Bacterial infections occurring in the first few days of neonatal life usually result from intrauterine pathogens which have ascended from the vagina. Long labors, prolonged rupture of membranes and intrapartal fevers are often associated with bacterial contamination of the amniotic fluid, with resulting infection of the endometrium, decidua and placenta, and fetal septicemia or aspiration pneumonia. The organisms causing toxoplasmosis, some fungus diseases, tuberculosis, syphilis, malaria, and listeriosis are disseminated through the fetus after entering the fetal blood stream from the mother through a placental lesion.

Hemolytic Disease of the Newborn
This disease induced by Rh isoimmunization, ABO incompatibility, or drug toxicity remains a significant cause of perinatal death, despite recent improvements in management which include fetal transfusions in utero. This technique of administering blood in utero attempts to sustain the fetus until reasonable maturity. Another recent advance, the administration of anti-Rh gamma-globulin to unsensitized postpartal women to suppress specific immunological responses to fetal Rh positive cells which have gained access to the maternal blood stream in the course of labor and delivery, offers the greatest hope for the future (17). It was assumed for years that no more than 5 percent of cases of hemolytic disease were due to factors other than Rh incompatibility, but active search for additional causes has shown that a variety of conditions in the mother and infant may be responsible (18).

Low Birth Weight
From the clinical and epidemiological standpoints, infants of low birth weight (those weighing 2,500 grams or less at birth) constitute a heterogeneous group. Among those who are truly premature, in the sense that they are delivered before term, the spontaneous premature delivery may be associated with a complication of pregnancy or some abnormality in the fetus, or the pregnancy may have been terminated early because of the mother's condition or to save the infant's life; others are related to multiple delivery. Some low

birth-weight infants are not truly premature in that they are born at or close to term, and for some of these infants a birth weight close to 2,500 grams only represents the lower end of the distribution of birth weights for normal pregnancies. A restricted group of very small, full-term infants suffer from what has been called "placental insufficiency," which results in retarded intrauterine fetal growth and development (19). An advanced degree of hypertensive cardio-vascular renal disease is the underlying cause in many cases.

At present, the role of specific etiological factors in explaining the occurrence of low birth weight remains unresolved for a large majority of the cases. Studies have included nutrition, birth inter-val, work during pregnancy, cigarette smoking, asymptomatic basteriuria, and heart volume. A critical review of available ma-terial has led one investigator to conclude that a great deal more evidence is needed before associations involving these factors are accepted as fully established (20).

The interest in asymptomatic basteriuria arises from the demon-stration that it occurs in 5 to 10 percent of pregnant women who otherwise appear normal, and during the puerperium the incidence is even higher (21). Although the presence of pathogenic organisms in the urine does not necessarily portend trouble, these patients exhibit a significantly increased susceptibility for acute urinary tract infection, a condition which appears to be accompanied by elevated rates of pregnancy loss and damage (22).

Cigarette smoking among mothers as an influence on infant birth weight has attracted increasing attention. A consistent finding in investigations of this relationship is the association between cigarette smoking during pregnancy and the risk of low birth weight (23–26).

However, no increase in infant mortality has been demonstrated for the offspring of mothers who smoke (25, 27). The challenge against the evidence on low birth-weight associations is that smok-ers may be self-selected and may have other characteristics respon-sible for the observed correlation (27,28). Also, the significance of low birth weight in the absence of increased mortality is questioned. These reservations have, in turn, been challenged recently (26).

Complications of Pregnancy and Delivery and Operative Procedures —Relationships Derived from Vital Statistics
A relatively untapped source of data on obstetrical difficulties has been the live birth and fetal death certificates. It is now over 25

years since some of the states added to these certificates a confidential section on complications of pregnancy, labor, and delivery, and on operative procedures during delivery. An important deterrent to the intensive use of the information has been the lack of reliability of the entries on the record (29, 30). Despite this problem, valuable insights have been obtained from these entries about the relation between pregnancy loss and damage and the more serious obstetrical complications and operative procedures at delivery (31–33). Interest in expanding the use of vital records for studying these complications is high, since they provide a basis for placing large well-defined populations under continuous observation for trend analysis. An alternative approach with the same objective is the pooling of data collected in a standard form from a number of hospitals (34, 35). However, the vital record offers the greatest possibilities for repetitive studies on the subject.

In the absence of data for the country as a whole, special analysis has been made of the records for upstate New York (36). The population studied is restricted to single births, mainly for two time periods, 1951–52 and 1960–62.[2] The data indicate the order of magnitude of the rate of selected obstetrical complications and obstetrical surgery, some of their correlates, and changes in the situation that occurred during a period of time when there were only small decreases in the perinatal mortality rate; also, the relation between these conditions and neonatal, fetal, and perinatal mortality.

For the purpose of this study, complications chosen include the following groupings: hypertensive disorders, including hypertensive cardiovascular disease, pre-eclampsia and eclampsia (referred to as toxemias of pregnancy); diabetes mellitus; placental complications, including premature separation and placenta previa; prolapsed umbilical cord; and dystocia, including contracted pelvis, fetal malpresentation, inertia, and other problems of labor. Data on operative procedures concern Caesarean sections primarily. Variables examined in relation to the obstetrical complications and Caesarean section include color, maternal age, birth order, and birth weight. Information on Caesarean section among

[2] Until the fall of 1951, live birth and fetal death certificates contained unstructured items on complications and operative procedures (for instance, "*complications*, if any, enter _____ "). New certificates, with check boxes provided for specific complications and procedures, were then introduced. By early 1952 these completely replaced the old forms, and the check-box format has been in effect since then.

women with a previous section is limited to 1962; comparable data were not available for the 1950 period. Throughout this chapter the term "births" includes live births and reported fetal deaths of 20 weeks or more gestation.

Complications of Pregnancy and Labor

Rates in 1960–62

Color

About 1 out of 12 white pregnant women (86 per 1,000) in 1960–62 had at least one of the specified complications of pregnancy and labor (Table 4.1). Dystocias, with a rate of 51 per 1,000, accounted for three-fifths of all the reported complications. The next most frequent set of complications consisted of placental problems; this was followed by toxemias of pregnancy (19 and 12 per 1,000 births, respectively). Diabetes and prolapsed umbilical cord appeared much less often as complications (2 per 1,000 births, each category).

The overall rate of complications was moderately higher among nonwhite pregnancies (100 per 1,000). The difference is almost entirely due to the great excess of toxemias of pregnancy in the nonwhite group. Diabetes and cord complications were also more frequent among the nonwhite, but because of their comparatively low rates the differentials in these complications had little influence on the margin between the overall rates. Placental problems occurred at about the same rate among white and nonwhite pregnant women, and the dystocia rates were also quite similar.

Age of Mother and Birth Order

For the selected conditions as a group, the complication rate was comparatively high among the very young mothers, those under 18 years of age, and highest at ages 40 and over (Table 4.1). This relationship was found among both white and nonwhite women. However, in the nonwhite group the low point in the rate occurred at 20–24 years, as compared with 25–29 years among white mothers. Also, advancing age appeared to carry with it a sharper increase in risk among the nonwhite and the peak at ages 40 and over was exceedingly high in this color group (214 per 1,000 births).

The pattern of the association between maternal age and com-

Table 4.1   Specified complications of pregnancy and delivery per 1,000 single births by age of mother and color and by birth order and color: Upstate New York, 1951-52 and 1960-62.

Age of mother, birth order, color	1960-62						1951-52					
	A–E[1]	A	B	C	D	E	A–E[1]	A	B	C	D	E
White												
Total[2]	86	12	2	19	2	51	113	12	1	17	2	80
Under 18	110	27	1	15	1	68	123	19	*	12	2	89
18-19	98	19	1	14	1	66	113	14	0	12	2	85
20-24	83	11	1	15	2	55	106	11	1	13	2	80
25-29	75	8	2	18	2	46	107	9	0	16	2	79
30-34	83	11	2	22	3	46	113	12	1	21	3	77
35-39	103	18	3	27	4	54	138	21	1	26	5	88
40 or over	133	32	5	34	5	65	170	34	2	33	7	100
Birth order[3]												
1	127	21	2	14	2	92	161	19	1	14	2	128
2 and 3	69	8	2	10	2	41	90	8	0	17	2	61
4 and 5	74	10	2	23	3	36	87	10	0	21	3	52
6 or more	91	15	2	32	4	39	113	19	2	31	5	58
Nonwhite												
Total[2]	100	28	3	21	4	46	111	22	1	22	3	66
Under 18	105	48	*	15	4	45	135	38	*	20	*	74
18-19	93	23	*	19	5	47	104	18	*	20	*	65
20-24	85	20	2	18	3	44	101	13	*	21	*	64
25-29	94	21	3	22	5	44	106	20	*	21	*	64
30-34	114	34	6	27	4	49	121	31	*	23	*	65
35-39	146	58	11	26	4	59	140	39	*	25	*	73
40 or more	214	98	*	37	*	75	160	65	*	*	*	76
Birth order[3]												
1	135	41	2	19	3	77	160	29	*	18	4	113
2 and 3	79	18	3	17	4	39	89	14	*	20	2	52
4 and 5	87	23	4	24	4	35	102	27	*	26	*	49
6 or more	115	40	6	30	5	39	99	29	*	29	*	39

Source: Special tabulations, New York State Department of Health.

Note: Included are live births and all reported fetal deaths of 20 weeks or more gestation or gestation not stated. Complications are as follows: A—pre-eclampsia, eclampsia and hypertension; B—diabetes; C—placenta previa and premature separation; D—prolapse of cord; E—dystocias.

[1]Sum of rates for individual complications is greater than the total because more than 1 complication was reported for some pregnancies.

[2]Not stated ages are included in totals but not distributed.

[3]Number of children ever born to mother including fetal deaths.

*Rates not computed, less than 10 cases.

plication rate differed from one complication to the next. Elevated rates at both ends of the reproductive age span were strongly evident in the toxemias of pregnancy for both white and nonwhite mothers. This type of relationship in a highly attenuated form was present in the white pregnancies complicated by dystocias. In the other complications, and particularly in placental complications, the rate tended to increase with maternal age, with the more important increases occurring generally after age 30.

Nonwhite mothers had a higher toxemia rate than white women at every age level. The nonwhite rates were double the white at ages 20–29 years and triple the white at ages over 30 years. Another interesting observation is that the dystocia rates among the white women were well above the figures for the nonwhite at the younger ages. Above age 25 the rates were very close.

In the aggregate the complication rate was highest at birth order 1, with a sharp decrease occurring at birth orders 2 and 3 and increases at the higher birth orders. The exceptionally high rate of complications associated with birth order 1 is primarily related to dystocias, but there also appears to be an elevated rate of toxemias in first pregnancies. In the case of dystocia, the rate does not rise in the higher birth orders. The toxemia rate is at a low point at birth orders 2 and 3 and increases in succeeding pregnancies. Placental complications depart from these patterns with the higher birth orders showing the largest rates. The relationships between the rates of complications of pregnancy and birth order are similar for white and nonwhite women.

Joint consideration of maternal age and birth order for white women modifies the impressions obtained when each of these variables is examined separately (Appendix Table I.22a). It is evident that at every birth order, the overall rate of the selected complications increases with maternal age, particularly after age 30. The earlier observation that young women have an elevated risk of complications seems to reflect heavy weighting of this group with first pregnancies which have comparatively high complication rates. In an analogous way, the data show clearly that once maternal age is taken into account and once the woman is past her first pregnancy, increasing birth order does not seem to influence the overall complication rate to any extent.

In the dystocias, as expected, the rate is substantially higher at birth order 1 than at any other birth order no matter what age group is looked at. Under 25 years of age, the rate among women in their first pregnancy is double the rate in later pregnancies. Beyond this age the margin is greater. It is also apparent that within each birth order, the risk of dystocia increases with age particularly among women over 30 years of age. In the toxemias of pregnancy the rate also tends to increase markedly in each birth order group with advancing age past 30 years. After the first pregnancy, birth order is of little consequence in the toxemia rate at each age level. In placental complications, however, the rate is lowest at birth orders 1 or 2 and 3, and increases in each succeeding birth order within a maternal age group.

The range in the magnitude of the risk of obstetrical complications associated with birth order and maternal age is very large. Among white mothers the combined rate for the selected complications varies from about 60 per 1,000 at ages under 30 in birth orders 2-5 to four and five times this figure in first pregnancies at ages 35-39 and 40 and over, respectively. Both the dystocias and toxemias contribute heavily to this differential. Actually, in each of these sets of complications, there is an eightfold to tenfold differential between the low-risk and high-risk groups of women.

Among nonwhite women the same general types of relationships are observed when maternal age and birth order are considered jointly as described for white women (Appendix Table I.22b). Maternal age, however, has an even more dramatic effect on changes in the overall rate of complications among nonwhite women. As a result, while the peak rates in this color group are found among first pregnancies at ages past 35 years, the risk among women over 40 years at all birth orders is extremely high. Other high-risk groups of nonwhite women consist of those aged 25-34 years who are in their first pregnancies.

Previous Child Losses
Women with a history of prior fetal or child losses have a markedly higher obstetrical complication rate during their current pregnancy than do other women who are in their second or later pregnancy (Fig. 4.1). The overall rate of complications rises sharply with increasing number of prior losses until the group of women with at least four previous losses is reached. The drop in the rate in the latter group must be viewed with caution because of the small numbers involved. Both the toxemia and placental complication

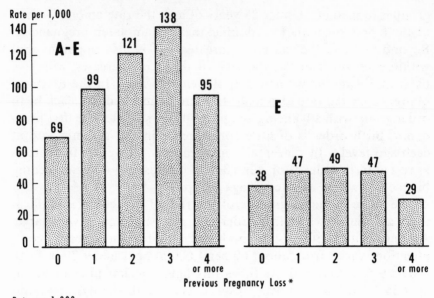

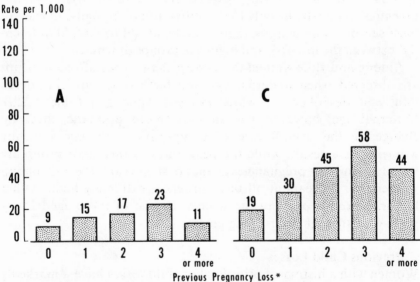

Fig. 4.1. Specified complications of pregnancy and delivery per 1,000 single white births by previous pregnancy loss (excludes first pregnancies): Upstate New York, 1960–62.

Source: Special tabulations by the New York State Department of Health.

Notes: Included are live births and all reported fetal deaths of 20 weeks' or more gestation. Complications are as follows: A—pre-eclampsia, eclampsia and hypertension; C—placenta previa and premature separation; E—dystocias. Complications B (diabetes) and D (prolapse of cord) included in "Complications A–E" but not shown separately.

*Previous loss refers to the number of children born alive to the mother who died plus the number of fetal deaths that the mother had.

rates exhibit strong associations with the number of prior losses. By comparison, the relationship between the dystocia rate and prior losses is insignificant.

These observations complement the findings presented in Chapter 2 concerning the elevation of pregnancy loss among women with a history of prior fetal loss or premature birth. It would add greatly to the interpretation of the associations involving complications in the current pregnancy if the rate of various types of complications in previous pregnancies were known. However, this information is not available from the birth records.

Birth Weight

Among both white and nonwhite women the risk of a pregnancy terminating in a birth at 2,500 grams or less was sharply raised in the presence of one or more of the selected obstetrical complications. Furthermore, as indicated below, the chances that a complicated pregnancy would end with a birth at the very low birth weights of 1,500 grams or less were several times the corresponding figure for all pregnancies combined.

	Percent of those in each category with specified birth weights (1960–62)			
	White		Nonwhite	
Complications	1,500 grams or less	1,501– 2,500 grams	1,500 grams or less	1,501– 2,500 grams
All single births	*1.3*	*5.5*	*3.3*	*10.7*
Total with specified complication	6.8	12.5	13.0	16.8
Pre-eclampsia, eclampsia, hypertension	3.7	12.9	6.1	18.5
Diabetes	4.5	10.2	2.8	13.2
Placental complications	19.9	27.6	33.3	29.3
Prolapse of cord	12.6	13.3	25.8	15.1
Dystocias	2.6	7.0	7.7	11.3

Exceptionally high proportions of the pregnancies with placental complications terminated with a low birth-weight child; almost half of the white births and three-fifths of the nonwhite births weighed 2,500 grams or less. The risk of low birth weight was also very high in pregnancies complicated by prolapse of cord. Excess risk remained high in the presence of toxemias and was only moderately elevated in the dystocia cases. Diabetes appeared to be followed by an unusually high proportion of births at the low weights in pregnancies among white mothers but not among nonwhite mothers. About 9 percent of the white and nonwhite women with diabetes had births weighing 4,500 grams or more; approximately 1 percent of the births to all women (with and without complications combined) were in this weight group.

The relation between birth weight and obstetrical complications may also be examined to determine the extent to which births of a particular weight were preceded by one or more of the specified complications. The data are given in Appendix Table I.23. Among white women almost half of the pregnancies terminating with a birth at 1,000 grams or less (46 percent) had a reported complication. The proportion was close to this figure in the next weight group, 1,001–1,500 grams (43 percent), but with increasing birth weight, it dropped rapidly. The low point (7 percent) was found in the weight groups 2,501–3,500 grams and 3,501–4,000 grams. The proportion was almost twice as great (13 percent) at the high birth weights of 4,501 grams or more.

While the patterns of the relation between birth weight and complications among white and nonwhite pregnancies were generally similar, they showed several differences of some importance. Smaller proportions of the nonwhite pregnancies ending with births at low weights were reported to have one of the specified complications. This is of interest in view of the earlier observation that nonwhite children at birth weights below 2,001 grams have lower neonatal mortality rates than corresponding groups of white children.

Another difference is that in the nonwhite group, an extraordinarily high proportion (25 percent) of the births over 4,500 grams were preceded by complications in pregnancy; the proportion for the white group was half this figure (13 percent). Again, this is of interest in relation to the observation that neonatal mortality at birth weights over 4,500 grams is considerably higher among the nonwhite. As mentioned later, however, a restriction on drawing far-reaching inferences about relations between complications and mortality is the possibility that the reporting of complications is more complete when death occurs soon after birth.

Each of the specified complications was present among pregnancies ending in low birth weights in considerable excess as compared with the situation for all pregnancies combined. Placental complications showed the greatest excess and accounted for exceptionally large proportions of the total complications, particularly at very low birth weights. At birth weights of 4,501 grams or more, all but the placental complications were in excess of the general averages. Dystocias were of considerable importance for this weight category, but in the nonwhite group especially, the excesses in the toxemia and diabetes complications were extraordinarily large.

Changes in Rates
There has been a moderate decrease in the reported overall incidence of selected obstetrical complications in upstate New York in the decade from 1951–52 to 1960–62 (Table 4.1). The decrease among white women was about twice that among nonwhite women. A major decline in the rate of dystocia accounted for virtually all of the total decline observed. In the white group the rates for the other complications were essentially the same in the two time periods, but the toxemia rate increased slightly among the nonwhite women.

Among white mothers a reduction in the complication rate was experienced at all age levels and in each birth-order group. Young women under 20 years of age showed the smallest relative change. In the nonwhite group the degree of change varied widely, with mothers over the age of 35 having at least as high a complication rate in 1960–62 as a decade earlier.

Caesarean Sections

Rates in 1960–62
The rate of Caesarean sections among both white and nonwhite women in upstate New York in 1960–62 was 39 per 1,000 births (Table 4.2). The Caesarean section rate bears a definite relation to maternal age, and to birth order when age is taken into account. Within each birth-order group the rate of Caesarean section increased consistently with maternal age, the highest rate among white women (313 per 1,000 births) occurring in the age group 40 and over with no previous births. At each maternal age, except

Table 4.2   Caesarean sections per 1,000 single births by age of mother, birth order and color: Upstate New York, 1951-52 and 1960-62.

Color and age of mother	1960-62					1951-52				
	Total	Birth order			6 or more	Total	Birth order			6 or more
		1	2 and 3	4 and 5			1	2 and 3	4 and 5	
White										
Total¹	39	37	39	40	38	37	40	39	28	26
Under 20	22	22	22	*	-	19	20	19	-	-
20-24	28	29	27	26	18	25	26	24	17	*
25-29	35	46	35	32	27	34	43	34	22	23
30-34	47	83	52	40	35	45	74	48	28	23
35-39	65	156	79	54	44	66	159	77	38	24
40 or more	90	313	118	66	60	93	294	120	49	42
Nonwhite										
Total¹	39	44	44	35	29	34	47	34	27	17
Under 20	26	25	27	*	-	25	28	19	*	-
20-24	31	37	31	23	20	32	41	31	24	*
25-29	42	78	50	34	24	33	70	32	22	*
30-34	51	126	69	44	34	44	107	46	44	*
35-39	73	240	132	57	38	45	*	81	*	*
40 or more	69	*	172	*	*	*	*	*	-	*

Source: Special tabulations, New York State Department of Health.

Note: Birth order refers to number of children ever born to mother including fetal deaths.

¹Not stated ages are included in totals but not distributed.

*Rates not computed, less than 10 cases.

under 20, the rate of Caesarean section was highest with the first birth, declining at higher birth orders. The decline was marginal among those 20–24 years of age; but in each successive age group the drop in the Caesarean section rate between first births and higher-order births became progressively larger. This may well result from a tendency for older women who have a Caesarean section not to become pregnant again.

Among white women the rate of Caesarean section was sharply elevated in pregnancies involving infants weighing 1,001–2,500 grams at birth (Table 4.3). The peak rate, 103 per 1,000 births, occurred at birth weights 1,501–2,000 grams. After declining from this figure as weight increased, the Caesarean section rate rose at birth weights over 4,500 grams. The pattern for nonwhite women differed considerably. Caesarean rates in this group were elevated at birth weights 1,001–2,500 grams but the highest point was reached at the heavy birth weights. Also, there was markedly less variation in the Caesarean section rates among nonwhite women than among the white. Furthermore, under 2,501 grams, the rates in the nonwhite group were substantially lower than in the white.

Almost one in four of the white women with one of the selected

Table 4.3 Caesarean sections per 1,000 single births by birth weight,
selected complication of labor and delivery, and color:
Upstate New York, 1951-52 and 1960-62.

Birth weight, complications	1960-62		1951-52	
	White	Nonwhite	White	Nonwhite
Total[1]	39	39	37	34
1,000 grams or less	30	22	37	*
1,001-1,500	82	57	82	*
1,501-2,000	103	58	104	55
2,001-2,500	76	48	73	53
2,501-3,500	39	36	36	31[2]
3,501-4,500	32	41	30[2]	32[2]
4,501 or more	48	76	57[3]	-
2,500 or less	76	47	76	51
2,501 or more	36	38	34	31
A-E[4]	225	206	199	201
A	123	89	154	94
B	363	284	342	*
C	290	210	318	187
D	215	182	62	*
E	227	281	187	255
None of above	21	21	16	13

Source: Special tabulations, New York State Department of Health.

Note: Included are live births and all reported fetal deaths of 20
weeks or more gestation or gestation not stated. Complications are as
follows: A--pre-eclampsia, eclampsia and hypertension; B--diabetes;
C--placenta previa and premature separation, D--prolapse of cord; E--dystocias.

[1]Not stated birth weights included in totals but not distributed.

[2]Birth weight 3,501-5,000 grams.

[3]Birth weight 5,001 grams or more.

[4]Sum of rates for individual complications is greater than the total
because more than 1 complication was reported for some pregnancies.

*Rates not computed, less than 10 cases.

complications of pregnancy and labor (225 per 1,000) had a Caesarean section. The highest rate of sections was associated with maternal diabetes; this was followed by the rate for placental complications, which figures prominently among deliveries involving very small babies. Rates of section in pregnancies complicated by prolapsed cord or dystocias were also high, involving one in five or one in four of these pregnancies. The section rate among women with toxemias lagged far behind (one in eight).

In general, the Caesarean section rates in the presence of specific complications vary among nonwhite women in much the same way as among the white, except that the rate for dystocias is as high as for diabetes. But, probing beyond this similarity reveals one of the more illuminating differences between white and nonwhite pregnancies demonstrated by vital statistics. In each of the complications, except dystocia, the Caesarean section rate is considerably higher among the white women. Inquiries into differences in sources of prenatal care and in management of labor and delivery would seem to be among the more important ways to understand this relationship.

Thus far the discussion has covered the rate at which women with various complications undergo Caesarean section. The issue may also be examined by determining the composition of the cases delivered by Caesarean section, particularly with regard to the history of previous section. Major complications of pregnancy and labor were reported for about half of all the white women delivered by Caesarean section in 1962. After the first pregnancy two-thirds of the sections were performed among women with a previous section. The proportion of cases with complications differed sharply in the presence or absence of a previous Caesarean section. In the absence of a previous section, 78 percent of the white mothers had recorded obstetrical complications, in contrast to only 20 percent when a previous section had been performed. This documents the well-known clinical observation that a high proportion of repeat Caesarean sections are elective.

Among white women of birth order 1 who were delivered by Caesarean section, dystocia was reported in 68 percent of the cases. This dropped to 27 percent among women of birth order 2 or more who had no previous section and to only 14 percent among those with previous sections. Placental complications were associated with section in about 10 percent of women of birth order 1, jumping to 38 percent among the women of birth order 2 or more who did not have a previous section. In contrast, placental complications were reported in only 3 percent of the women of higher birth order who had had a previous section. Similar relationships were found for the nonwhite women.

Changes in Rates

Among white women the rate of Caesarean sections increased very slightly between 1951–52 and 1960–62 (Table 4.2). This increase in Caesarean sections was compensated for by a similar decrease in the rate of mid-forceps deliveries (Fig. 4.2). In both time periods 6 percent of the mothers were delivered by Caesarean section or mid-forceps, with most of the cases being sections. The only category of women for which mid-forceps were used more frequently than Caesarean sections consisted of primiparous women. In succeeding pregnancies the rate for mid-forceps was substantially lower than the rate for sections. These relationships were stronger in 1960–62 than 10 years earlier.

Although the Caesarean section rate for all white mothers combined changed little, important shifts took place in some of the subgroups. For example, the decline in the Caesarean section rate with increasing birth order was more pronounced at all maternal age levels in 1951–52 than in 1960–62 (Table 4.2). This change assumes added meaning when it is realized that the Caesarean section rate in first pregnancies was about the same in both time periods. In view of this, it might be concluded that the current, less rapid, decrease in Caesarean section rates after the first pregnancy reflects a greater likelihood among women with a prior section to become pregnant again and/or a greater tendency among obstetricians to repeat sections.

There was a moderate increase in the Caesarean section rate among nonwhite women between 1951–52 and 1960–62, so that the small difference in the earlier period in the overall rates for the two color groups was wiped out by the later date. Increases in the section rate occurred among nonwhite women at all ages above 25 years.

No change of consequence occurred over the decade in the Caesarean section rate related to any birth-weight grouping among either white or nonwhite women (Table 4.3). The story is somewhat different when attention is directed to Caesarean sections associ-

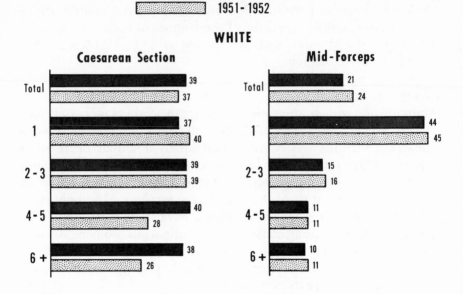

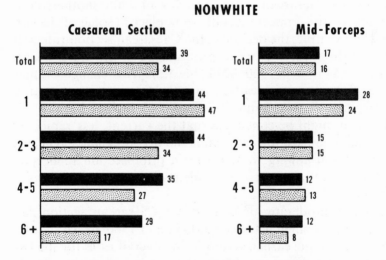

Fig. 4.2. Caesarean section and mid-forceps deliveries per 1,000 single births by birth order and color: Upstate New York, 1951–52 and 1960–62.

Source: Special tabulations by the New York State Department of Health.

Notes: Included are live births and all recorded fetal deaths of 20 weeks' or more gestation. Birth order refers to number of children ever born to mother, including fetal deaths.

ated with complications. Within the groups of white women suffering obstetrical complications a slightly greater proportion had sections in 1960–62 than in 1951–52. The increase in the rate of Caesarean section as the mode of delivery in the presence of prolapsed umbilical cord was striking. In 1960–62 the rate of Caesarean section among white mothers with prolapsed cord was 21 percent, in contrast to only 6 percent in 1951–52. This dramatic shift in mode of management probably reflects the increased concern about fetal distress and intrauterine hypoxia during the past decade. Although the numbers are small and subject to large chance variation, it would appear that a sharp increase in the section rate for prolapsed cord also occurred among nonwhite women.

Changes in Caesarean section rates related to the other complications have not been marked, although some increase seems to have occurred in the dystocia cases. Minor reductions in Caesarean section rates among women with toxemia and placental complications and a slight increase in relation to diabetes can not be construed as reflecting changes in clinical attitudes.

The proportion of pregnant women with none of the specified obstetrical complications who underwent Caesarean sections increased over the 1950 decade in both the white and nonwhite groups. This is consistent with the earlier observation that there may now be a greater tendency or opportunity to perform repeat sections than in 1951–52. The increase in the section rate among uncomplicated cases was greater in the nonwhite group and the rates in 1960–62 were identical for the two groups.

Perinatal Mortality Associated with Obstetrical Complications

Rates in 1960–62

In 1960–62 the perinatal mortality rate associated with obstetrical complications among white women in upstate New York was 122 per 1,000 births as compared with the overall perinatal mortality rate of 25 per 1,000 (Appendix Table I.24). The rates were highest in complications of the placenta (312 per 1,000) and prolapse of the cord (342 per 1,000). These were followed by rates of 223 per 1,000 for diabetes, 86 per 1,000 for toxemias, and 50 per 1,000 for dystocia. Before proceeding with further discussions of losses associated with complications, a word of caution is needed. Since the data are derived from reports on birth and fetal death certificates, there may be an increased tendency to enter one of the obstetrical complications on the certificates when a death occurred or the prognosis for the child is poor. Although it is not known to what extent this does occur, it may be assumed that the mortality rates in complicated cases may be somewhat higher than would be obtained in a study conducted with uniformly applied criteria for classifying births. Similarly, the extremely low perinatal mortality rate for cases without the selected complications, 16 per 1,000, may understate the true situation.

Comparison of neonatal and fetal death rates indicates that the timing of the loss, intrauterine versus extrauterine, differs greatly from one type of complication to another. Among white women with one or more of the specified complications the fetal death rate is moderately higher than the neonatal death rate; the differential is more significant among nonwhites. Fetal mortality is substantially higher than neonatal mortality in the toxemias, diabetes, and prolapsed cord. In the placental complications the difference was in the same direction but much smaller. The only complication in which the risk of loss after birth was greater than the risk of fetal mortality was dystocia, and here the difference was large.

Generally, the relationships described for white births were also found in the nonwhite group. An important exception was the exceptionally high loss rate in the dystocia category, for which the perinatal mortality rate was close to the rate for toxemias. As seen below, in the mortality rates per 1,000 single births, 1960–62, the loss rate in cases without the selected complications was well below the rate for all births combined.

Complications	White			Nonwhite		
	Neonatal	Fetal	Perinatal	Neonatal	Fetal	Perinatal
All single births	*12*	*13*	*25*	*22*	*22*	*44*
Total with specified complications	57	68	122	85	119	194
Pre-eclampsia, eclampsia, hypertension	22	65	86	23	98	119
Diabetes	87	149	223	*	146	118
Placental complications	162	179	312	225	291	451
Prolapse of cord	100	269	342	157	321	428
Dystocias	31	20	50	70	48	114
None of specified complications	8	8	16	16	11	27

White and nonwhite perinatal mortality rates for 1960–62 differed by about the same relative amounts in pregnancies with one or more complications and in those without the reported complications. The greatest relative difference was evident in the dystocias, in which the rate among the nonwhite women was about two and a half times the rate among the white women. The only complication in which the rate was not higher among the nonwhite was diabetes. These patterns were present in both the fetal and neonatal mortality rates. However, among complicated cases the differential between the white and nonwhite rates was larger in fetal mortality than in neonatal mortality (75 percent compared with 49 percent); and among cases without the selected complications the differential was greater in neonatal mortality (100 percent compared with 38 percent).

Changes in Rates
Between 1951–52 and 1960–62 the perinatal mortality rate among the offspring of white women decreased by 17 percent. The rate in the presence of major complications of pregnancy and delivery increased slightly (Appendix Table I.24). There was a sharp decrease in the perinatal mortality rate for prolapse of cord and a lesser decrease in each of the other obstetrical complications, except for dystocia, which experienced an increase in the rate.

The increase in the perinatal mortality rate related to the dystocias, although very small, bears further scrutiny. It was previously pointed out that the rate of reported dystocias decreased markedly during the 1950's in the white group. In view of this change, it is necessary to entertain the possibility that the nature of reported dystocias may also have changed and that the rise in the perinatal mortality rate in the dystocia cases may reflect a shift towards more severe cases in this category. Another consequence of the lowered incidence of dystocias is that these complications represented a smaller proportion of the total complications under study in 1960–62 than in 1951–52 (60 percent and 72 percent in the two periods, respectively). Taking this reduction into account results in an adjusted[3] perinatal mortality rate of 103 per 1,000 births

[3] Perinatal mortality rates for 1960–62 in each specified complication category were applied to the distribution of births with complications in 1951–52. The total number of deaths derived in this calculation was reduced to allow for the fact that for a small proportion of pregnancies more than one complication was reported. After this step, the number of perinatal deaths was divided by the total number of births with one or more complications.

for the total group of complications in 1960–62, which is slightly lower than the rate 113 per 1,000 births in 1951–52. It is apparent that the improvement in perinatal mortality in the presence of most types of complications was large enough to counteract increased losses in the dystocias despite the fact that the dystocias were considerably more numerous than all other complications combined.

Among the nonwhite, the 1950 decade was a period of no reduction in the perinatal mortality rate (44 per 1,000 births in both 1951–52 and 1960–62). Losses increased in the group with complications from 149 per 1,000 to 194 per 1,000; while the rate in pregnancies with no reported complications changed little (31 per 1,000 in 1951–52 and 27 per 1,000 in 1960–62). Adjustment for changes in the incidence of the various complications does not alter the conclusion that the perinatal mortality rate in the presence of complications rose (the adjusted rate for 1960–62 was 188 per 1,000 births). The increase in mortality among complicated cases seems to have been greater in the neonatal mortality rates than in the fetal death rates. This may reflect an increased likelihood that poor-risk infants survive birth only to succumb shortly afterwards. While this speculation is important, within the context of understanding the lack of improvement in perinatal mortality, the more significant observation is that both the fetal and neonatal mortality rates in complicated cases rose. On the other hand, both components of the perinatal mortality rate decreased slightly when none of the selected complications was present.

Perinatal Mortality in Caesarean Sections

Rates in 1960–62
Perinatal mortality among white births delivered by Caesarean section was two and a half times the rate for all births (61 per 1,000 as against 25 per 1,000). This excess is deceptive. In the presence of the obstetrical complications under study in this chapter, the group of women that underwent Caesarean sections had lower loss rates (Appendix Table I.24). This held for each of the complications other than toxemia. Especially noteworthy is the extraordinarily low rate in the dystocia cases with sections. When perinatal mortality rates are examined for cases with none of the complications,

the Caesarean section group is found to have twice as high a rate as the total group. Data for 1962 on repeat sections indicate that a large majority (82 percent) of the Caesarean sections with no obstetrical complications were performed among multiparous women who had a prior Caesarean section (discussed later). This, however, does not explain the elevated rate. More complete information would be required than is available regarding other difficulties or circumstances present during labor and delivery to assess the meaning of the comparatively high rate in this Caesarean section group.

The neonatal mortality rate in the white group with Caesarean sections was almost twice the corresponding fetal death rate. This represents a major shift in the timing of the perinatal deaths as compared with the situation in the total group of births, in which most of the deaths were intrauterine. The shift is most extreme among Caesarean section cases with none of the specified obstetrical complications. In this group the neonatal death rate was three and a half times the fetal mortality rate. Large relative differentials also occurred in the diabetes and dystocia cases. Prolapsed cord was the only complication not associated with a higher neonatal mortality rate.

Among nonwhite births the perinatal mortality rate was higher in the Caesarean section category than in the total group; but the differential was far less than among the white. Actually, the difference between perinatal mortality rates for nonwhite and white births with sections was only about 24 percent as compared with 74 percent for all births. Unlike the situation among the white, the neonatal and fetal mortality rates among the nonwhite with sections were very close.

Changes in Rates
The perinatal mortality rate among white births associated with Caesarean section showed a small decrease from 72 to 61 per 1,000 total births between 1951–52 and 1960–62 in upstate New York (Appendix Table I.24). This paralleled the decline in perinatal mortality for all births during the same period. Most of the decline in perinatal mortality among the Caesarean section births was in the fetal mortality component, with only a very slight drop in neonatal mortality.

In each of the major complications of labor and delivery with Caesarean sections the perinatal mortality decreased in the white group. A particularly large decline was evident in the rate when Caesarean section was performed in the presence of prolapsed cord. In this complication, the several-fold increase in the use of Caesarean section may have been the decisive factor. One of the smaller proportionate decreases in mortality occurred in the group with dystocias. Adjustment of the 1960–62 rate for changes in the distribution of complications among the Caesarean section cases indicates that if there had been no such change, the perinatal mortality rate would have been lowered from 89 per 1,000 in 1951–52 to 78 per 1,000 in 1960–62.

In the white group with Caesarean sections fetal death rates declined by almost a third during the 1950's, while neonatal death rates remained stationary for all practical purposes. This raises once again the possibility that some of the infants who in 1951–52 might have died before or during delivery were born alive in 1960–62, only to succumb during the neonatal period. Support for this possibility is found in the rates for women with the specified complications. Among these women the fetal death rate associated with Caesarean sections decreased slightly, while the neonatal death rate increased. Changes in the distribution of complications over the 1950 decade do not explain the preceding observations.

In the nonwhite group the number of births is too small to support the type of exploration conducted for the white births. However, both the neonatal and fetal death rates for births with Caesarean sections changed very little over the decade.

Rates by Previous Caesarean Section
Of special interest are the perinatal mortality rates in 1962 according to history of previous Caesarean section (Appendix Table I.25). Birth and fetal death certificates provide information on prior abdominal delivery only if a Caesarean section has been performed in the current pregnancy, and the discussion is accordingly limited to this group. Despite this restriction the data are extremely useful in clarifying perinatal mortality risks associated with Caesarean sections. All rates are for white births; frequencies are too small for nonwhite births.

Women with a repeat Caesarean section had a much lower perinatal mortality rate among their offspring than those subjected to abdominal delivery for the first time. This is to be expected, since an overwhelming majority of primary sections are performed in the presence of obstetrical complications. However, even when the rates are confined to Caesarean sections in the presence of reported obstetrical complications, the perinatal mortality rate in the repeat sections was substantially lower than the rate in the primary section group. In fact, the risk of perinatal mortality in the repeat group of sections (1962) was only moderately higher than the risk among all births, with and without sections in 1960–62 (30 per 1,000 as compared with 25 per 1,000).

Increasing birth order sharply elevated the risk of perinatal mortality in primary Caesarean sections. First pregnancies with sections had a perinatal mortality rate of 41 per 1,000; this rate more than doubled at birth orders 2 and 3 (108 per 1,000) and increased further at higher birth orders (137 per 1,000). The doubling of the perinatal mortality rate at birth orders 2 and 3 runs counter to the reduction in mortality found at these birth orders in the total group of births. In large measure, this relationship reflects the more serious nature of the complications in second and third pregnancies that lead to primary sections.

Three out of four of the perinatal deaths in repeat sections occurred among children born alive. A preponderance of neonatal deaths was found among repeat sections in the presence of obstetrical complications (68 percent) and in the absence of these complications (85 percent). This is to be expected as a consequence of the timing of the intervention in abdominal deliveries to minimize the likelihood of a fetal death, and the fact that a section may not be undertaken in some cases if the fetus is already known to be dead. The proportion of perinatal deaths in the primary section group that consisted of neonatal deaths (57 percent) was considerably lower than in the repeat sections. It was, however, somewhat above the proportion for all births in 1960–62 (48 percent).

5 / INTERNATIONAL COMPARISONS

Concern about the failure of the infant mortality rate in the United States to show a major decline during the 1950's and early 1960's was sharpened by the realization that the rate in other countries continued to decrease long after it started to level off here and that increasing numbers of countries are experiencing lower rates than the United States. In this chapter the relative position of the United States is considered with regard to trend and level of infant loss from 1935 to 1964. Much of the material is drawn from an earlier analysis of the situation (1) and from documents prepared for an international conference on the problem convened by the National Center for Health Statistics May 13–14, 1965 (2). Both the earlier analysis and the conference were interested in the nature of the differences and similarities in trends between the United States and other countries, the reality of the relative position of the rate in this country, and the prospects for further significant reductions in the rate here as judged by experience elsewhere. The discussion that follows is concerned with similar issues (3).

Most of the comparisons involve Australia, Canada, Denmark, England and Wales, Finland, the Netherlands, New Zealand, Norway, Sweden, and Switzerland. These countries have been characterized by comparatively low infant mortality rates for a long period of time.[1] All of them have had for many years a well-developed vital registration system, and the definition of live birth and the reporting requirements for early infant deaths have been comparatively stable.

Data for these countries represent the most favorable set of statistics for studying trends. However, there are certain problems of interpretation of the levels of mortality arising from differences in definition of live birth and fetal death, and from differences in statistical practice. These problems are considered later. At this point it should be noted that although variations in definitions, registration, and data-handling are serious enough to qualify statements about the magnitude of differences between the infant loss rate in the United States and in other countries, they do not explain

[1] Another country which has recorded low infant mortality rates for years is Iceland. Because of the small frequency of infant deaths (64 in 1960), the rates are subject to wide variations. Therefore, data for this country are not included in this discussion.

this country's relative position in infant mortality or the differences between the trends in the rates in the United States and abroad.

Infant Mortality

Infant mortality rates in all of the countries mentioned above were at a much lower level in the early 1960's than in the mid-1930's (Table 5.1). The progress in the reduction of infant loss does not reflect consistent and continuous decreases over the whole period. World War II was a period of increase in infant mortality for some countries but other periods of stability or increase in the rate are also found. This makes it difficult to assess infant mortality rates over a short run. Nevertheless, certain time periods stand out as being of particular importance in interpreting the course of the infant mortality rate.

During the prewar period, 1935–39, most countries experienced significant reductions in infant mortality. This downward trend was interrupted by the war in many of the belligerent nations. The wartime increases in the infant mortality rate were particularly severe for the Netherlands, Finland, and Norway, and to a lesser extent, for England and Wales. Major reductions in the infant mortality rate occurred in many countries the year after the war ended. This was followed by a period (1946–50) of important decreases in all areas. Relatively, the greatest reductions occurred in Denmark, England and Wales, and the Netherlands; the smallest in Canada, New Zealand, and the United States.

The leveling off of the infant mortality rate in the United States very early during the 1950's was not matched at the time by the experience of any other country (Fig. 5.1). A slowing down or cessation in the decline of the rate did set in later in the decade in most of these countries. However, in several of them, impressive additional decreases were recorded in the early 1960's. Whether this is a temporary situation or not, it is significant that by 1964 no sharp dip in the rate, even of a temporary nature, had occurred in the United States. The fact is that the infant mortality rate for the United States would have to start decreasing much more sharply to modify the strong impression that the United States is lagging behind many countries in reducing the loss in infancy.

Furthermore, the comparisons include countries that already

Table 5.1   Infant mortality rates per 1,000 live births: Selected countries, 1935-64.

Year	Australia[1]	Canada[2]	Denmark[3]	England and Wales	Finland	Netherlands[4]	New Zealand[5]	Norway	Sweden	Switzerland	United States
1964	----	24.7	18.7[6]	19.9	----	14.8	19.1	----	14.2	----	24.8
1963	19.5	26.3	19.1	21.1	18.2	15.8	19.6	16.9	15.4	20.5	25.2
1962	20.4	27.6	20.1	21.7	20.5	17.0	20.4	17.7	15.4	21.2	25.3
1961	19.5	27.2	21.8	21.4	20.8	17.0	22.8	17.9	15.8	21.0	25.3
1960	20.2	27.3	21.5	21.8	21.0	17.9	19.7	18.9	16.6	21.1	26.0
1959	21.5	28.4	22.5	22.2	23.6	18.1	19.9	18.7	16.6	22.2	26.4
1958	20.5	30.2	22.4	22.5	24.5	18.5	19.4	20.0	15.9	22.2	27.1
1957	21.4	30.9	23.4	23.1	27.9	18.4	20.0	20.5	17.8	22.9	26.3
1956	21.7	31.9	24.9	23.6	25.4	20.2	19.4	21.2	17.3	25.8	26.0
1955	22.0	31.3	25.2	24.9	29.7	21.6	20.1	20.6	17.4	26.5	26.4
1954	22.5	31.9	26.9	25.5	30.6	22.6	20.0	21.4	18.7	27.2	26.6
1953	23.3	35.6	27.2	26.8	34.2	23.7	20.1	22.0	18.7	29.8	27.8
1952	23.8	38.2	28.9	27.5	31.8	24.1	21.8	23.7	20.0	29.1	28.4
1951	25.2	38.5	28.9	29.8	35.4	26.7	22.8	25.7	21.6	30.1	28.4
1950	24.5	41.5	30.7	29.9	43.5	26.7	22.7	28.2	21.0	31.2	29.2
1949	25.3	43.3	34.5	32.7	48.3	26.8	23.8	27.7	23.3	34.3	31.3
1948	27.8	43.7	35.3	34.5	51.9	29.3	21.9	29.6	23.2	35.9	32.0
1947	28.5	45.5	40.4	41.8	58.5	33.5	25.0	34.6	25.4	39.3	32.2
1946	29.0	46.7	45.8	40.9	56.2	38.7	26.1	34.6	26.5	39.2	33.8
1945	29.4	51.3	48.3	47.0	63.2	79.7	28.0	36.4	29.9	40.7	38.3
1944	31.3	54.7	47.7	44.5	68.6	46.3	30.1	36.7	31.1	42.2	39.8
1943	36.3	53.7	44.8	48.9	49.5	40.1	31.4	35.4	28.9	39.8	40.4
1942	36.5	53.8	47.0	49.5	67.2	39.5	28.7	35.9	29.3	38.3	40.4
1941	39.7	59.7	55.0	59.7	59.2	43.6	29.8	43.0	37.0	41.1	45.3
1940	38.4	56.4	50.2	57.4	88.3	39.1	30.2	38.7	39.2	46.2	47.0
1939	38.2	60.7	58.1	50.8	69.6	33.7	31.1	37.2	39.5	42.6	48.0
1938	38.3	63.3	58.7	52.7	67.8	36.5	35.6	37.3	42.5	42.8	51.0
1937	38.1	75.8	66.1	57.6	68.5	38.1	31.2	42.0	45.2	46.7	54.4
1936	41.2	66.1	67.3	58.5	65.9	38.9	31.0	42.0	43.4	46.5	57.1
1935	39.8	71.0	71.0	56.9	66.8	40.0	32.3	44.2	45.9	47.9	55.7

Sources: Files of the Statistical Office of the United Nations and annual volumes <u>Vital Statistics of the United States</u>, National Center for Health Statistics, Public Health Service, Washington.

[1]Excludes full-blooded aborigines. Data tabulated by year of registration rather than occurrence.

[2]For 1935-1949, data exclude Yukon, Northwest Territories; Newfoundland which became the tenth province April 1, 1949 is excluded prior to 1950.

[3]Excluding Faeroe Islands 1932-1948; Faeroe Islands and Greenland starting 1949.

[4]For 1935-1949, live-born infants of less than 28 weeks gestation who died before registration were not registered as either live births or deaths.

[5]By year of registration rather than year of occurrence. Excludes Maoris 1935-1960. Includes Maoris 1961-1964. In 1961, excluding Maoris, rate is 19.1.

[6]Provisional

Rate per 1,000 Live Births

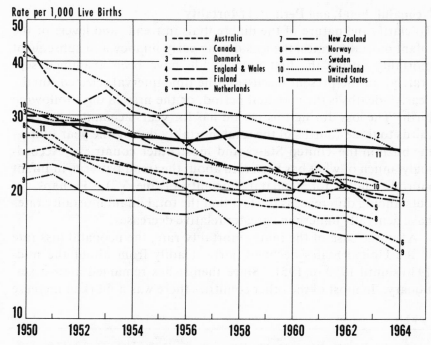

Fig. 5.1. Infant mortality rates: Selected countries, 1935–64.

Source: Files of the Statistical Office of the United Nations; National Center for Health Statistics, *Vital Statistics of the United States*, annual volumes.

have lower infant mortality rates than the United States. Otherwise, one might be tempted to attribute the greater decline in the rates for the other countries to a period of "catching up." While differences in definition and reporting practices create certain difficulties for international comparisons, the infant mortality rates for Australia, Denmark, England and Wales, Finland, New Zealand, and Switzerland are almost certainly lower than that for the United States, and the rates for the Netherlands, Norway, and Sweden are definitely lower. Canada appears to be moving into the group of nations with a lower rate than the United States. Several other countries, not shown in Table 5.1, have either already overtaken the United States or are close to doing so. These include Czechoslovakia, Japan, Belgium, and France, where the infant mortality rate was considerably higher than in the United States not too many years ago.

Neonatal, Fetal, and Perinatal Mortality

To clarify the nature of the differentials in trends and levels of the infant mortality rates, the loss during early infancy and subsequent mortality during the first year of life have been examined separately. In the present discussion the time interval selected for the "early" deaths is the neonatal period, or the first 28 days following birth. The loss during this period has for years accounted for two-thirds to three-fourths of the total mortality during the year following birth in the United States and most other countries. Accordingly, much of what has been said about the trend patterns in infant mortality holds for neonatal mortality (Table 5.2). Perhaps the outstanding difference is the fact that the total infant mortality rates have generally undergone greater relative decreases.

As in the case of the infant mortality rate, the neonatal loss rate in the United States declined fairly steadily from about the mid-1930's until 1950 or 1951. Since then it has remained almost stationary. In most of the other countries there was a marked increase

Table 5.2   Neonatal mortality rates per 1,000 live births: Selected countries, 1935-64.

Year	Australia[1]	Canada[2]	Denmark[3]	England and Wales	Finland	Netherlands[4]	New Zealand[5]	Norway	Sweden	Switzerland	United States
1964	---	17.3	---	13.8	---	11.6	12.4	---	11.7	---	17.9
1963	14.3	18.1	14.7	14.3	13.7	12.0	12.8	11.9	12.3	15.6	18.2
1962	14.7	18.7	15.2	15.1	15.8	12.8	12.7	12.0	12.4	16.1	18.3
1961	14.0	18.0	16.5	15.3	15.3	12.8	14.5	12.3	12.8	16.0	18.4
1960	14.6	17.6	16.1	15.5	14.4	13.5	14.5	11.7	13.9	16.0	18.7
1959	15.3	18.4	16.2	15.9	15.7	13.3	13.9	12.4	13.0	16.6	19.0
1958	14.5	19.3	16.1	16.2	15.4	13.3	13.6	13.3	12.1	16.4	19.5
1957	15.4	20.2	16.3	16.5	16.6	13.1	13.9	13.3	13.5	16.6	19.1
1956	15.6	20.1	17.7	16.8	16.4	14.2	13.3	12.4	13.2	18.9	18.9
1955	15.5	19.3	17.9	17.2	18.6	15.6	14.0	12.5	12.9	18.9	19.1
1954	16.2	19.3	18.0	17.7	19.3	16.2	14.3	11.8	13.8	19.9	19.1
1953	16.5	21.4	18.6	17.7	19.7	16.5	14.3	12.6	13.8	21.2	19.6
1952	16.6	22.7	19.3	18.3	19.1	16.6	15.1	14.1	14.9	20.2	19.8
1951	17.5	22.6	18.3	18.9	19.7	18.4	16.2	14.4	15.8	21.3	20.0
1950	17.4	24.4	18.2	18.5	21.8	17.9	16.6	14.7	15.2	21.1	20.5
1949	18.0	24.1	19.1	19.3	23.1	16.8	17.0	14.5	16.1	23.6	21.4
1948	19.6	25.6	19.1	19.8	23.6	17.4	15.8	15.7	16.8	24.9	22.2
1947	20.5	26.5	22.0	22.8	24.9	18.5	18.1	17.5	17.5	25.8	22.8
1946	21.2	27.2	23.6	24.2	25.9	20.9	19.1	16.9	18.1	25.9	24.0
1945	21.8	28.6	24.9	24.9	26.0	29.8	19.6	18.1	19.1	26.4	24.3
1944	22.0	29.1	24.2	24.2	26.4	23.0	20.6	18.3	19.7	25.8	24.7
1943	24.0	29.6	22.9	25.2	22.9	20.4	21.3	18.0	18.4	25.8	24.7
1942	25.3	28.1	23.6	27.1	24.5	21.0	18.7	17.8	17.9	25.1	25.7
1941	26.6	30.6	23.7	28.9	24.7	22.7	20.0	20.0	21.4	27.9	27.7
1940	25.5	29.7	25.2	29.7	30.4	21.4	22.0	20.5	23.5	27.0	28.8
1939	25.8	30.7	27.5	28.3	28.0	19.8	21.8	18.3	24.2	27.7	29.3
1938	26.0	31.7	27.2	28.3	29.7	20.5	24.1	20.2	25.2	26.2	29.6
1937	26.3	34.2	29.0	29.8	29.4	20.9	22.2	22.9	25.0	28.0	31.3
1936	27.5	33.5	29.1	30.2	27.3	21.5	22.3	22.3	23.2	28.2	32.6
1935	27.5	35.0	29.1	30.4	30.2	22.5	22.0	21.6	25.6	29.3	32.4

Sources: Files of the Statistical Office of the United Nations and annual volumes Vital Statistics of the United States, National Center for Health Statistics, Public Health Service, Washington.

[1]Excludes full-blooded aborigines. Data tabulated by year of registration rather than occurrence.

[2]For 1935-1949, data exclude Yukon, Northwest Territories; Newfoundland, which became the tenth province April 1, 1949 is excluded prior to 1950.

[3]Excluding Faeroe Islands 1932-1948; Faeroe Islands and Greenland starting 1949.

[4]For 1935-1949, live-born infants of less than 28 weeks gestation who died before registration were not registered as either live births or deaths.

[5]By year of registration rather than year of occurrence. Excludes Maoris 1935-1960. Includes Maoris 1961-1964.

in the rate of decline near the end of or immediately after World War II, although the drop was not as sharp as for the total infant mortality rate. The decline persisted, in general, well beyond the year in which the rate leveled off in the United States.

Because of the differences in rates of decline there has been a major shift in the relative levels of the neonatal mortality rates. When the decline in the United States rate started to taper off (1950–51), the neonatal rate in five countries (Canada, Denmark, England and Wales, Finland, and Switzerland) closely approximated the figure here. By the early 1960's the neonatal rates for all the foreign countries shown in Table 5.2, except for Canada, were well below the rate for the United States. Substantially the same situation is found when mortality rates are restricted to the first week after birth.

As discussed later, some care has to be taken in interpreting the significance of the large margin between the mortality rate in early infancy in the United States and the rate elsewhere because of variations in registration requirements and practices. In this connection, it is useful to consider the relative levels of fetal mortality rates (28 weeks' or more gestation) and then to examine the perinatal mortality rates (defined in terms of first-week mortality and fetal mortality).

It has been customary to make the observation that the fetal mortality ratio in the United States is substantially below the ratios in all the other countries under discussion here. This statement is no longer true (Table 5.3). While the ratio in the United States has been almost stationary since the year 1956, it has decreased in practically all of the other countries, and now in several of them the ratio is very similar to the figure for the United States. The closeness of these ratios does, however, seem to be anomalous in light of the wide divergence among the mortality rates in the period shortly after birth. It is not certain whether differences in registration requirements and definitions are entirely responsible for this situation. It may be that some of the pregnancies that are destined to end in a neonatal or first-week death in the United States terminate in a fetal death in other countries. The perinatal mortality rate takes care of both sources of incomparability. What it cannot do is to make allowance for differential rates in completeness of reporting of fetal deaths.

The range of perinatal mortality rates among most of the

Table 5.3   Fetal death ratios: Selected countries, 1940-64.

(Fetal deaths of at least 28 weeks gestation or unknown gestation per 1,000 live births.)

Year	Australia[1]	Canada[2]	Denmark[3]	England and Wales	Finland[4]	Netherlands	New Zealand[5]	Norway	Sweden[6]	Switzerland[7]	United States[8]
1964	---	---	---	16.7	---	13.6	13.0	---	11.3	---	12.3
1963	---	12.3	11.5	17.6	11.6	14.5	12.7	12.7	12.1	11.4	11.8
1962	---	12.5	12.0	18.4	12.6	14.8	12.9	13.8	12.7	12.2	11.5
1961	14.2	12.7	12.7	19.4	13.5	15.1	13.9	13.2	12.8	12.0	11.6
1960	14.4	13.5	12.6	20.2	12.7	15.1	14.4	14.1	13.9	11.5	11.6
1959	14.2	13.7	14.8	21.2	13.4	16.0	14.6	13.3	15.0	12.0	11.7
1958	14.3	14.3	15.7	22.0	13.6	17.0	15.2	14.5	15.9	12.6	11.9
1957	15.6	14.6	15.5	23.0	14.3	17.2	16.1	14.9	15.9	14.3	12.0
1956	15.5	15.5	17.8	23.4	15.3	17.2	17.0	15.4	17.0	13.7	12.1
1955	15.4	15.6	18.2	23.7	14.6	17.3	16.0	15.2	17.0	14.5	12.6
1954	16.0	16.6	19.6	24.0	18.0	17.7	18.0	14.6	17.2	15.6	12.9
1953	16.7	16.7	19.3	22.9	17.9	17.7	19.1	15.7	18.2	15.3	13.4
1952	17.3	18.0	17.8	23.2	19.2	18.6	18.2	15.5	18.6	15.3	13.8
1951	19.0	18.4	18.6	23.6	18.4	18.6	18.0	16.4	19.6	16.0	14.3
1950	19.4	19.3	18.8	23.1	18.9	19.6	19.5	16.4	20.3	17.1	14.6
1949	19.6	19.9	17.1	23.2	17.6	19.7	18.1	16.7	20.5	16.9	15.1
1948	20.7[1]	19.7	18.2	23.7	18.0	19.3	18.9	18.0	19.8	17.3	15.5
1947	21.8[1]	20.8	17.8	24.7	19.5	20.5	20.3	18.7	21.6	16.2	16.1
1946	---	21.5	19.1	27.9	19.6	20.6	22.2	19.2	22.1	15.8	17.2
1945	28.0	23.1	19.8	28.4	21.5	19.6	23.4	20.3	24.6	16.3	18.5
1944	28.0	23.6	20.0	28.4	20.7	18.8	23.8	20.0	23.6	16.7	19.0
1943	28.1	24.0	21.7	31.1	21.3	18.8	27.0	21.1	22.3	16.8	19.3
1942	28.5	26.2	21.3	34.4	22.6	19.7	26.5	20.6	22.9	16.8	20.1
1941	28.2	27.0	23.6	36.0	21.4	21.7	27.7	21.1	25.1	18.9	---
1940	27.8	27.2	25.9	38.6	21.0	25.7	29.4	22.5	29.4	20.9	---

Sources: Files of the Statistical Office of the United Nations and annual volumes Vital Statistics of the United States, National Center for Health Statistics, Public Health Service, Washington.

[1]Excludes full-blooded aborigines. Data tabulated by year of registration rather than occurrence. Excludes Northern Territory in 1947 and 1948.

[2]For 1935-1949, data exclude Yukon, Northwest Territories; Newfoundland, which became the tenth province April 1, 1949, is excluded prior to 1950.

[3]Excluding Faeroe Islands 1932-1948; Faeroe Islands and Greenland starting 1949.

[4]Prior to 1955, data according to age of fetus not available; figures assumed to include gestations of less than 28 weeks.

[5]By year of registration rather than year of occurrence. Excludes Maoris 1935-1960. Includes Maoris 1961-1964.

[6]Fetal death is defined as "measuring at least 35 cm. in length."

[7]Fetal death is defined as "height more than 30 cm."

[8]For 1942-1964, data include fetal deaths of at least 28 weeks gestation and a proportionate number of fetal deaths of unknown gestation. For 1940-1941, available data include all reported fetal deaths and are therefore not shown.

countries studied, including the United States, has been small for years (Table 5.4). In view of the possible variation in registration completeness, it is difficult to attach great importance to some of the observed differences. However, it is significant that whereas the rate for the United States in 1950-51 was at the lower end of the range of perinatal mortality rates, by 1962-64 it was at the upper end of the range. (In 1950-51 the rate was lower only in Norway; in 1962-64 the rate was higher only in England and Wales and possibly in Canada.)

The primary reason for examining perinatal mortality rates has been to search for artifacts that might explain the comparatively high mortality rate in early infancy for the United States. From the preceding, it seems reasonable to conclude that only part of the excess is attributable to registration practices, and it is highly likely that the United States actually has a less favorable mortality experience shortly after birth than most of the other countries studied.

Post-neonatal Mortality

All the qualifications inherent in any discussion of differences in the loss in early infancy may be discarded when considering events after the first month of life. Straightforward comparisons can be made not only of relative rates of decline but of the rates themselves. A major reduction in the rate started several years before this country's entry into World War II (Table 5.5). Little change occurred during the war years, but in the year immediately after the war (1945–46) the rate dropped by about 30 percent. The decline definitely slowed down thereafter and has been almost at a standstill since about 1954.

Major reductions in the post-neonatal mortality rates have been quite general. The outstanding exception is New Zealand, where the rate in the years around 1940 was the lowest in the world. The rate of decline in New Zealand has been negligible compared with what has been happening elsewhere, although its loss rate is still one of the lowest in the world.

Aside from New Zealand, patterns of change in the post-neonatal mortality rate have varied appreciably among most of the countries. One similarity in several countries is the sharp drop in the rate immediately following World War II. The fundamental difference between the course of the rate in the United States and its course in most of the other countries is that while the rate of decline slowed down here toward the end of the 1940's and finally came to a halt in the mid-1950's, the decline continued at a brisk pace in these other countries to the end of the 1950's.

As a result of the greater relative decreases elsewhere during the 1950's, the post-neonatal mortality rate in the United States by 1964 ranked close to the highest among the low infant mortality countries. The rates for the Netherlands and Sweden were less than half the figure for the United States. This is in sharp contrast to what existed in 1950, when Canada, Denmark, England and Wales, Finland, Norway, and Switzerland recorded substantially higher rates than the United States.

In assessing the differences among countries in their post-neonatal rates, it might be asked whether these rates have not already reached such a low point in most countries that small absolute differences appear large when expressed in relative terms. This holds for some of the differentials found. Nevertheless, the gap between the rate for the United States and those for a few countries is substantial even on an absolute basis.

Table 5.4   Perinatal mortality rates: Selected countries, 1940-64 (Deaths under one week plus fetal deaths of
at least 28 weeks gestation or unknown gestation per 1,000 live births plus specified fetal deaths.)

Year	Australia[1]	Canada[2]	Denmark[3]	England and Wales	Finland[4]	Netherlands[5]	New Zealand[6]	Norway	Sweden[7]	Switzerland[8]	United States[9]
1964	---	---	---	28.2	---	23.4	23.7	---	21.6	---	28.0
1963	---	28.0	24.3	29.3	23.6	24.5	---	22.5	22.8	25.3	27.9
1962	---	28.6	24.9	30.8	26.2	25.7	---	23.7	23.5	26.5	27.7
1961	26.1	28.1	26.9	32.0	26.7	25.9	26.3	23.2	23.9	26.3	28.0
1960	26.8	28.4	26.2	32.8	25.0	26.6	26.9	23.7	25.9	25.6	28.2
1959	27.3	28.9	28.2	34.1	26.7	27.1	26.3	23.6	25.9	26.5	28.4
1958	26.5	30.2	28.9	35.0	26.6	28.0	26.5	26.1	26.1	26.9	28.9
1957	28.6	31.0	29.1	36.2	27.4	28.1	28.0	24.8	27.3	28.5	28.5
1956	28.7	31.7	32.4	36.7	28.7	29.0	28.1	25.5	28.3	29.8	28.6
1955	28.5	31.0	33.3	37.4	29.6	30.2	27.2	25.6	27.9	30.4	29.3
1954	29.8	31.9	34.4	38.0	32.7	31.2	30.0	24.3	28.8	32.5	29.5
1953	30.3	33.1	34.9	36.9	33.2	31.5	30.7	25.8	29.8	33.5	30.3
1952	31.3	35.2	34.0	37.5	34.0	32.4	30.7	27.1	31.0	32.4	30.8
1951	33.5	35.8	33.9	38.7	33.3	33.4	32.1	27.7	32.8	34.1	31.5
1950	33.9	37.9	33.7	37.4	34.5	34.2	33.5	27.8	32.9	34.7	32.2
1949	34.5	37.5	32.5	38.0	34.0	33.0	---	28.1	33.8	36.6	33.1
1948	36.8[1]	38.3	33.1	38.5	34.1	32.4	32.0	30.4	33.5	37.3	34.1
1947	38.3[1]	39.9	34.3	40.3	34.6	34.2	35.1	31.9	35.5	37.1	35.1
1946	---	41.1	36.4	44.3	35.1	34.8	37.5	31.2	36.2	36.6	36.9
1945	45.2	42.8	37.6	45.2	37.2	35.0	38.8	32.7	39.1	36.8	37.8
1944	45.1	43.7	38.1	44.5	34.9	33.6	39.5	31.6	38.3	35.7	38.6
1943	45.7	45.1	41.2	47.9	34.9	32.4	43.5	33.0	36.4	36.6	38.8
1942	47.2	45.6	38.7	52.1	36.1	33.6	41.1	31.8	36.3	36.5	40.5
1941	48.6	48.0	41.3	54.7	36.9	37.5	42.8	34.3	40.6	40.5	---
1940	47.4	48.0	44.7	57.7	39.8	40.7	46.6	37.3	46.3	41.9	---

Sources: Files of the Statistical Office of the United Nations and annual volumes Vital Statistics of the United States,
National Center for Health Statistics, Public Health Service, Washington.

[1]Excludes full-blooded aborigines. Data tabulated by year of registration rather than occurrence. Excludes Northern Territory
in 1947 and 1948.

[2]For 1935-1949, data exclude Yukon, Northwest Territories; Newfoundland which became the tenth province April 1, 1949 is excluded
prior to 1950.

[3]Excluding Faeroe Islands 1932-1948; Faeroe Islands and Greenland starting 1949.

[4]Prior to 1955, data according to age of fetus not available; figures assumed to include gestations of less than 28 weeks.

[5]For 1935-1949, live-born infants of less than 28 weeks gestation who died before registration were not registered as either
live births or deaths.

[6]By year of registration rather than year of occurrence. Excludes Maoris 1935-1960. Includes Maoris 1961-1964.

[7]Fetal death is defined as "measuring at least 35 cm. in length."

[8]Fetal death is defined as "height more than 30 cm."

[9]For 1942-1964, data include fetal deaths of at least 28 weeks gestation and a proportionate number of fetal deaths of unknown
gestation. For 1940-1941, available data include all reported fetal deaths and are therefore not shown.

Table 5.5   Postneonatal mortality rates per 1,000 live births: Selected countries, 1935-64.

Year	Australia[1]	Canada[2]	Denmark[3]	England and Wales	Finland	Netherlands[4]	New Zealand[5]	Norway	Sweden	Switzerland	United States
1964	---	7.4	---	6.1	---	3.2	6.7	---	2.6	---	6.9
1963	5.2	8.3	4.4	6.9	4.5	3.8	6.8	5.0	3.1	4.9	7.0
1962	5.7	8.9	4.9	6.6	4.8	4.2	7.8	5.7	3.0	5.1	7.0
1961	5.5	9.2	5.3	6.1	5.5	4.2	8.2	5.6	3.0	5.0	6.9
1960	5.5	9.3	5.4	6.3	6.7	4.5	5.1	7.2	2.7	5.1	7.3
1959	6.2	9.9	6.3	6.3	7.8	4.8	6.0	6.2	3.7	5.6	7.4
1958	6.0	10.9	6.4	6.4	9.1	5.2	5.8	6.7	3.8	5.9	7.6
1957	6.0	10.7	7.0	6.7	11.3	5.2	6.1	8.2	4.3	6.3	7.3
1956	6.1	11.8	7.3	6.8	9.2	6.0	6.0	8.9	4.1	7.0	7.1
1955	6.5	12.0	7.2	7.6	11.1	6.1	6.1	8.0	4.5	7.6	7.3
1954	6.3	12.7	8.9	7.7	11.3	6.4	5.7	9.6	4.9	7.3	7.5
1953	6.8	14.2	8.6	9.1	14.5	7.2	5.8	9.4	4.9	8.6	8.2
1952	7.1	15.5	9.6	9.2	12.7	7.5	6.7	9.5	5.1	8.9	8.6
1951	7.7	15.9	10.5	11.0	15.7	8.3	6.6	11.3	5.7	8.8	8.4
1950	7.1	17.1	12.5	11.3	21.7	8.8	6.2	13.5	5.7	10.1	8.7
1949	7.3	19.2	15.4	13.4	25.2	10.1	6.8	13.2	7.1	10.7	9.9
1948	8.1	18.0	16.2	14.8	28.3	11.9	6.2	13.8	6.4	11.0	9.8
1947	8.0	19.0	18.4	19.0	33.6	15.0	7.0	17.1	7.9	11.5	9.4
1946	7.8	19.5	22.3	16.7	30.3	17.8	7.0	17.6	8.4	13.3	9.7
1945	7.6	22.8	23.4	22.1	37.2	49.9	8.4	19.2	10.9	14.3	13.9
1944	9.3	25.5	23.5	20.3	42.2	23.3	9.5	18.3	11.4	16.4	15.1
1943	12.2	24.1	21.9	23.6	26.5	19.7	10.1	17.4	10.5	13.9	15.6
1942	14.2	25.7	23.4	22.4	42.7	18.5	10.0	18.1	11.4	13.2	14.7
1941	13.1	29.1	31.3	30.7	34.4	20.9	9.8	23.0	15.5	13.3	17.7
1940	12.9	26.7	25.0	27.8	57.9	17.8	8.2	18.2	15.7	19.2	18.3
1939	12.4	30.1	30.6	22.4	41.6	13.9	9.3	16.8	15.3	14.9	18.7
1938	12.3	31.6	31.5	24.4	38.0	16.1	11.5	17.1	17.3	16.6	21.4
1937	11.8	41.6	37.0	27.9	39.1	17.2	9.0	19.0	20.1	18.7	23.2
1936	13.7	32.6	38.2	28.4	38.6	17.3	8.7	19.8	20.1	18.4	24.6
1935	12.3	36.0	41.9	26.5	36.6	17.6	10.2	22.6	20.3	18.6	23.3

Sources: Files of the Statistical Office of the United Nations and annual volumes Vital Statistics of the United States, National Center for Health Statistics, Public Health Service, Washington.

[1]Excludes full-blooded aborigines. Data tabulated by year of registration rather than occurrence.

[2]For 1935-1949, data exclude Yukon, Northwest Territories; Newfoundland which became the tenth province April 1, 1949 is excluded prior to 1950.

[3]Excluding Faeroe Islands 1932-1948; Faeroe Islands and Greenland starting 1949.

[4]For 1935-1949, live-born infants of less than 28 weeks gestation who died before registration were not registered as either live births or deaths.

[5]By year of registration rather than year of occurrence. Excludes Maòris 1935-1960. Includes Maòris 1961-1964.

Cause of Death

One might hope that cause-of-death information would help in the search for clues to the circumstances that underly the increasingly adverse position of the United States in infant mortality. However, the previously discussed difficulties in interpreting cause-of-death data for the United States are compounded when international comparisons are involved. This is particularly true for the neonatal period. Nevertheless, it is apparent that the comparatively high neonatal rate in this country cannot be attributed to a few causes. In fact, except for congenital malformations and birth injuries, the rates for all cause groupings are substantially above the corresponding rates in most of the other countries shown in Table 5.6.[2]

[2] Included are the seven countries from which the data were obtained for the international conference (2). Scotland is the only country not in the group for which trends have been discussed, and it is the only country included in this section that has a higher infant mortality rate than the United States.

The post-neonatal situation is somewhat clearer. Differences in the rates of mortality from infectious diseases of the respiratory and digestive systems and from accidents[3] account for almost the entire gap between the post-neonatal rate in the United States and most other countries. The margins are exceedingly large when comparisons are made with the Netherlands and the Scandinavian countries. For respiratory diseases, which account for almost 40 percent of the post-neonatal deaths in the United States, the rate in this country is about four times as high as the rate in Sweden and the Netherlands.

There is evidence that the post-neonatal mortality rate from respiratory conditions has not been as favorable in the United States as in Sweden and the Netherlands for a long time.[4] In 1950, however, the rate was substantially lower here than in England and Wales, Denmark, and Norway. The leveling off in the post-neonatal mortality rate from influenza and pneumonia that started in the early 1950's in the United States was not paralleled in other countries. Instead, in all but one of the other countries the rate continued sharply downward throughout the 1950's and into the 1960's. The only exception was England and Wales, where the rate flattened out in the late 1950's at about the same level as in the United States.

Evidence of the difference between the United States and other countries in post-neonatal mortality attributed to respiratory conditions is also found in the cause group consisting of all other diseases of the respiratory system. The rate for these causes rose markedly in the United States during the 1950's and stayed high in 1960–63. Although there are problems in interpreting the increase because of changes in cause-of-death reporting and classification, it would appear that at least part of it is real. In all the other countries, with the exception of England and Wales, the mortality rate for these conditions was substantially lower in 1960–62 than 10 years earlier.

Congenital malformations accounted for a larger proportion of

[3] Many of the deaths attributed to accidents are believed to be instances of "sudden death" or "crib death" syndrome, the causes of which are unknown.

[4] Cause-of-death data are shown in this chapter only for 1959–61. Statements about trends in cause-of-death rates are based on data prepared for background documents for the international conference on perinatal and infant mortality (4).

the post-neonatal deaths outside the United States. About two out of five deaths in Sweden and the Netherlands are attributed to these causes, compared with 17 percent here. The relative prominence of congenital malformations as a cause of death in these other countries is related, of course, to the very low mortality from respiratory diseases. The mortality rate from congenital malformations in the United States is actually not too different from the rates in Norway and Sweden.

Comparisons Involving Demographic and Other Factors

Few opportunities exist to determine the role of various demographic circumstances in explaining the comparatively high infant mortality rate in the United States. There is no direct way to take into account differences in economic, cultural, or ethnic background, or the effect of geography. However, it is useful to see if there are subgroups in this country that have attained the low infant mortality rates in Northern European countries (5).

No major geographic subdivision of the United States has an infant mortality rate as low as Scandinavia or the Netherlands, although the rate is slightly below 20 per 1,000 among the white population in a few states. The extraordinarily large racial differences in infant mortality in the United States are of special interest. At the high end of the range, among Negroes and Indians, the rates are two to three times as high as in the other countries. At the low end, among infants of Oriental stock, the rate is at the same level as in Sweden and the Netherlands. In the United States the rate among white children is only about 10 percent below the figure for all races combined and it stands well above the rate in many of the low mortality countries.

Geographic variability in infant mortality exists within all countries. For example, in England and Wales the infant mortality rate varied during 1960–62 from 18.1 to 25.6 among its standard regions; in the Netherlands the rates ranged from 14.3 to 18.6 among the provinces during the same period; and in Sweden county rates varied from 13.6 to 20.6 in 1959–61.

Other variables are found to be more productive than race and geography in throwing light on the nature of the gap between the infant mortality rates in the United States and elsewhere. It is

Table 5.6   Average annual infant mortality rates per 10,000 live births for selected causes of death by age at death: Selected countries, 1959-61.

Cause of Death (7th Revision International Classification of Diseases)	Denmark	England and Wales	Netherlands	Norway	Scotland	Sweden	United States
Under 1 year							
All causes	219.2	218.1	162.3	184.7	268.6	163.4	259.0
Infective and parasitic diseases (001-138)	2.9	2.3	1.6	3.3	3.2	1.2	3.4
Influenza and pneumonia, including pneumonia of newborn (480-493,763)	14.4	30.2	11.0	19.3	35.3	8.2	31.0
All other diseases of respiratory system (470-475,500-527)	--	5.8	1.3	2.6	4.5	1.6	6.2
Gastritis, duodenitis, enteritis and colitis, including diarrhea of newborn (543,571,572,764)	4.3	4.5	1.5	3.7	8.1	2.0	6.9
All other diseases of digestive system (530-542, 544-570,573-587)	2.7	4.3	2.7	3.6	4.1	3.4	3.8
Congenital malformations (750-759)	44.7	45.0	43.0	33.1	54.3	34.3	36.4
Birth injuries (760,761)	25.9	24.4	32.0	20.5	27.2	25.2	23.9
Postnatal asphyxia and atelectasis (762)	48.3	34.3	12.8	19.2	53.9	33.3	45.7
Hemolytic disease of newborn (770)	4.4	4.6	4.2	2.8	5.1	2.5	5.0
Immaturity unqualified (776)	--	36.5	18.8	36.1	35.9	28.9	45.4
Neonatal disorders arising from certain diseases of mother (765-769,771-774)	--	12.2	14.2	13.5	11.9	14.1	27.5
Symptoms and ill-defined conditions (780-793,795)	3.6	0.4	6.4	13.8	3.5	0.1	5.8
Accidents (E800-E962)	3.6	5.9	3.4	3.9	13.5	2.0	8.8
Residual (140-468,590-749,E963-E985)	--	8.0	9.5	9.3	8.1	6.6	9.2
Under 28 days							
All causes	162.5	155.7	117.3	121.4	185.0	131.8	187.1
Infective and parasitic diseases (001-138)	0.7	0.2	0.1	0.1	0.0	0.3	0.5
Influenza and pneumonia, including pneumonia of newborn (480-493,763)	2.5	9.4	5.4	5.1	9.0	2.9	8.6
All other diseases of respiratory system (470-475,500-527)	--	0.6	0.2	0.2	0.1	0.2	0.7
Gastritis, duodenitis, enteritis and colitis, including diarrhea of newborn (543,571,572,764)	0.7	0.7	0.2	0.4	1.5	0.4	1.1

Birth injuries (760,761)	25.8	24.4	31.7	20.4	27.1	25.1	23.9
Postnatal asphyxia and atelectasis (762)	47.7	33.9	12.7	18.7	53.6	32.8	45.0
Hemolytic disease of newborn (770)	4.2	4.5	4.1	2.5	5.0	2.4	5.0
Immaturity unqualified (776)	--	36.4	18.7	35.3	35.9	28.7	45.1
Neonatal disorders arising from certain diseases of mother[1] (765-769,771-774)	--	11.6	11.3	11.8	10.9	13.3	25.0
Symptoms and ill-defined conditions (780-793,795)	0.7	0.2	3.0	5.6	0.3	-	2.4
Accidents (E800-E962)	0.3	1.2	0.4	0.3	1.9	0.2	1.4
Residual (140-468,590-749,E963-E985)	--	2.1	2.5	1.1	2.2	2.2	2.5
28 days - 11 months							
All causes	56.7	62.4	45.0	63.2	83.6	31.6	71.9
Infective and parasitic diseases (001-138)	2.2	2.1	1.4	3.2	3.2	1.0	2.9
Influenza and pneumonia, including pneumonia of newborn (480-493,763)	11.9	20.8	5.5	14.2	26.4	5.3	22.4
All other diseases of respiratory system (470-475,500-527)	--	5.2	1.1	2.4	4.4	1.4	5.5
Gastritis, duodenitis, enteritis and colitis, including diarrhea of newborn (543,571,572,764)	3.6	3.8	1.3	3.3	6.7	1.6	5.8
All other diseases of digestive system (530-542, 544-570,573-587)	1.3	2.1	1.1	1.9	2.3	1.4	1.4
Congenital malformations (750-759)	18.9	16.6	17.5	14.7	18.5	12.8	12.5
Birth injuries (760,761)	0.1	0.0	0.3	0.2	0.0	0.2	0.0
Postnatal asphyxia and atelectasis (762)	0.6	0.3	0.2	0.5	0.4	0.5	0.7
Hemolytic disease of newborn (770)	0.2	0.1	0.1	0.3	0.1	0.1	0.0
Immaturity unqualified (776)	--	0.1	0.2	0.8	0.1	0.2	0.3
Neonatal disorders arising from certain diseases of mother[1] (765-769,771-774)	--	0.6	2.9	1.7	1.0	0.8	2.6
Symptoms and ill-defined conditions (780-793,795)	3.0	0.1	3.4	8.2	3.2	0.1	3.4
Accidents (E800-E962)	3.3	4.7	3.0	3.6	11.6	1.8	7.4
Residual (140-468,590-749,E963-E985)	--	5.9	7.0	8.3	5.9	4.4	6.7

Source: Chase, Helen C., International Comparison of Perinatal and Infant Mortality: The United States and Six West European Countries, National Center for Health Statistics, Series 3, No. 6, March 1967.

[1] Includes neonatal disorders arising from certain diseases of the mother during pregnancy; ill-defined diseases peculiar to early infancy; immaturity with mention of other subsidiary condition; and other diseases peculiar to early infancy not already shown.

known that age-of-mother and birth-order distributions of live births in this country differ from those in other countries. To assess the effect of this circumstance on international differences in mortality, neonatal mortality rates in the United States and the Netherlands have been standardized (indirect method) by applying age-of-mother birth-order rates in the United States for January–March 1950. The Netherlands was selected for the comparison principally because this country's distributions differ markedly from those of the United States. As indicated in the following figures, the standardized rates for the two countries are closer than the observed rates, but there is still a wide margin:

	United States (1960–61)	The Netherlands (1961)	Difference
Observed neonatal rates	18.6	12.8	45 percent
Standardized neonatal rates	17.7	13.6	30 percent

Birth weight is by far the most important variable in considering differences between the rate in the United States and elsewhere. Comparable information is unavailable for comprehensive analysis of this variable, but what is known suggests that a major factor accounting for the comparatively high neonatal mortality rate in the United States is the proportion of infants whose birth weight is 2,500 grams or less. This can be seen clearly from the experience in England and Wales, the only country besides the United States where national data on birth weight have been collected routinely (this practice is being adopted by additional countries).

In 1963 the proportion of newborn with low birth weights was 8.2 percent in the United States and 6.6 percent in England and Wales. The neonatal mortality rates during the year were 18.2 and 14.3 per 1,000 live births in these two countries, respectively. The expected rate in the United States, obtained by applying birth-weight-specific mortality rates in England and Wales[5] to the birth-

---

[5] Neonatal mortality rates per 1,000 live births by birth weight were as follows in England and Wales during 1963:

Birth weight	Neonatal rate
1,500 grams or less	626
1,501–2,000 grams	162
2,001–2,500 grams	40
2,501 grams or more	6.7

weight distribution here, is 18.4, which is very close to the observed rate (18.2). It is therefore apparent that the difference between the two countries in their birth-weight distributions accounts for the large margin between the neonatal mortality rates for the United States and England and Wales.

Estimates of the proportion of live births at 2,500 grams or less are available for the Netherlands and Norway, and in both instances the figures are below the proportion in the United States. In the Netherlands a special study in 1954 indicated that 5.5 percent of the infants had low birth weights; in Norway it is estimated that 5–6 percent of the live-born had birth weights under 2,501 grams.

Problems of Comparability

International comparisons of infant and perinatal mortality rates have been plagued by problems related to differences in definition, reporting and registration requirements, and statistical practices. These sources of incomparability have already been examined from several standpoints. A review of definitions and registration practices among the various countries with which infant mortality in the United States has been compared showed that there are some differences in the criteria for the registration of an event as a live birth. The effect of these differences is to register an event in some countries as a live birth and an infant death, whereas in others a similar event would be registered and counted as a stillbirth. Although this difference has little effect on the live-birth statistics, it could affect the infant mortality rate and particularly the neonatal rate.

In most countries "any sign of life" is taken as one of the criteria. In the United States the criteria for registration specify a range of alternative evidence, such as breathing, heart action, pulsation of umbilical cord, and movement of voluntary muscle, whereas in most of the other countries the definitions lack specificity. Whether or not the specification of the various signs affects registration of live births is not known, but it is probably minimal in comparison with other registration problems. A more important problem is the more restrictive definition used in Sweden, wherein breathing is taken as the only criterion of life. An infant born that did not breathe but showed other evidence of life would have been counted as a stillbirth in Sweden until 1960.[6] In the other countries represented in the study this infant would be counted as a live birth and an infant death.

In a survey of lying-in hospitals in Sweden in 1956 reported by Soop (6) some 17 percent of the registered stillbirths showed other signs of life but did not breathe. This represented about 0.1 percent of the live-birth total, which is almost identical with the proportion found in about 20,000 live births that occurred in 1959–61 in selected hospitals in the United States (7).

On the basis of these figures, the infant mortality rates for Sweden would be at least one point higher if the more inclusive definition of live birth adopted by other countries were used. For example, on a comparable definition of live birth, the infant mortality rate for Sweden in 1959 may be 17.6 per 1,000 live births rather than the rate of 16.6 which was recorded for that year. The effect may actually be greater, but the maximum is probably not much more than two or three points.

In the Netherlands the practice of excluding from birth or death registration a live-born infant of less than 28 weeks' gestation that dies before registration results in a moderate understatement in the infant mortality rate based on registered events. Adjustments have been made for this factor starting with 1950 rates.

Another problem relates to differences in the registration requirements for fetal deaths. All of the states in the United States require registration of all fetal deaths or those of 20 weeks' or more gestation, whereas the other countries confine registration to dead fetuses of 28 weeks' or more gestation. Other things being equal, the effect of this difference in definition would generally be to record fewer fetal deaths in other countries because of the tendency to underestimate gestation age which is slightly over 28 weeks to avoid registration of the fetal death.

One indication of this may be found in the experience of states that have changed the requirements for the reporting of fetal deaths. Since 1950 nine states have revised their laws to make reportable all products of conception regardless of gestation age, and

---

[6]This situation may also have been true until recent years in several of the provinces of Canada. However, the effect on the rates for Canada as a whole is believed to be negligible.

in one state the change was to require reports for fetal deaths of 16 or more weeks' gestation. Prior to this, the laws in these states called for the registration of dead fetuses after at least 20 weeks of gestation. The effect of such changes in registration requirements have varied. Generally, the number of fetuses of 20 weeks' and over gestation increased after the change in the definition of a reportable fetal death. For the ten states referred to above, it is estimated that the resulting increase in the number of fetal deaths at these gestation ages averaged 4.35 percent (8).

It is difficult to assess precisely how many more fetal deaths of 28 weeks' or more gestation would be registered in other countries if registration requirements covered deaths below this gestation age. However, the experience in the United States suggests that a 4–5 percent increase in the fetal death rates of these countries might well result. On the other hand, there is indication of substantial under-registration of fetal deaths in the United States. This may very well also be true for other countries, but no study of fetal death registration has been made elsewhere.

It would appear reasonable to conclude from the preceding that differences in reporting requirements and practices could account for only a minor part of the gap between the infant mortality rate for the United States and the rates in other low mortality countries. Also, only a small part of the gap between perinatal mortality rates is probably attributable to these factors.

Other Comparisons

The discussion in this chapter is focused on comparisons involving countries with traditionally low mortality rates. In most of the rest of the world, the rate has consistently been far greater than the loss in these countries even on the basis of registered births and deaths— at least five to ten times the figures in the United States and Northern European countries.

Between these two extremes is a group of countries that until quite recently had intermediate infant mortality rates. Although their rates were considerably below the figures in the high mortality countries, they were well above the figures in the low mortality countries. As recently as the early 1950's their rates were approximately double the rates in the United States. A startling change in this relationship has occurred since then. During the 1950's and early 1960's, while the rate in the United States leveled off, infant mortality continued to decline in a number of these countries. As a result, the rates in Czechoslovakia, France, and Japan fell below the rate in the United States by 1963 or 1964.

6 / REVIEW AND PERSPECTIVES

What about the future course of infant and perinatal mortality rates in the United States? Is there a potential for a sustained, major downward trend in these rates, or is this an experience peculiar to the past, with little likelihood of being repeated? The framework for considering this issue is available data on trends and present status of infant and perinatal mortality. A summary of the most relevant elements follows.

Summary
1. Until about 1950 there were large reductions in infant mortality. The decreases were greater after the first few weeks of life than shortly after birth, but the improvement in mortality at all ages was significant. Every area of the country and both the white and nonwhite populations shared in the sizable reductions in the loss rate. A major contributory factor to the sharp decline in the death rate was the lowering of mortality from infectious diseases of all types.

2. During the 1950's and the early 1960's the decline in the infant mortality rate slowed down appreciably. The specific year when this change occurred differed by age at death, but the general conclusion is the same—the major declines that formerly characterized the mortality rates were no longer being experienced at any stage during infancy. This reflects lack of change in the rates for most of the important causes of death. There were, however, continued declines in the rates for infective and parasitic diseases and for infections of the digestive system. Increases occurred in the rate for respiratory diseases other than influenza and pneumonia. The rates for both white and nonwhite infants leveled off, but the slowdown in the rate of decline was more marked among the nonwhite infants.

3. Decreases in the infant mortality rate during the 1950's were small in all geographic areas. Nevertheless, areas that were comparatively high in their rates at the beginning of the decade showed a larger decrease in their infant death rates. The gap between rates in the metropolitan and nonmetropolitan areas narrowed, and the rates in geographic divisions (representing aggregates of states) varied less at the end of the 1950 decade than previously.

Infant mortality increased in many large cities. Nonwhite infants especially were affected by this increase, but in some cities white infants also had a higher rate in 1960–61 than 10 years earlier. The widespread increase in infant mortality among nonwhite births in cities appears to be related to the movement of many nonwhite persons to major cities during the 1950's. Large-scale migration was common in all population groups, but among white persons the movement frequently was from the central city to the suburban areas.

4. Changes in racial or geographic composition of births do not explain the slow decline in the U.S. infant mortality rate. More important is the increase in the proportions of births in the comparatively high-risk groups of very young mothers and women with many pregnancies. However, if this factor were eliminated, the decrease in the mortality rate during the 1950's would still lag far behind the decrease in the 1940's.

The distribution of births by birth weight has changed slightly since 1950 for the country as a whole. Among white babies the proportion weighing 2,500 grams or less at birth has changed only slightly; among nonwhite infants the proportion increased markedly, a circumstance that exerted a strong brake on the rate of decline in the neonatal mortality rate among nonwhite infants.

5. High-risk groups identifiable through vital statistics for the United States or local areas showed little improvement in the 1950's in the infant mortality rates. This held for low birth-weight groups, children born to mothers who had previously had a fetal death, and nonwhite infants. Perinatal mortality rates did not improve significantly in the presence of major complications of pregnancy and delivery or in deliveries with Caesarean sections. Among nonwhite pregnancies with major complications, the perinatal loss rate actually increased (upstate New York).

6. More specific comparisons between high-risk groups and the more favored groups indicate that:

a. Nonwhite infants have almost twice as high a death rate as white infants. The differential is relatively small shortly after birth, but it rapidly increases as postnatal environmental conditions become the dominant factors. The loss rate in every part of the country is greater among nonwhite than white infants.

b. Infants weighing 2,500 grams or less at birth have a neonatal death rate that is about 22 times the rate for the other babies, and they account for two-thirds of all neonatal deaths. Chances of survival improve with increasing weight, reaching an optimum in the birth-weight class 3,501–4,000 grams.

c. Pregnancies among women who previously had a pregnancy which terminated in a fetal death are at least twice as likely to end in a neonatal or fetal death as are pregnancies among other women. Very young mothers and women with many prior pregnancies also represent high risks with respect to neonatal and fetal mortality.

d. The risk of perinatal mortality among white and nonwhite births is elevated four to five times in the presence of major obstetrical complications. A significant proportion of the pregnancies have such complications (about 1 in 12 in upstate New York); the figure was moderately higher in the early 1950's. The rate of complications is relatively high in first pregnancies, among very young mothers, among women near the end of the child-bearing ages, and among women with a history of prior fetal or child loss. Pregnancies terminating with very low birth-weight infants (1,500 grams or less) have extremely high complication rates (40 to 50 percent).

e. Perinatal mortality among white births involving Caesarean sections is two to three times higher than the loss rates for all births; among nonwhite births the differential is about 70 percent. Strongly influencing the increased risk is the high proportion of Caesarean section cases with major obstetrical complications. Repeat Caesarean sections are associated with a much lower perinatal mortality rate than primary sections; the risk of perinatal mortality in the former group is only moderately higher than the risk among all births. Caesarean section is the mode of delivery in about 4 percent of the pregnancies (upstate New York); this represents a slight increase during the 1950's. The rate increases with maternal age, and within each group (except for women under 20 years) it is highest among first births. Relatively large proportions of the births in Caesarean section deliveries are at the low and very high birth weights.

f. Infant mortality varies inversely with socioeconomic status as measured by occupation of father. The gradient is considerably larger in the post-neonatal rates than in the perinatal rates.

7. Many of the countries with traditionally low infant mortality rates have continued to show significant improvement in their rates

since 1950, in contrast to the slowdown in the downward trend in the United States. As a result, the number of countries that have lower infant mortality rates than the United States has increased. Furthermore, several other countries, which not too long ago had substantially higher rates than in the United States, had lower rates by 1964 than this country.

Perspectives

Why is it that during the 1950's and early 1960's years of great economic advancement and expanding allocation of economic resources to medical care, the infant mortality rate decreased only moderately? Contrasting economic and medical care advances in this period with what happened to the infant mortality rate poses a difficult paradox. Reductions in the proportion of the population in the low socioeconomic classes and migration of population groups from rural areas with high mortality rates and relatively poor medical facilities to large urban centers where highly trained physicians and large medical institutions are located could logically have been expected to result in major decreases in infant mortality. In the 1940's, when similar demographic changes were experienced, infant mortality did decline markedly. There were a number of differences, however, between these two periods.

During the 1940's maternal and child health programs at the state and local levels were greatly strengthened, and infant mortality was a prime target of health department activities. The Federal Emergency Maternity and Infant Care Program, designed to meet the urgent needs of wives and infants of men in the Armed Forces during World War II, helped bring regular prenatal and infant health supervision to broad segments of the population. This program ended after World War II. A large part of the reduction in infant loss was concentrated in the control of infectious diseases, whose toll was still substantial at the beginning of the 1940's. In some areas the introduction of special programs for the care of prematurely born infants also had an impact on the mortality rate.

In the 1950's a general attitude that significant progress in reducing infant mortality required, above all, new insights into basic biological processes tended to dampen the fervor for action programs. The 1950's might also be characterized as a decade in which earlier medical and program advances in maternal and child health continued without significant innovations. This occurred in the absence of major scientific breakthroughs that could have been expected to produce broad effects through immediate application.

Finally, some of the very conditions which, on the surface, might be taken as harbingers of improvement had the reverse result. An outstanding example is the migration of nonwhite persons to large metropolitan areas; in many of these areas, infant mortality increased instead of decreasing. The explanation encompasses many social, economic, and program issues. High on the list would be a lag in community facilities in providing for the change, difficulties experienced by the in-migrant group in taking advantage of their new medical care environment, overcrowding, and low income.

For years there was pessimism about the possibility of a resumption of a significant downward trend in infant mortality. Decreases in 1966 and 1967 have tempered this point of view but there is still considerable caution in interpreting the change as the beginning of a progression to substantially lower rates than in the past. The reason relates generally to the fact that most of the losses occur in early infancy, many of the underlying mechanisms are poorly understood, and reduction in the incidence of low birth weight is central to the problem.

The importance of such considerations cannot be denied, but there are other circumstances that would seem more decisive in assessing the potential for large-scale improvement in infant mortality. Although the relevant biological processes will be incompletely understood for some time, many of them may well be subject to change through alteration of environmental conditions broadly defined to include not only general socioeconomic circumstances but family planning, organization and availability of high quality medical care, and personal health practices. Furthermore, there are groups in the population with extraordinarily high loss rates. Also, many other countries now have infant mortality rates that are far below the rate in the United States, thereby providing concrete evidence that the current level of infant mortality in the United States is considerably above the level possible with present-day knowledge.

In considering prospects for additional reduction in the infant mortality rate, it is also necessary to bear in mind that close to 30 percent of the infant deaths are still attributed to factors related to identifiable environmental conditions and to conditions that may reflect quality of medical and hospital care. Decreases in the frequency of deaths from these causes alone would have a significant effect on the level of the infant mortality rate. If mortality from infectious diseases of all types (respiratory and digestive, principally), accidents, and such conditions as hemolytic disease of the newborn and neonatal conditions arising from maternal disorders (diabetes and toxemia, for example), and ill-defined diseases of the newborn were cut in half, the infant mortality rate would show approximately a 10-percent decline.

Additional reductions would have to be sought primarily through decreases in the frequency of prematurity and in mortality attributed directly or indirectly to immaturity. The potential for such reductions is, of course, uncertain. But only slight improvements in the rates among low-risk groups, if accompanied by a moderate closing of the gap between high-risk and low-risk groups, would result in lowering the overall mortality rate another 10 percent.

Attainment of an infant mortality rate of 18–20 per 1,000 in the United States appears to be a realistic short-term goal—a longer-term goal of 15 per 1,000 can well be entertained. General conditions that are expected to contribute to the movement toward these goals are continued improvements in standard of living, strengthening of medical and hospital resources, and the likely shift over the next few years to more favorable age-of-mother birth-order distributions resulting from the large numbers of women who were born during the war period and will soon be in their mid-20's.

Specific efforts aimed at increasing the rate of decline in infant mortality are focused today on community action programs directed at high mortality risk groups identified by their concentrations in economically depressed areas and by illegitimacy, prior pregnancy loss, and racial origin. Many questions remain in the development of these action programs. For example, are there better methods than are now available of identifying subgroups which should be given concentrated attention, and if so, how is this knowledge to be applied in the appropriate areas? In the face of personnel shortages described in Chapter 13, who is to become the focal point for the coordination of health services in the community, and how are available health personnel at all levels of professional and technical competence to be used effectively? What measures are needed to relieve the overcrowded clinics and ward services in metropolitan areas and to bring specialized health services into the rural areas? Issues related to personnel and facilities are paralleled by problems of a situational, cultural, and economic nature that adversely affect health practices of many in the high-risk groups. It is increasingly being recognized that these factors must receive concentrated attention in community programs if the benefits expected of improved personnel and facilities are to be realized.

There is also a growing conviction that in the long run concern with pregnancy outcome begins with preventive care during the adolescent period, since young people establish many health habits and attitudes that influence their physical status and medical care behavior later in life. This concept includes guidance in preparing for family life, and later, family planning. It has relevance not only for those who are potentially a high-risk group but also for segments of the population that may never be directly involved in the community programs that are currently evolving.

Part II
Maternal Mortality

Part II
Material Synthesis

7 / TRENDS AND RECENT STATUS

The risk of maternal mortality has undergone a most remarkable transformation within the lifetime of most Americans. In the short space of 30 years the maternal mortality rate had dropped almost 95 percent by 1964, a decrease that exceeded even the large-scale changes that have occurred in the death rate at all ages from infectious diseases. During this period the chances of a pregnant woman dying from causes related to the pregnancy went from 1 in about 150 to 1 in 3,000. Maternal deaths accounted for 10–15 percent of all deaths among women in the child-bearing ages in the early 1930's but for only 2–3 percent 30 years later, despite the increase in the birth rate.

Progress in reducing maternal mortality is one of the truly gratifying accomplishments in modern medicine. Nevertheless, several aspects of the problem of maternal mortality are still disturbing. The rate of decline in the death rate has slowed down appreciably and attainment of the goal of virtual elimination of maternal deaths appears to be remote. Also, there are major differentials in maternal mortality among various groups within the population.

Maternal mortality rates in this chapter are derived primarily from vital statistics sources. Deaths are classified as maternal only if the delivery or a complication of pregnancy, childbirth, or puerperium is given on the death certificate as the underlying cause. It is recognized that the number of deaths so classified does not represent all deaths related to pregnancy. Evidence on the possible magnitude of the resulting discrepancy comes from a study in one state based on death certificates matched with birth records (1). About 30 percent of the deaths among women during or shortly after pregnancy were found to be coded to causes other than maternal. This circumstance, however, is not believed to be sufficiently important to affect a consideration of trends in maternal mortality or the relative risks associated with population characteristics, particularly when the differentials or changes are large, as is often the case.

Another issue relevant to maternal mortality arises from the definition of the rate. Customarily the rate is calculated by relating the number of maternal deaths to the number of live births in the same period of time. Strictly speaking this is not a rate, since the denominator does not represent the group "at risk" for maternal deaths. Pregnancies terminating in multiple live births are counted more than once; and pregnancies terminating in a fetal death are excluded from the denominator. A "true" rate of maternal mortality would be defined in terms of total pregnancies regardless of gestation age. This definition would theoretically result in a maternal mortality rate that is probably one-fifth below the rate as usually determined. However, since reporting of fetal deaths in most areas is restricted to pregnancies of 20 weeks' gestation or more and fetal deaths that occur below 20 weeks' gestation are grossly under-reported in most other areas, national rates based on all reported pregnancy terminations would be indistinguishable from the customary rate.

Trends

Consideration of the long-term trend in the maternal mortality rate starts with 1915, the year the birth registration area was formed (Fig. 7.1). Expansion of the birth registration area from ten states and the District of Columbia to full coverage of the United States in 1933, with the comparatively high mortality states coming in late, exerted a slightly dampening effect on the rate of decrease in the maternal mortality rate between 1915 and 1933. Improvement in registration completeness of live births had the reverse effect until the early 1950's, when completeness closely approximated 100 percent. Changes in the classification of causes of death in 1939 also resulted in a modest overstatement of the decrease in maternal mortality that occurred immediately after the change.[1]

It should be emphasized that all of these circumstances are minor compared with the strong currents that influenced the trend of the maternal mortality rate. Between 1915 and 1928 or 1929 the maternal mortality rate followed a desultory course not only in the expanding registration area as a whole but in all geographic subdivisions. The rate skyrocketed during the influenza pandemic of 1918 and remained high during the influenza epidemic of 1919–20. It then dropped back to the pre-epidemic level. Toward the end of

---

[1] During the period 1939–48 rules were in effect under which the cause of death was classified as maternal if conditions associated with pregnancy were recorded on the certificate even though the physician did not consider them to be the underlying cause of death. Accordingly, maternal mortality rates for this period are estimated to be 9 percent higher than they would have been under the rules in effect after 1948.

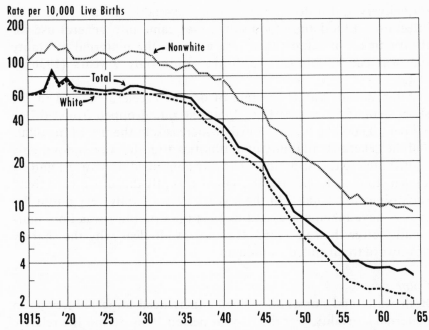

Fig. 7.1. Maternal mortality rates by color: Birth registration states or United States, 1915–64.

Source: National Center for Health Statistics, *Vital Statistics of the United States,* annual volumes.

Notes: Rates relate to the birth registration states through 1932 and to the total United States for later years. Alaska included from 1959 and Hawaii from 1960. New Jersey excluded from data by color for 1962–63.

the 1920's the first signs of a downward trend in maternal mortality appeared. The rate decreased from 69.5 per 10,000 live births in 1929 to 56.8 in 1936. This could not be interpreted as a major change, especially since the 1929 figure was high even for the 1920's. However, it did represent a break from the past.

After 1936 the rate of decline in maternal mortality became precipitous. A combination of factors was responsible for this situation. Impatience with the course of the maternal mortality rate had been building up for years. The publication in 1933 of the New York Academy of Medicine's historic study of the causes of maternal mortality aroused the medical profession and hospital authorities (2). It led to the formation of hospital committees to investigate the cause of each maternal death and fix responsibility for the death. Simultaneously there was a rapid increase in hospitalization for delivery and sulfonamides became available for the control of infections. Blood and blood substitutes came into general use for the treatment of hemorrhage. As a result, the maternal mortality rate was cut by almost two-thirds within only 9 years (1936 to 1945).

After World War II the rate of decline accelerated, and in the short span of 5 years, 1945 to 1950, the rate dropped from 20.7 to 8.3 per 10,000 live births. Further increases in the use of hospitals and the general availability of antibiotics after the war undoubtedly contributed to this situation. The rate continued downward and by 1956 it stood at 4.1 per 10,000. Quite abruptly this downward trend came almost to a halt. In the 8 years 1956–64 only very minor decreases have taken place, and in 1964 the rate (3.3) was only marginally lower than in 1956. It is not at all clear why the sharply downward trend ended so suddenly.

Color

Both white and nonwhite women experienced large reductions in maternal mortality over the 20-year period 1936–56 but the relative magnitude of the decrease was far smaller among the nonwhite women. In 1936 the rate among nonwhite mothers was not quite double the rate in the white group; in 1956 the margin was almost fourfold; and in 1964 the rates for the two color groups were relatively further apart (2.2 per 10,000 for white women as compared with 9.0 per 10,000 for the nonwhite). The unfavorable position of the nonwhite group is more marked in maternal mortality than in all but a few nonmaternal causes of death. The 1964 rate among nonwhite mothers was at about the same level as the rate among white mothers 16 years earlier (1948). Furthermore, the downward trend in the maternal mortality rate has slowed down somewhat more among nonwhite women than among white since the mid-1950's. Unless there is a change, nonwhite mothers will soon be a full generation behind white mothers in mortality due to conditions arising in pregnancy (Appendix Table II.1).

Age of Mother

The risk of maternal mortality is lowest at ages 20–24 years (20.1 per 100,000 in 1959–61) (Table 7.1). It is slightly higher under 20 years of age; from 25 years of age on, increasing age is associated with a steep rise in maternal mortality. At 40–44 years of age the

Table 7.1   Average annual maternal mortality rates per 100,000 live births by age of mother and color: United States, selected decennium period.

Age	Total			White			Nonwhite		
	1959-61	1949-51	1939-41	1959-61	1949-51	1939-41	1959-61	1949-51	1939-41
All ages	37.1	82.7	363.9	25.5	61.3	311.3	100.0	218.8	736.5
Under 20	23.4	71.8	355.2	14.7	47.0	267.7	53.4	149.9	629.0
20-24	20.1	47.6	238.9	14.0	35.3	201.1	55.7	124.3	508.5
25-29	29.7	64.8	288.9	20.4	47.2	246.7	86.6	206.8	699.9
30-34	52.3	106.1	442.3	34.4	77.7	385.5	158.6	342.1	1009.6
35-39	90.1	180.6	708.3	64.5	132.3	630.0	238.4	519.2	1318.3
40-44	143.3	323.7	982.7	104.7	280.7	898.8	366.8	602.9	1700.7
45 & over	280.3	627.2	1481.0	162.9	537.2	1331.3	819.1	1035.9	2365.4

Source: Annual volumes Vital Statistics of the United States, National Center for Health Statistics, Public Health Service, Washington, and special tabulations.

Note: Alaska and Hawaii included in 1959-61 deaths. Deaths for age not stated distributed among age groups.

rate is seven times the loss at 20–24 years; at the oldest age in the reproductive age span, 45 years or older, it is 14 times the low figure.

In earlier decennium periods maternal mortality among young mothers under 20 years of age was definitely higher than at ages 20–29 years. A major change occurred between 1949–51 and 1959–61, when the rate at ages under 20 was reduced by 67 percent as compared with about a 57 percent decrease in the rates at ages 20–29 years. Rates for women at the high-risk ages over 40 years dropped by 56 percent in this period. The general pattern of the association between age of mother and maternal mortality is very similar for white and nonwhite mothers. In 1959–61 the differential was approximately fourfold in every age group except 45 years of age and over, when few pregnancies occur. A three- to fourfold margin was found 10 years earlier at each 5-year age level under 40 years of age.

Cause of Death

Reduction in mortality from toxemias of pregnancy was the largest single element responsible for the reduction in the total maternal mortality rate, from 82.7 per 100,000 live births in 1949–51 to 37.1 in 1959–61 (Table 7.2). Next in importance came the lowering in mortality from hemorrhage and sepsis in cases other than abortion. Mortality attributed to ectopic pregnancies also dropped, although the decrease was a minor factor in the reduction in the overall ma-

Table 7.2   Average annual maternal mortality rates per 100,000 live births for selected causes of death by color: United States, selected decennium periods.

Cause of Death	Total			White			Nonwhite		
	1959-61	1949-51	1939-41	1959-61	1949-51	1939-41	1959-61	1949-51	1939-41
Deliveries and complications of pregnancy, childbirth, and the puerperium (640-689)	37.1	82.7	363.9	25.5	61.3	311.3	100.0	218.8	736.5
Sepsis of pregnancy, childbirth and the puerperium (640, 641, 681, 682, 684)	4.0	11.7	91.1	3.1	9.4	79.9	8.9	26.4	170.4
Toxemias of pregnancy and puerperium, except abortion with toxemia (642, 685, 686)	7.1	26.8	87.4	4.4	19.0	69.5	21.5	76.0	213.9
Hemorrhage of pregnancy and childbirth (643, 644, 670-672)	6.3	14.6	46.3	4.5	11.2	42.6	15.8	36.3	72.1
Ectopic pregnancy (645)	2.6	5.3	15.7	1.2	3.2	13.4	10.3	18.8	32.6
Abortion without mention of sepsis or toxemia (650)	2.1	2.5	11.7	1.4	1.7	9.6	6.0	7.6	26.6
Abortion with sepsis (651)	4.6	5.9	52.4	2.6	4.0	44.7	15.6	18.0	106.7
Abortion with toxemia, without mention of sepsis (652)	0.3	0.9	3.8	0.1*	0.7	3.4	1.1	2.4	6.8
Other complications of pregnancy, childbirth, and puerperium and delivery without mention of complication (646-649, 660, 673-680, 683, 687-689)	10.1	15.0	55.5	8.1	12.2	48.1	20.9	33.2	107.5

Source: Annual volumes Vital Statistics of the United States, National Center for Health Statistics, Public Health Service, Washington, and special tabulations.

Note: Alaska and Hawaii included in 1959-61 deaths. Numbers after causes of death are category numbers of the Seventh Revision of the International Classification of Diseases, 1955. Deaths are classified according to the Sixth Revision, 1948 for 1949-51 and Fifth Revision, 1938 for 1939-41. Comparability between rates for the 1939-41 period and rates for later decennium periods was affected by the change in the rules for classifying a death as "maternal" that was adopted in the 1948 revision of the I.C.D. For 1939-41, the major factor was whether the death occurred before, during or after childbirth. Since the 1948 revision, the classification has been based on whether the condition arose during pregnancy, or was noted before delivery; whether the delivery occurred with complications; or whether there were some complications of the puerperium. These classification procedures result in about 9 per cent fewer deaths assigned to deliveries and complications of pregnancy, childbirth and the puerperium, principally because certain complications of childbirth and the puerperium are often mentioned as a contributory cause rather than as an underlying cause of death. Also, the 1939-41 rates for "Other complications of pregnancy, etc." include "Other diseases and accidents of pregnancy with mention of septic conditions" which in the later revisions were included with "Sepsis of pregnancy, childbirth and the puerperium."

*Rate based on less than 20 deaths.

ternal death rate because of the relatively small number of deaths from this cause.[2]

The mortality rate for abortion with sepsis remained almost unchanged during the 1950's. This is quite different from what happened during the 1940's. Although there are problems of comparability between maternal cause-of-death data for 1939–41 and cause data in succeeding decennium periods, it is clear that the vast reduction in mortality that occurred in the 1940 decade was to a large extent due to a remarkable decrease in mortality from sepsis, which affected cases involving abortions as well as cases in which abortion was not mentioned. Mortality due to toxemias, hemorrhage, and ectopic pregnancies also fell sharply in the 1940's but not to the same degree as the rates for infections.

In 1959–61 toxemias ranked first among the causes of maternal

[2] In this section, the discussion of causes of maternal death is confined to the more specific causes for which trend data are available. This excludes the residual category, other complications of pregnancy, childbirth, and puerperium and delivery without mention of complication. In 1959–61 the rate for this category was 10.1 per 100,000, or 27 percent of all maternal deaths.

mortality; this cause was closely followed in order by abortions of all types combined and hemorrhages, and then by sepsis (other than in abortions). These four sets of conditions encompassed two-thirds of the maternal deaths. Ten years earlier, 1949–51, the fre-

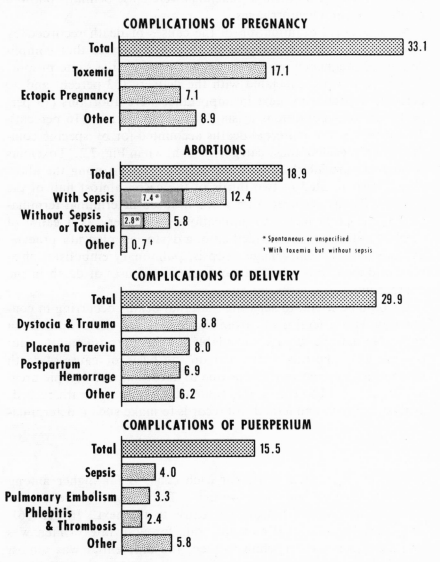

Fig. 7.2. Percent of maternal deaths by specified causes: United States, 1959–61.

Source: National Center for Health Statistics, special tabulations.

quency of maternal deaths from toxemias far exceeded the loss from any other cause, and in fact, the number of toxemia deaths was almost as large as the number attributed to hemorrhages and sepsis combined. In 1939–41, before the changes described above occurred, sepsis ranked first; toxemias were close behind, followed by abortions and hemorrhages.

More detailed examination of the causes of death recorded by physicians on death certificates in 1959–61 indicates that complications of pregnancy were responsible for about the same proportion as difficulties associated with the delivery (33 percent and 30 percent, respectively); next in importance were abortions (19 percent); and then conditions arising in the puerperium (16 percent). The proportion of maternal deaths accounted for by specific complications in each of these categories is shown in Fig. 7.2. Toxemias loom as a particularly significant cause group. Among the abortions, sepsis is cited in two-thirds of the cases; almost half of the abortion deaths occurred after a self-induced or criminal termination of the pregnancy. Complications of delivery as a cause of death are about evenly divided among dystocias, placenta praevia, and postpartum hemorrhage. Sepsis, pulmonary embolism, phlebitis, and thrombosis are the most common causes of death in the puerperium.

It would be useful to separate maternal deaths occurring in conjunction with a fetal death from those in which the child is born alive. No national data are available for this purpose and it is not possible to make this distinction on the basis of cause-of-death information. Except for deaths due to abortions and ectopic pregnancy, it would be necessary to match the maternal death records against live birth and fetal death records to make such a determination.

Color

The maternal mortality rate for each cause is far higher among nonwhite than among white women. The margin between rates varies greatly, however, from one cause to the next. In 1959–61, when the total maternal mortality rate for nonwhite women was four times the rate for white women, the differential was almost fivefold for toxemias (no mention of abortion), four to fivefold for abortion (no mention of sepsis or toxemia), sixfold for abortion with sepsis, and eight to ninefold for ectopic pregnancies (Table

7.2). There were lesser differentials for sepsis (no mention of abortion) and hemorrhages. For no cause was the differential significantly smaller than 10 years earlier. In fact, for toxemia, ectopic pregnancies, and abortion with sepsis the margin increased by 20 percent or more during the 1950's.

Age of Mother

In general, maternal mortality during 1959–61 for each cause-of-death group increased with age beyond 25 years, with the gradient becoming especially large after 30 years of age (Appendix Table II.2). Maternal mortality experienced under 20 years of age is of special interest because in more recent years the rate in this age group for all causes combined has come close to the low figure at ages 20–24 years. The one cause of death for which there is still a substantially higher rate among women under 20 years of age than at ages 20–24 or 25–29 years is the toxemias. The differential (80 percent) is about the same relative magnitude as found in the incidence of toxemias of pregnancy discussed in Chapter 4 for upstate New York women. Among women above 35 years of age the increase in the rate is considerably greater than the rise in the incidence rates for toxemias in upstate New York.

The relative margin between the mortality rate for toxemias under 20 years of age and the loss among women 20–24 years of age in 1959–61 was much smaller than in earlier decennium periods. Actually, the toxemia mortality rate for those under 20 was reduced by 94 percent in the period 1939–41 to 1959–61, a decrease that rivaled the 96 percent drop in the rate for sepsis.

Geographic Area

Every geographic area in the United States underwent a major change in maternal mortality during the 1940's and 1950's.[3] Nevertheless, in 1959–61 there were large differences among the states in their maternal mortality rates (Appendix Table II.3). In six states the rates were below 22 per 100,000 live births and in four states and the District of Columbia they exceeded 60 per 100,000.[4] The

---

[3] Trend data by geographic area are not shown; the basis for this statement is an examination of data in annual volumes, *Vital Statistics of the United States* (National Center for Health Statistics).

[4] Excluded from this discussion are states in which there were fewer than ten maternal deaths during 1959–61.

range is reduced, but by no means eliminated, when rates are examined separately for the white population. In seven states the maternal mortality rate for white women was below 20 per 100,000. Eleven states had rates above 30 per 100,000. Six of these 11 states were in the East and West South Central divisions of the country and two were in the Mountain division of states.

Because of small frequencies it is difficult to make similar comparisons among the states for nonwhite women. However, an examination of the rates for geographic divisions indicates clearly that among nonwhite mothers maternal mortality also varied widely from one area of the country to another. In three geographic divisions, Middle Atlantic, South Atlantic, and East South Central, the rates were above 110 per 100,000. The lowest rates were in the West North Central division (64 per 100,000) and Pacific division (60 per 100,000). The rate in the Pacific area is heavily influenced by the high proportion of nonwhite women who are of Oriental stock and who have a lower rate than Negroes. However, even when the rates are examined separately for Negroes, the Pacific division's rate is comparatively low (74 per 100,000).

Within each geographic division maternal mortality among nonwhite women was three or four times the rate of loss among white mothers. Furthermore, the lowest maternal mortality rates attained by nonwhite women in any area (Pacific and West North Central, 60 and 64 per 100,000, respectively) were substantially higher than the rate in the area with the highest loss among white women (East South Central, 35 per 100,000).

Maternal mortality among women living in metropolitan areas is appreciably lower than among residents of nonmetropolitan areas. In 1959–61 the respective rates were 33.0 and 44.3 per 100,000 live births for the country as a whole (Table 7.3). Similar relative differences were found in the white and nonwhite groups. The pattern of lower rates in metropolitan areas was sharply reversed in the Northeast geographic region. Here, the metropolitan maternal mortality rate was almost 40 percent higher than the nonmetropolitan. The reversal was greatly influenced by the heavy weighting of the population of metropolitan areas in the Northeast with nonwhite population. When rates are examined only for white women in this region, losses in metropolitan and nonmetropolitan areas are approximately the same. Among nonwhite mothers in the Northeast the mortality rate is higher in metropolitan areas. The

Table 7.3   Average annual maternal mortality rates per 100,000 live
             births by color, in metropolitan and nonmetropolitan
             counties: United States and each geographic region, 1959-61.

Color and area	United States[1]	Northeast	North Central	South	West[1]
Total	37.1	34.4	28.1	51.8	28.2
Metropolitan counties	33.0	36.4	27.6	39.7	26.9
Nonmetropolitan counties	44.3	26.4	28.9	63.9	31.4
White	25.5	25.9	23.0	29.2	24.0
Metropolitan counties	22.7	26.3	20.0	22.0	22.1
Nonmetropolitan counties	30.5	24.5	27.3	36.6	28.4
Nonwhite	100.0	108.9	75.6	113.3	62.6
Metropolitan counties	87.6	110.2	73.8	92.2	62.9
Nonmetropolitan counties	123.4	88.1*	91.9	132.1	61.5

Source: Special tabulations of the Division of Vital Statistics, National
Center for Health Statistics, Public Health Service, Washington.

[1]Includes Alaska and Hawaii.

*Rate based on less than 20 deaths.

largest excesses in maternal mortality associated with residence in
nonmetropolitan areas are in the South. This holds for both white
and nonwhite women.

An interesting set of differentials in causes of maternal mortality
exists between women in metropolitan areas and those in nonmetropolitan areas (Appendix Table II.4). To a large extent, the
greater loss rate among women in nonmetropolitan areas in
1959–61 was due to considerably higher mortality attributed to
toxemias and hemorrhage. Rates for these causes were at least
twice as high in nonmetropolitan areas as in metropolitan areas.
A moderately higher rate in nonmetropolitan areas was also found
for sepsis. The direction of these differentials was the same for both
white and nonwhite women but the magnitude was greater in the
nonwhite group. Among nonwhite women in nonmetropolitan
areas the mortality rate for toxemias alone exceeded the total
maternal mortality rate for white women, and their rate for
hemorrhage was almost identical with the overall figure for white
women.

Not all maternal causes of death are at a higher rate in nonmetropolitan areas. Mortality due to ectopic pregnancies is relatively as frequent among white mothers in metropolitan and nonmetropolitan areas; but among nonwhite women the rate is higher
in metropolitan areas. The possibility that ectopic pregnancies are

inadequately diagnosed in nonmetropolitan areas severely qualifies these observations. The other cause of maternal deaths that is of special interest is abortion, for which both white and nonwhite women in metropolitan areas have a substantially higher rate than their counterparts in nonmetropolitan areas. This cannot be explained by an exceptionally large differential in one particular area; a higher mortality rate for abortion is found in most metropolitan areas. Before speculating about the reasons for the curious reversal between metropolitan and nonmetropolitan rates found in this cause-of-death group, it would be desirable to examine more closely residence information reported on the vital records and also the legitimacy status of the births.

Clinical Assessment of Selected Causes of Death

As the mortality rate from toxemia, hemorrhage, and infection has decreased, other conditions resulting in maternal deaths have attracted increased clinical attention. Studies based on hospital experience provide more extensive information about these causes than is possible through recourse to the death certificate. The discussion that follows is based on such special studies.

Cardiac disease, a condition significantly aggravated by pregnancy, seems destined to become one of the foremost causes of maternal mortality. In some hospitals heart disease already accounts for as much as one-quarter of all maternal deaths (3). In the 1940's rheumatic heart disease was found in more than 90 percent of the heart disease cases (4). However, in two recent series, congenital heart disease accounted for 19 percent and 44 percent of the pregnant women with heart disease (5, 6). Hypertensive cardiovascular disease and arteriosclerotic heart disease are uncommon in the reproductive period and are rarely associated with maternal mortality.

Cardiac patients who have a limited functional capacity (Class III or IV), especially those of higher age or who have had a previous episode of decompensation, constitute the gravest maternal risk. Similarly, patients with active myocarditis, atrial fibrillation or some coexisting medical disorder, such as infection, anemia, or hypertension, are under a special hazard in pregnancy. Depending upon the general condition of the patient, the mortality rate for pregnant patients with unfavorable lesions may reach 10–20 percent. Although these women comprise only about 20 percent of all patients with cardiac disease, they account for 85 percent of the deaths among cardiac patients (7). Congenital heart disease is responsible at present for a small but significant number of deaths in this category. The patient known to have patent ductus arteriosus or atrial defects may succumb to systemic hypotension, since a right-to-left shunt of blood can develop in this situation. In addition to the deaths which bear a relation to the functional incapacity of the heart, certain cardiovascular complications, such as vascular accidents and bacterial endocarditis, may take an extra toll.

Vascular Accidents
Currently between 10 and 20 percent of all maternal deaths (8) are considered secondary to vascular catastrophes which may take the form of embolism (nonseptic thrombi, air or amniotic fluid), hemorrhage from arterial rupture (mainly subarachnoid and intra-cerebral; rarely, subdural), and thrombosis (cerebral vein or coro-nary artery). Diffuse petechial hemorrhages in the cerebral cortex occur in about one-third of patients with eclampsia who die within 48 hours (9). Less commonly, small hemorrhages within the depth of the cerebrum or brain stem occur, and occasionally these may rupture into the ventricles. Rarely, massive intracranial hem-orrhage develops following rupture of a major artery, especially when acute toxemia is superimposed on underlying chronic vas-cular disease. However, most spontaneous intracranial hemor-rhages of this magnitude are due to rupture of congenital aneurysms (10, 11, 12).

Anesthesia
Maternal deaths directly or indirectly related to complications of anesthesia have made up a small but important proportion of all deaths related to pregnancy (13). Aspiration of vomitus in associa-tion with general anesthesia in the improperly prepared patient and overdosage of spinal anesthesia represent the principal risks. Other prime offenders in fatal cases are apnea, anoxia, and cerebral injury; inadequate, delayed or improper fluid, electrolyte, and blood replacement; administration of incompatible drugs; and in-fection. The wider use of conduction anesthesia in recent years, particularly peridural, paracervical and pudendal blocks, combined

with improved general supportive measures, has resulted in greater maternal safety (14, 15).

Acute Infectious Hepatitis
This disease shows a predilection for the younger age groups, and hence it is not uncommon among pregnant women. In areas where malnutrition is prevalent, mortality rates among women with this condition during pregnancy may be as high as 15 percent (16, 17).

Other Medical Disorders
The majority of patients with nonobstetric hypertension and renal disease are women with essential vascular hypertension, chronic glomerulonephritis, and chronic pyelonephritis. The major risk to a woman who becomes pregnant while suffering from one of these conditions is the development of toxemia. A great variety of other medical disorders—that is, pulmonary, urinary tract, reproductive tract, and metabolic diseases, appendicitis, and sickle cell disease— may be masked, altered, or aggravated by pregnancy.

Correspondence between Maternal Mortality and
Infant and Prenatal Loss
It seems reasonable to assume that many of the same forces, economic, social, and medical, that influence the level of infant and perinatal mortality affect the rate of maternal mortality. This is strongly supported by the relationships discussed above and in earlier chapters. The trends in infant, perinatal, and maternal mortality were all sharply downward during the late 1930's and throughout the 1940's. There has been a slowdown in the downward course of all of these rates; starting in 1950–51 for infant mortality, a few years later for perinatal and maternal mortality. The nonwhite group has consistently had higher pregnancy and maternal losses than the white group, and the differentials have widened. Also, the risk of neonatal and fetal mortality as well as of maternal mortality increases as age advances beyond 20–24 years. Finally, geographic areas with comparatively high infant and perinatal mortality rates are also high in maternal mortality.

These similarities should not obscure the fundamental difference between pregnancy loss and maternal mortality in the relative magnitude of the changes that have occurred and the variability that still exists among population subgroups. Maternal mortality has responded better than infant mortality to improvement in medical and environmental circumstances. Between 1935 and 1950, for example, the maternal mortality rate decreased by 86 percent, infant mortality rate by 48 percent. Differentials between population groups are greater in maternal mortality. This holds for color comparisons, where the margin between the white and nonwhite populations is twice as large in maternal mortality rates as in the infant or perinatal mortality rates. Similarly the increased risk associated with age beyond 30 years is several times greater in maternal mortality, and geographic variability is far more pronounced in maternal death rates.

These comparisons emphasize that as the means for achieving control over particular causes of death become available, the hard-core problems assume relatively greater importance and the ability to profit from the potential to control mortality lags in groups with comparatively poor economic and medical resources. This is seen in connection with the increasing divergence in infant and maternal mortality rates between the white and nonwhite groups. The fact that in maternal mortality, which has approached a controlled situation, there is a fourfold differential between the rates for these two groups suggests that the present large color differential in infant mortality can become even larger as the overall rate goes down.

International Comparisons

The sharp decline in maternal mortality experienced by the United States after 1935 was shared by all Northern European countries,

Table 7.4 Maternal mortality rates per 10,000 live births: Selected countries, 1950-64.

Year	Australia[1]	Canada	Denmark[2]	England and Wales	Finland	Netherlands	New Zealand[3]	Norway	Sweden	Switzerland	United States
1964	3.3	---	---	2.6	4.2[4]	3.3[4]	3.2	---	---	---	3.3
1963	2.7	3.5	2.5	2.9	5.0	3.3	4.0	2.1*	2.7	3.5	3.6
1962	3.6	4.1	2.1*	3.6	5.2	3.3	2.9*	2.1*	1.3*	5.7	3.5
1961	4.5	4.6	2.2*	3.4	5.5	3.8	3.8	2.7*	2.1	4.9	3.7
1960	5.3	4.3	3.0	3.9	7.2	3.9	3.4*	6.5	3.7	5.7	3.7
1959	4.6	5.5	4.3	3.9	6.7	5.0	4.4	3.9	2.4	6.7	3.7
1958	5.0	5.6	4.4	4.4	10.0	4.1	4.1	5.4	3.0	7.5	3.8
1957	6.3	5.4	4.1	4.8	8.9	6.0	6.7	5.1	3.6	7.6	4.1
1956	5.6	6.2	4.8	5.7	11.1	6.7	4.0	6.9	3.4	7.5	4.1
1955	6.4	7.6	4.6	6.6	10.5	6.1	10.6	6.8	4.9	10.4	4.7
1954	6.9	7.2	6.8	---	10.7	6.8	5.2	6.2	5.4	10.7	5.2
1953	6.2	7.8	8.3	7.7	13.3	8.0	5.4	7.3	6.2	12.3	6.1
1952	9.4	9.3	5.8	7.4	12.5	7.8	7.1	7.8	---	11.3	6.8
1951	10.5	10.7	8.0	8.4	12.1	8.2	6.9	9.6[5]	8.6	24.2[5]	7.5
1950	10.9	11.4	7.8[5]	8.8	14.6[5]	10.5	9.0[5]	10.3[5]	6.2[5]	14.0[5]	8.3

Source: Files of the Statistical Office of the United Nations and annual volumes Vital Statistics of the United States, National Center for Health Statistics, Public Health Service, Washington.

[1]Excludes full-blooded aborigines. Data tabulated by year of registration rather than occurrence.
[2]Excluding Faeroe Islands and Greenland.
[3]Excludes Maoris prior to 1961. Data tabulated by year of registration rather than occurrence.
[4]Provisional
[5]Deaths classified according to Fifth Revision of the International Classification of Diseases, 1938.
*Rates based on less than 20 deaths.

Canada, Australia, and New Zealand. Most of these countries are also undergoing a slowdown in the rate of decline in the maternal mortality rate, although this change in trend generally started later than in the United States.

In 1961–63 the maternal mortality rate covered a narrow range among the low mortality countries, with the United States falling in the middle. Norway, Sweden, and Denmark have rates close to 2 per 10,000 (Table 7.4). In England and Wales the maternal mortality rate has also dropped below 3 per 10,000 (2.9 and 2.6 in 1963 and 1964, respectively). The lowest mortality rate attained by the United States is 3.3 per 10,000 (1964).

8 / REVIEW AND PERSPECTIVES

The large reduction in maternal mortality since the mid-1930's occurred during an era impressive for its record of rapid development and of changing concepts of obstetrics and public health. It is generally agreed that this achievement in saving lives reflects not only the striking advances in medical knowledge and clinical practices but also the effectiveness of maternal health programs throughout the country. Some of the more important medical advances responsible for improved survival rates warrant special mention. Others will be reviewed in a broader historical context in a subsequent discussion of community resources in Chapter 12.

Factors Promoting Improved Maternal Mortality Rates
A particularly noteworthy factor has been the expansion of facilities for prenatal care in almost every state (1). Programs have been developed in some states to screen pregnant women for significant abnormalities and to refer them to well-staffed and well-equipped clinics where they can receive intensive supervision and specialized obstetric care. The sharp reduction in the frequency with which pre-eclampsia progresses to eclampsia may well be the principal dividend of expanded prenatal care. The dramatic increase in hospital deliveries has also added to the safety of child-bearing, since multiple safeguards can be provided in that setting, especially in emergency situations.

During the past several decades there has been a vast expansion of training and educational programs in obstetrics, which have provided more and better qualified specialists, and at the same time, more competent general practitioners.

Establishment of the American Board of Obstetrics and Gynecology, which has now certified more than 6,000 specialists, has spearheaded the drive to elevate standards of obstetric care (1). Also, the American College of Obstetricians and Gynecologists, since its inception a decade and a half ago, has strongly emphasized postgraduate education at the district as well as the national level. Through its various committees and activities, it has sponsored a continuous search into the problems of providing comprehensive care for the obstetrical patient, of stimulating research and of suggesting rules and regulations to be used as a guide in establishing and conducting obstetrical services. These stimuli have brought about an increase in the number of approved residency training programs in obstetrics and gynecology.

Many of the considerations relevant to the reduction in maternal mortality and morbidity are identical with those of concern in improving the likelihood that a normal child will be born. For both, the modern concept of good medical care entails a continuity of supervision during childhood, the teenage period, and the reproductive era. By the same token, it encompasses diagnosis and treatment prior to pregnancy of conditions inimical to maternal health, effective family planning, intensive prenatal care when pregnancy ensues, adequate postpartal follow-ups to assure proper involutionary changes, and the institution of effective preventive and therapeutic measures to assure a favorable health status in anticipation of subsequent child-bearing. More physicians than ever before appreciate the scope and magnitude of these efforts, and facilities are becoming available in some urban areas to receive high-risk individuals where appropriate specialized investigations can be performed.

The recognition that the solution of maternal health problems necessitates a joint effort of multiple health agencies, as well as representation by multiple disciplines, is broadening the base of effective programs within communities. It is becoming apparent that an effective attack upon the residual problems related to maternal mortality is contingent upon a proper liaison among all professional groups interested in maternal and child health. It must be acknowledged, however, that cooperation among professional personnel and institution of appropriate mechanisms for rallying the health resources within the community has been realized only to a limited extent.

A most powerful deterrent to poor medical care practices has been the maternal mortality conference. Although the format is variable, the conference's general objective is to obtain a broad spectrum of information relevant to individual maternal deaths. Deaths are usually classified as direct obstetric, indirect obstetric, or nonobstetric; the extent of preventability is judged; and factors of responsibility are assigned to the physician, patient, hospital, or other agent. Maternal welfare studies derived from these investigations have made a valuable contribution to better maternal care and will continue to play an important role in reducing maternal and perinatal mortality and morbidity. They serve as an educational force in improving hospital and medical standards (2).

The unprecedented advances in medical facilities, knowledge, and the therapeutic armamentarium in the last three decades have been discussed briefly in relation to trends in maternal mortality. Some have had a particular impact upon obstetrical practices and improved survival rates and deserve further elaboration:

1. The availability of blood and its liberal use probably transcends all other advances in the management of hemorrhage (3). Concurrently during the past three decades, the routine use of ergot preparations and oxytocic agents as a means of improving uterine tone and of minimizing postpartal hemorrhage has been a significant advance (4).

2. A reduction in traumatic obstetrics has resulted not only in a reduction of hemorrhage and lacerations but also in puerperal sepsis, which develops in devitalized tissues (5).

3. The availability of an increasing variety of chemotherapeutic agents for specific as well as prophylactic use has made it possible to prevent or control intrapartal or postpartal infections to a large extent. The expansion of proper technical facilities and insistence upon aseptic techniques in the hospital have similarly reduced the incidence of serious infections on the obstetrical wards. Strict rules and regulations have been enforced by governmental agencies, as well as by obstetrical organizations, to assure the establishment and maintenance of appropriate control measures for maternity and newborn services. In addition, most hospitals now have a standing infection committee, whose primary function is to survey and study these problems within the institution.

4. Caesarean section has become increasingly safe for the mother, so that this operation can now be performed at the optimal time in a variety of medical and obstetrical conditions, as an alternative to long, complicated labors and difficult vaginal deliveries (6). In addition, X-ray pelvimetry has greatly augmented knowledge of pelvic anatomy, and its proper use has proved a valuable adjunct in the detection and proper management of pelvic contraction.

5. The advances in conduction anesthesia, including local pudendal blocks, have added a significant dimension of safety in the conduct of labor and delivery. The increasing emphasis upon the education of the patient, her emotional support, the use of

minimum analgesia, and upon "physiological" childbirth has minimized the necessity for deep narcosis and general anesthesia (7).

Unsolved Problems of Maternity Care

Although there has been a dramatic reduction in maternal mortality in the past three decades, there are disturbing elements in the picture. These were discussed in detail in Chapter 7. Briefly, the more important are:

1. The rate of progress in reducing maternal mortality has diminished in recent years and the mortality rate in 1964 (3.3 per 10,000) was not far below the figure for 1956 (4.1).

2. Nonwhite women have four times the maternal mortality rate found among white women (9.0 and 2.2 per 10,000 in 1964 for the two color groups, respectively); there is a lag of 16 years in the level of mortality among nonwhite women as compared with white.

3. Women at the more advanced reproductive ages are still at exceptionally high risk for maternal mortality.

4. Geographic areas vary greatly in maternal mortality, several states having had rates above 60 per 100,000 in 1959–61, which is far above the rate for the country as a whole (37 per 100,000).

5. Despite the vast reductions in mortality from toxemias, hemorrhage, and sepsis, these still represent significant causes of maternal death; comparatively little progress was made during the 1950's in lowering mortality attributed to abortions with sepsis.

Major changes in population composition in the past decade, which have tended to concentrate the unsolved problems of maternity care in densely populated geographic areas, have complicated the problem of providing comprehensive care to the groups most in need. Rapid growth of the population, shortages of professional personnel, inadequate educational, social, and economic opportunities for significant segments of the population, influx of rural population into large metropolitan areas, expansion of inner city slums, inadequate expansion of facilities, and actual deterioration of some existing facilities have exerted heavy pressures on standards and depth of maternity services in these areas.

In the municipal hospitals of many of our large cities about one-half of the pregnant women receive either late or no prenatal care (8). By contrast, on the private services of voluntary hospitals

in the same cities, only 5 percent or less of the patients fail to receive prenatal care prior to the last few months of pregnancy.

Reaching women subject to special maternal hazards earlier in
pregnancy or between pregnancies is a pressing issue. Without
adequate services, provided in a manner meaningful to the intended
recipients, educational programs designed to motivate women to
make full use of such services can hardly be expected to meet with
success. Related obstacles to prenatal care, such as transportation
problems and care of other children in the family, must also receive
close attention. Early sex education and instruction in family
planning are increasingly being accepted as a community responsibility, but new approaches must, and are being, developed to
reach sectors of the population that in the past have had little
access to constructive approaches in these areas.

Much still needs to be done to make good prenatal care a uniform experience throughout the country, even among those women
who are under supervision. When the case records of women who
have died in the course of pregnancy or the puerperium are subjected to individual scrutiny, too often it is found that many of
them received poor obstetrical supervision and care. It is reasonable to assume that the clinical course of many of these patients
might well have achieved a more favorable outcome if each one had
received the best possible management. These indications of
marked variations in the quality of professional care emphasize the
need to intensify and broaden postgraduage educational programs
in maternity care, stressing preventive measures, maternal safeguards, detection of the early signs and symptoms of disease, and
fundamentals of management and therapeutics. Wider application
of what is now known about sound obstetrical practice should lead
to significant reductions in maternal mortality.

Part III
Childhood Mortality

9 / TRENDS AND RECENT STATUS

Childhood[1] is the most favorable period for survival over the entire life span. Decreases in the risk of mortality in succeeding age periods during infancy continue beyond the first birthday. The death rate in the preschool age groups, 1–4 years, has always been a small fraction of the infant mortality rate—in recent years it has been less than 5 percent of the rate under 1 year of age. Beyond infancy, adverse circumstances during fetal development and delivery and deleterious genetic factors continue to exert their influence on mortality and morbidity, but to a diminishing degree. Excess mortality associated with low birth weight decreases throughout infancy, but it is still manifest to some degree after the first birthday (1).

Further reductions in mortality occur at ages 5–14 years, and it is at these school ages that the lowest mortality rates at any age have always been found. Exceedingly favorable mortality rates are experienced throughout this 10-year age span, but the 10–14-year-olds have the lowest mortality risk of all.

Trends

Age

Significant decreases in childhood mortality rates were scored during the early 1900's. The influenza epidemic and its sequelae during and immediately after World War I interrupted the downward trend in the mortality rate only temporarily (Figs. 9.1 and 9.2, Appendix Tables III.1 and III.2). In the preschool ages and school ages, the death rates in 1921–22 dropped to levels consistent with what might have been expected if there had been no interruption in the pre-World War I downward trends. Decreases continued throughout the 1920's and well into the 1930's. Starting about 1937 the rates of decline in both age groups increased sharply, and the decrease in mortality that followed for about 15 years can well be characterized as precipitous. The sharp drop during this period was in striking contrast to the subsequent per-

---

[1] In the discussion that follows, childhood is synonymous with the age period 1–14 years, the preschool period with 1–4 years, and the school-age period with 5–14 years.

Rate per 1,000 Population

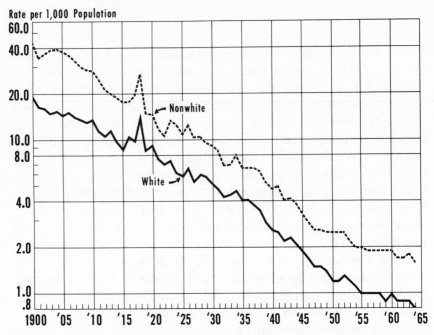

Fig. 9.1. Mortality rates at ages 1–4 years by color: Death registration states or United States, 1900–1964.

Source: National Center for Health Statistics, *Vital Statistics of the United States,* annual volumes.

Notes: Rates based upon population enumerated as of April 1 for 1940, 1950, and 1960, and estimated as of July 1 for all other years. Rates relate to the death registration area through 1932 and to the total United States for later years. Alaska included from 1959 and Hawaii from 1960. New Jersey excluded from date by color for 1962–63.

sistent slow decline that set in during the mid-1950's. This change in the rate of decline has been linked to the more general observation that the mortality rate is leveling off to varying degrees among all age groups of the population (2).

An interesting feature of the decline in the mortality rates among preschool children is that in every period the rate of decline has been far more rapid than that in the infant mortality rate. This holds for the years when sharp decreases in mortality occurred (prior to 1950) and subsequently when the rates leveled off. School-age children have also experienced somewhat steeper rates of decline in their mortality rates than infants, but these have lagged behind the relative decreases among the 1–4-year-olds. Comparative rates of decline follow.[2]

[2] All rates of decline given here and elsewhere in the chapter are derived by fitting least square lines to death rates and are on a per annum basis.

	Period of rapid decline	Period of slow decline
Under 1 year	4.7% (1935–50)	0.9% (1951–64)
1–4 years	7.5% (1937–54)	1.9% (1955–64)
5–14 years	5.7% (1936–55)	1.3% (1956–64)

More rapid decreases in mortality at the preschool ages have apparently been underway even longer than the above data suggest. In the early 1900's mortality rates at ages 1–4 years were four to five times the rates at ages 5–14 years; in the mid-1930's the differential was threefold; in the early 1950's it was slightly more than twofold.

While the rates of decline are informative, the full importance of the changes in mortality rates cannot be appreciated unless the rates themselves are examined. In the first decade of this century

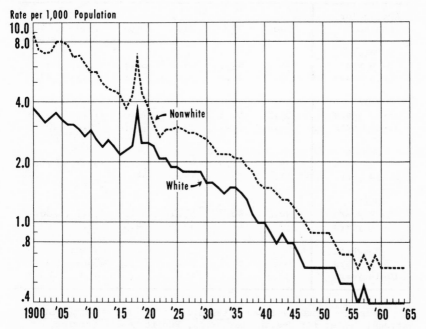

Fig. 9.2. Mortality rates at ages 5–14 years by color: Death registration states or United States, 1900–1964.

Source: National Center for Health Statistics, *Vital Statistics of the United States*, annual volumes.

Notes: Rates based upon population enumerated as of April 1, for 1940, 1950, and 1960, and estimated as of July 1 for all other years. Rates relate to the death registration area through 1932 and to the total United States for later years. Alaska included from 1959 and Hawaii from 1960. New Jersey excluded from data by color for 1962–63.

mortality among children 1–4 years of age varied between 13 and 20 per 1,000; by the mid-1930's the rate was cut to about one-fourth of these figures and stood at about 4 per 1,000; by the mid-1950's the rate was reduced to about 1 per 1,000, or less than 10 percent of the rate at the beginning of the twentieth century. In the 10-year period from 1955–64 the rate went from 1.14 per 1,000 in 1955 to 0.96 per 1,000 in 1964, a decrease of only 16 percent.

Among the 5–14-year-olds the annual rate was reduced from 3 to 4 per 1,000 prior to 1910 to 1.5 per 1,000 in the mid-1930's and then to about 0.5 per 1,000 in the 1950's. Between 1956 and 1964 the rate decreased by 9 percent (0.47 per 1,000 and 0.43 per 1,000 in the two years, respectively).

Table 9.1   Childhood mortality rates by age, color and sex per 100,000 population*: United States, selected years.

Age, color and sex	1963	1960	1955	1950	1948	1945
Total						
5- 9 years	45.2	49.0	49.2	61.7	67.2	89.3
10-14 years	41.5	44.0	47.4	58.1	65.2	87.8
Male						
5- 9 years	51.8	56.3	57.3	71.0	77.7	102.6
10-14 years	51.2	55.0	59.8	70.7	78.4	105.3
Female						
5- 9 years	38.4	41.5	40.7	52.2	56.4	75.4
10-14 years	31.5	32.6	34.5	44.9	51.6	69.9
White						
5- 9 years	42.2	46.2	47.0	58.0	64.7	86.4
10-14 years	39.3	41.4	44.9	54.5	60.8	82.0
Nonwhite						
5- 9 years	63.6	66.7	64.2	89.1	83.9	107.8
10-14 years	57.2	61.5	65.2	82.5	93.6	128.0

Source: Annual volumes Vital Statistics of the United States, National Center for Health Statistics, Public Health Service, Washington.

Note: Alaska and Hawaii included in 1960 and 1963. New Jersey excluded from data by color in 1963.

*Enumerated as of April 1 for 1950 and 1960 and estimated as of July 1 for other years.

Very similar decreases have been occurring in the mortality rate among the 5–9-year-olds and those 10–14 years of age. Starting from almost identical rates in 1945 (89.3 and 87.8 per 100,000, respectively), the rates have diverged only slightly; in 1963 the rates were 45.2 and 41.5 per 100,000 in these two age groups (Table 9.1).

Color and Sex
During the early decades of this century the gap between the mortality rates among nonwhite and white children of preschool age appeared to be narrowing (Fig. 9.1). Precise measures of changes in the difference between these rates cannot be made because of the changing composition of the death registration area and the possibility that completeness of registration of deaths among young children may have varied. Nevertheless, it seems clear that in all years 1900–1910, the nonwhite rate at the preschool ages was more than double the white rate. This margin decreased during the next two decades, and in the early 1930's the nonwhite rate was 60 to 80 percent higher than the white. The period of rapid decrease in the mortality rate among preschool children that started in the mid-1930's extended without significant interruption over a somewhat longer period among the white children and the gap widened once more. By 1950 the nonwhite rate was again double the white. Since the mid-1950's decreases in the mortality rates in both color groups have slowed down to almost the same extent (the rates of decline were 2.2 and 2.1 percent per year for the period 1955–64 among white and nonwhite preschool children, respectively). Accordingly, for about 15 years the relative margin between the rates for the two color groups has been the same; in 1964 the rates were 0.84 per 1,000 and 1.62 per 1,000 for white and nonwhite children.

Among children of school age excess mortality in the nonwhite group in the early 1900's was almost as great as that observed among preschool-age children (Fig. 9.2). However, the differential quickly narrowed, and for many years the nonwhite rate was 50–60 percent higher than the white rate. During the period of rapid decline (1936–55) the nonwhite rate dropped somewhat more rapidly (6.1 percent per year as compared with 5.6 percent for white children) and the gap dropped below 50 percent by the end of this period. In the years that followed, the rate of decline has been the same for the two color groups, 1.2 percent per year, and the differential between the white and nonwhite mortality rates has usually been 40 to 45 percent. This margin is substantially smaller than at ages 1–4 years or in any period during infancy after the first week of life.

Since about 1945 the mortality rate among white children has been slightly higher at the early school ages (5–9 years) than at ages 10–14 years (Table 9.1). Among the nonwhite children, on the other hand, the mortality rate was higher at 10–14 years of age in the middle and late 1940's. A greater decline in the risk of mortality in this age group since then has brought the rate for the 10–14-year-olds below the mortality rate at 5–9 years of age. The differential between the rates in these two age groups among nonwhite children has at times exceeded that among white children.

During the early 1900's the preschool mortality rate among males differed slightly from the rate for females; in most years the differential was less than 10 percent (Fig. 9.3). Subsequently, mortality reductions were greater for girls and by the mid-1930's the margin rose to 14–15 percent. Both sexes experienced rapid rates of decline in mortality until the mid-1950's, when the rates for each started to level off. Differences in the mortality rates between the sexes have been between 14 and 22 percent since about 1950. In 1964 the rates were 1.05 and 0.87 per 1,000 for males and females, respectively.

In the school-age group there was very little difference in the mortality rates by sex during the early 1900's (Fig. 9.4). As a result of a slower decline in the mortality among school-age boys, their rate gradually exceeded the female rate by an increasing margin. In the mid-1930's the mortality risk among males was about one-third higher than among females. Both sexes experienced sharp decreases in their rates until the mid-1950's, but the rate of decline was greater among females and at the point where the rates started to level off there was about a 50 percent margin. The slowdown in the rate of decrease in mortality has been similar for males and females, and the gap between their mortality rates has remained at about 50 percent. In 1964 their respective mortality rates were 0.52 per 1,000 and 0.34 per 1,000.

Among the 5–14-year-old girls the mortality rates have been consistently higher for the 5–9-year group than the 10–14-year group; since 1950 the differential has been 20 to 30 percent. The situation

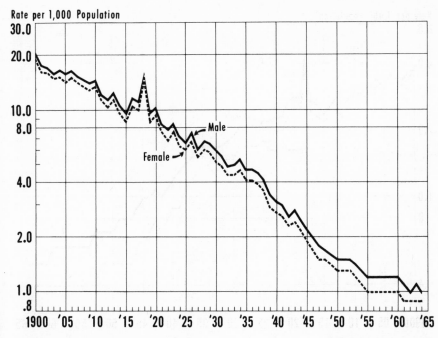

Fig. 9.3. Mortality rates at ages 1–4 years by sex: Death registration states or United States, 1900–1964.

Source: National Center for Health Statistics, *Vital Statistics of the United States*, annual volumes.

Notes: Rates based upon population enumerated as of April 1 for 1940, 1950, and 1960, and estimated as of July 1 for all other years. Rates relate to the death registration area through 1932 and to the total United States for later years. Alaska included from 1959 and Hawaii from 1960.

among boys has been quite different. Their mortality at ages 10–14 years has been very close to the rate at ages 5–9 years; and there were years during the 1940's and 1950's when it slightly exceeded the loss rate at the younger ages.

Examination of trends and comparative rates among the four color-sex groups at preschool and school ages produces no major surprises (Appendix Tables III.1, III.2, and III.3). In general, all of these categories went through periods of sharp decrease in mortality and are now in a prolonged period of slow decline. No one subgroup stands out as having had a trend uniquely different from the others. Among preschool children the relative excess of mortality for boys as compared with girls has generally been slightly higher for white than for nonwhite children. The dif-

Rate per 1,000 Population

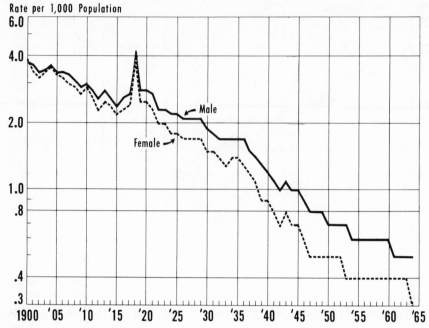

Fig. 9.4. Mortality rates at ages 5–14 years by sex: Death registration states or United States, 1900–1964.

Source: National Center for Health Statistics, *Vital Statistics of the United States*, annual volumes.

Notes: Rates based upon population enumerated as of April 1 for 1940, 1950, and 1960, and estimated as of July 1 for all other years. Rates relate to the death registration area through 1932 and to the total United States for later years. Alaska included from 1959 and Hawaii from 1960.

ferential is more significant at the school ages. Here, the ratio of male to female death rates has been consistently greater among white children.

Changes in Leading Causes of Death

In considering the causes of death in childhood in this section, emphasis is placed on the leading groups of causes of death as indicators of major public health problems. In addition, specific causes of death have been selected for discussion for one of several reasons: they may be responsible for comparatively large numbers of deaths; they may be of particular historical significance; or, because of their preventability or other factors, they are of special public health or medical interest. For example, gastroenteritis and tuberculosis have been singled out for special consideration because of their preventability and historical significance, and cystic fibrosis, although responsible for a very small segment of childhood mortality, has received a good deal of attention in public health programs for handicapped children.

Age

Comparison of the mortality rates at ages 1–4 years for successive 3-year periods centering around 1940, 1950, and 1960 shows marked changes in the rates themselves and in their relative ranks (Fig. 9.5). In the 1940 period infectious diseases, as represented by influenza and pneumonia, gastroenteritis, and tuberculosis, were first, third, and fourth in rank and were responsible for about 36

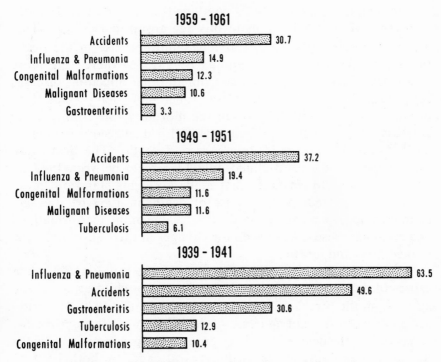

Fig. 9.5. Five leading causes of death at ages 1–4 years: United States, 1939–41, 1949–51, and 1959–61.

Source: National Center for Health Statistics, Vital Statistics of the United States, annual volumes.

Notes: Rates per 100,000 population. Alaska and Hawaii included for 1959–61.

percent of all deaths. Accidents and congenital malformations ranked second and fifth, respectively, among the leading causes of death.

Within a decade, influenza and pneumonia dropped to second place, to follow accidental causes, even though the death rate from accidents had declined 25 percent during the interval. Deaths from gastroenteritis fell so sharply that they were no longer among the five leading causes of death. The death rate from malignant diseases increased slightly, and they now appeared, for the first time, among the five leading causes of death in the preschool group with a rate equal to that of congenital malformations.

During the 1950 decade, death rates from infectious causes showed a further decline. However, the relative decline was considerably smaller than in the previous period, and deaths from all infectious diseases (infective and parasitic disease, influenza and pneumonia, and gastroenteritis combined) still represented nearly 25 percent of the total deaths in this age group in 1959–61. This was due chiefly to the comparatively small decrease in the death rate from influenza and pneumonia. By 1959–61 there were more deaths from these conditions than from all other infectious diseases combined. Since the death rate from tuberculosis fell precipitously during the decade and the drop in the mortality rate from gastroenteritis was relatively small, gastroenteritis displaced tuberculosis in fifth rank among the leading causes of death. The death rate from accidental causes declined only 17 percent between 1949–51 and 1959–61, a circumstance that made accidents stand out more sharply as the predominant cause of death; in 1959–61 they accounted for 29 percent of the deaths. Congenital malformations and malignant diseases, with minor changes in their absolute rates, ranked third and fourth.

During the 1940's and 1950's changes in the ranking of leading causes of death have been less dramatic among children of school age than in the preschool group (Fig. 9.6). In the 1939–41 period accidents were the leading cause of death and were responsible for 28 percent of the deaths in this age group. The proportion of deaths due to accidents rose in the ensuing two decades (in both 1949–51 and 1959–61 the proportion was approximately 40 percent), despite the fact that the actual death rate from accidents dropped more than one-third between 1939–41 and 1959–61. Influenza and pneumonia, which ranked second as a cause of death in 1939–41,

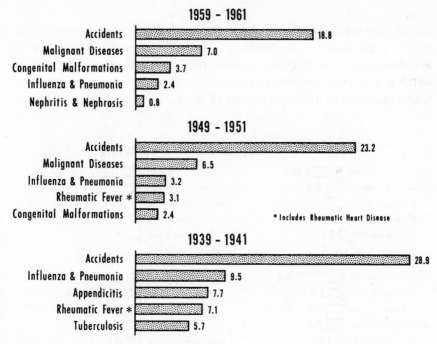

Fig. 9.6. Five leading causes of death at ages 5–14 years: United States, 1939–41, 1949–51, and 1959–61.

Source: National Center for Health Statistics, *Vital Statistics of the United States*, annual volumes.

Notes: Rates per 100,000 population. Alaska and Hawaii included for 1959–61.

dropped to third place in 1949–51, and to fourth by 1959–61. In the two most recent decennium periods influenza and pneumonia were the only infectious diseases remaining among the leading causes of death. Appendicitis, in third place in 1939–41, and tuberculosis, then in fifth place, both disappeared as leading causes of death within a decade. Rheumatic fever and rheumatic heart disease, in fourth place in both 1939–41 and 1949–51 (although the rate dropped 56 percent between these two periods), no longer appeared among the five leading causes of death in 1959–61. Nephritis and nephrosis appeared in fifth place in 1959–61. On the other hand, the malignant diseases and congenital malformations, which did not appear among the five leading causes of death in 1939–41, showed moderate increases in their recorded death rates over the two decades that followed and rose to second and third, respectively, in the rank of causes of death in 1959–61.

Color

For the preschool age group as a whole, the shift away from the infectious diseases as the leading causes of mortality in favor of accidents and noninfectious conditions has been pointed out. This pattern was even clearer and the shift more advanced among the white children in this age group (Fig. 9.7). Influenza and pneu-

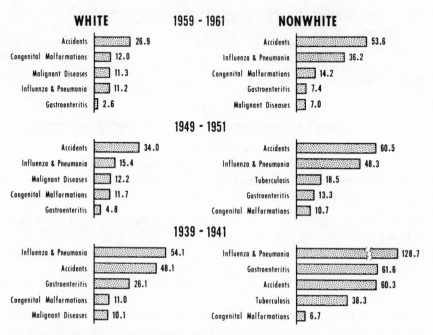

Fig. 9.7. Five leading causes of death at ages 1–4 years by color: United States, 1939–41, 1949–51, and 1959–61.

Source: National Center for Health Statistics, *Vital Statistics of the United States*, annual volumes.

Notes: Rates per 100,000 population. Alaska and Hawaii included for 1959–61.

monia, for example, ranked fourth as a cause of death among white children in 1959–61, whereas it was still the leading cause, after accidents, among the preschool children of all color groups combined. Among white preschool children the death rate from tuberculosis had fallen to such a low point by 1939–41 that it did not appear as one of the five leading causes of death at that or any subsequent time. The total group of infectious diseases, which were responsible for nearly half of all the deaths among these children in 1939–41, caused only 22 percent of the deaths in 1959–61.

The causes of death among nonwhite and white preschool children differed sharply during each time period. In general, the pattern of leading causes of death among the nonwhite children tended to resemble the pattern among white children at least a decade earlier. This is most demonstrable by comparing the leading causes of death among the nonwhite group in 1959–61 with those among the white preschool children in 1949–51. Influenza and pneumonia and gastroenteritis ranked second and fourth during the more recent period among nonwhite children, and they ranked second and fifth in the earlier period among white children. Among the white children in 1959–61, on the other hand, the two infectious disease groups ranked fourth and fifth, with the rate for gastroenteritis being distinctly below the rates for the other leading causes. Viewed in another way, infectious diseases among the nonwhite preschool children were responsible for 43 percent of all deaths in 1949–51; this approached the nearly 50 percent of all deaths ascribed to infectious causes among the white group in 1939–41. In 1959–61, 32 percent of the deaths among preschool nonwhite children were reported as due to infectious diseases, whereas the corresponding proportion of all deaths from infectious diseases among the white children in 1949–51 had already fallen to 30 percent.

The temporal pattern of the leading causes of death among white children in contrast to nonwhite children has also been evident in the school-age group (Fig. 9.8). Tuberculosis, which did not appear as one of the five leading causes of death among white children even in 1939–41, still ranked fourth as a cause of death among nonwhite children in 1949–51. Rheumatic fever and rheumatic heart disease, which may be considered closely related epidemiologically to the infectious diseases, followed much the same pattern. Among nonwhite children rheumatic fever and rheumatic heart disease ranked second among the causes of death in 1949–51, while it ranked fourth among the white children at that time. By 1959–61 it no longer appeared among the five leading causes of death among white children, but it ranked fifth among nonwhite children. Accidents ranked as the leading cause of death among both white and nonwhite children in all three time periods under study.

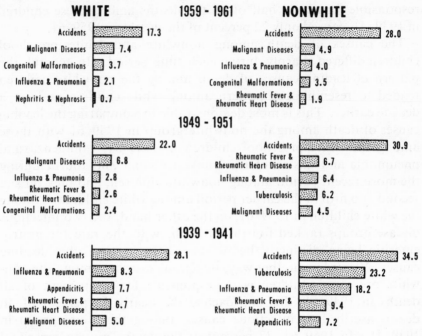

Fig. 9.8. Five leading causes of death at ages 5–14 years by color: United States, 1939–41, 1949–51, and 1959–61.

Source: National Center for Health Statistics, *Vital Statistics of the United States*, annual volumes.

Notes: Rates per 100,000 population. Alaska and Hawaii included for 1959–61.

Sex

The pattern in the leading causes of death among boys and girls of preschool age has been almost identical for many years (Fig. 9.9). While the death rate for accidents has been consistently higher among males than among females, the relative position of accidents among the causes of death has been identical in the two sexes, and its pre-eminence as a cause of death was evident in 1949–51 and in 1959–61. During these two periods accidents were the cause of about 30 percent of the deaths among males and about 25 percent of the deaths among females. As a result of the somewhat lower death rate from malignant diseases among females, the only difference in the order of causes of deaths between the two sexes in the three periods under study occurred in the 1949–51 period. At that time malignant diseases appeared as the third leading cause of death among preschool males, just above congenital malformations, whereas the order was reversed among females.

Minor differences are to be noted in the leading causes of death among boys and girls of school age in the three time periods under study (Fig. 9.10). Although accidents are consistently the leading cause of death in both sexes they constitute a far higher proportion of all deaths among males than among females. Conversely, greater death rates from rheumatic fever and rheumatic heart disease placed these conditions higher on the list of leading causes of deaths among females during 1939–41 and 1949–51, but these conditions no longer appeared among the five leading causes of death in either sex in 1959–61. The slightly higher death rate from tuberculosis among females accounted for its inclusion among the five leading

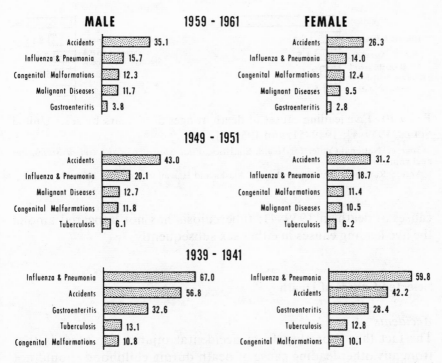

Fig. 9.9. Five leading causes of death at ages 1–4 years by sex: United States, 1939–41, 1949–51, and 1959–61.

Source: National Center for Health Statistics, *Vital Statistics of the United States*, annual volumes.

Notes: Rates per 100,000 population. Alaska and Hawaii included for 1959–61.

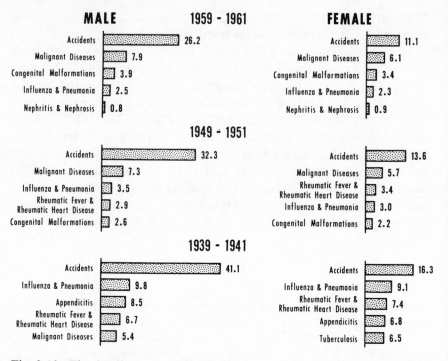

Fig. 9.10. Five leading causes of death at ages 5–14 years by sex: United States, 1939–41, 1949–51, and 1959–61.

Source: National Center for Health Statistics, *Vital Statistics of the United States*, annual volumes.

Notes: Rates per 100,000 population. Alaska and Hawaii included for 1959–61.

causes of death in 1939–41; tuberculosis has not appeared among the five leading causes in either sex subsequently.

Selected Causes of Death

Accidents
The fact that mortality from accidental injuries far exceeds that from any other leading cause of death during childhood should not obscure the gains in reducing losses over the past decades. In the decade ending with the 1959–61 period the death rate from accidents in the preschool group declined 17 percent, from 37.2 to 30.7 per 100,000 children (Fig. 9.11). While this was a significant gain, it was less than the decrease of 25 percent, from 49.6 to 37.2 per

100,000, during the preceding decade. In the school-age group the decline was about 20 percent during each of these 10-year intervals, with a drop in the death rate from 28.9 to 18.8 deaths per 100,000 over the two decades (Fig. 9.12).

Not only has the death rate from accidents been much higher among nonwhite than white children (53.6 versus 26.9 per 100,000 preschool children and 28.0 versus 17.3 in school-age children in 1959–61) but the decline in their death rate from these causes has been far smaller (Figs. 9.13 and 9.14). Among the white preschool group the death rate declined 21 percent in the decade ending 1959–61 and 29 percent in the previous decade. Among the non-white children a decline of only 11 percent was registered in the recent decade, with no reduction at all during the previous decade.

At the school ages the white children showed about a 22-percent decline in the death rate from accidents during each of the two

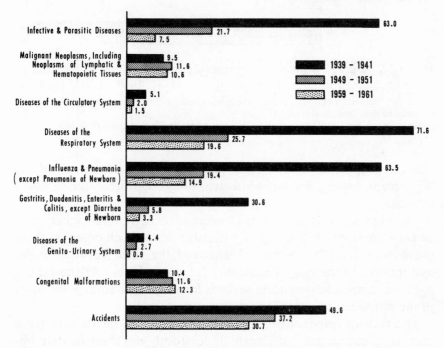

Fig. 9.11. Average annual death rates at ages 1–4 years for selected cause-of-death groupings: United States, 1939–41, 1949–51, and 1959–61.

Source: National Center for Health Statistics, special tabulations and *Vital Statistics of the United States,* annual volumes.

Notes: Rates per 100,000 population. Alaska and Hawaii included for 1959–61.

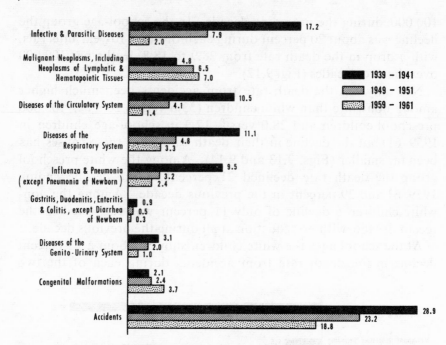

Fig. 9.12. Average annual death rates at ages 5–14 years for selected cause-of-death groupings: United States, 1939–41, 1949–51, and 1959–61.

Source: National Center for Health Statistics, special tabulations and *Vital Statistics of the United States,* annual volumes.

Notes: Rates per 100,000 population. Alaska and Hawaii included for 1959–61.

10-year periods studied, in comparison with a decline of about 10 percent among the nonwhite school-age children during these decades.

Throughout childhood, boys have consistently had higher rates of accidental death than girls. Similar relative changes in these death rates have left almost unchanged the ratio between males and females in the risk of mortality from accidents. At the school ages the margin between the sexes is large enough to explain most of the difference in overall mortality.

The factors responsible for the decline in the death rate from accidental causes are not clearly understood, and their relative importance is problematical. Reduction in the death rate can be achieved by preventing the incidents leading to bodily injury (through education, resulting in behavioral change, or through elimination of environmental hazards) and by improved immediate and subsequent treatment of the injury after its occurrence. The number of accidental injuries, no matter how defined, vastly exceeds the deaths from accidental causes; and the number of incidents which may result in bodily injury similarly exceeds the actual number of injuries (3). Certainly, with the major advances in pediatric surgery and pediatric care in general since 1940, part of the decline in the death rate from accidental causes during childhood must be ascribed to care after the occurrence of the injury,

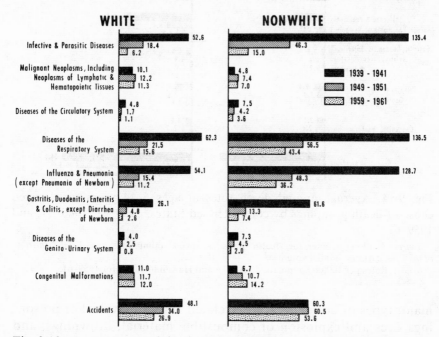

Fig. 9.13. Average annual death rates at ages 1–4 years for selected cause-of-death groupings by color: United States, 1939–41, 1949–51, and 1959–61.

Source: National Center for Health Statistics, special tabulations and *Vital Statistics of the United States*, annual volumes.

Notes: Rates per 100,000 population. Alaska and Hawaii included for 1959–61.

rather than solely to the elimination of environmental hazards and other preventive approaches.

Types of Accidents.

Among preschool children in the decade ending 1959–61 there was a decline of about 17 percent in the death rates from most of the

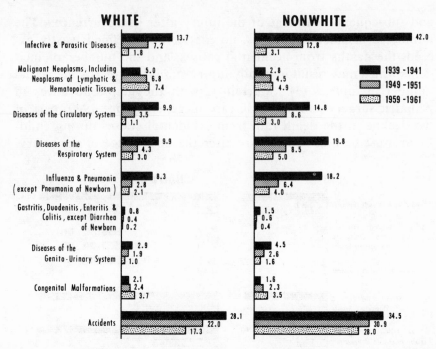

Fig. 9.14. Average annual death rates at ages 5–14 years for selected cause-of-death groupings by color: United States, 1939–41, 1949–51, and 1959–61.

Source: National Center for Health Statistics, special tabulations and *Vital Statistics of the United States*, annual volumes.

Notes: Rates per 100,000 population. Alaska and Hawaii included for 1959–61.

major types of accidents (those related to motor vehicles, poisonings, fires and explosion of combustible material, drownings, and firearms), but accidental fatalities related to falls showed no decrease (Appendix Table III.4). Another point of interest is that the death rate from poisonings during the preschool period, which received major attention in recent years, declined only to the same extent as the rate for total accidents during the decade.

During the 1940's, when there was a greater decrease in the death rate among preschool children from all accidents combined, a much wider fluctuation in the extent of the decrease by type of accident was observed. The death rate from fire and explosions was cut in half and the rate from poisonings was reduced by one-quarter, but the decline from motor vehicle accidents was only 11 percent.

In the 1959–61 period motor vehicle accidents, with a rate of 9.7

per 100,000, led all other types of accidents as a cause of death among preschool children and constituted 32 percent of all accidental deaths in this age group (Fig. 9.15). Deaths from fires and explosions, with a rate of 6.5 per 100,000, were 21 percent of the total. Deaths from drownings (4.2 per 100,000) and poisonings (2.6 per 100,000) followed next in order.

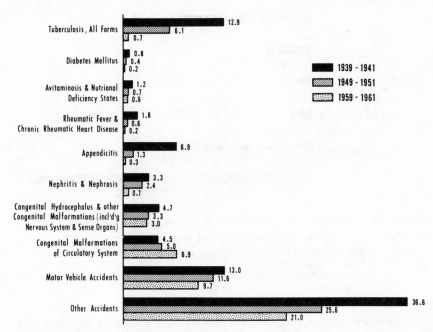

Fig. 9.15. Average annual death rates at ages 1–4 years for selected causes: United States, 1939–41, 1949–51, and 1959–61.

Source: National Center for Health Statistics, special tabulations and *Vital Statistics of the United States*, annual volumes.

Notes: Rates per 100,000 population. Alaska and Hawaii included for 1959–61.

Among the school-age children during the same period the death rate from motor vehicle accidents (7.8 per 100,000) was 20 percent less than among preschool children (9.7 per 100,000) (Fig. 9.16). Children of school age are presumably more exposed to the hazards of motor vehicles than are preschool children, so that the lower rate among school-age children may be a reflection of their greater experience in avoiding motor vehicle hazards. Even so, motor vehicle deaths were responsible for 41 percent of all accidental

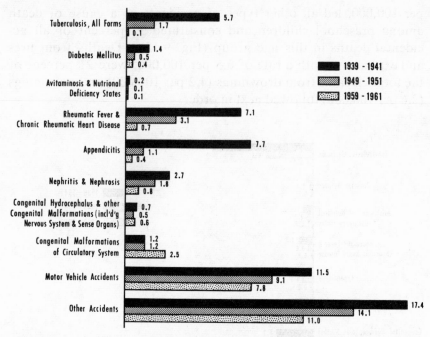

Fig. 9.16. Average annual death rates at ages 5–14 years for selected causes: United States, 1939–41, 1949–51, and 1959–61.

Source: National Center for Health Statistics, special tabulations and *Vital Statistics of the United States*, annual volumes.

Notes: Rates per 100,000 population. Alaska and Hawaii included for 1959–61.

deaths among school-age children, and motor vehicle accidents, by themselves, constituted the leading cause of death in this age group.

Deaths from drownings (3.6 per 100,000) and fires and explosions (2.2 per 100,000) followed in second and third places. The death rate from firearm accidents, although more than twice as high as in the preschool group, was fourth among all types of accidents among the school-age group. Accidental poisonings were insignificant as a cause of death among school-age children, with a death rate only 8 percent as high as in the preschool group. During the decade ending 1959–61 the death rate from motor vehicle accidents among school-age children declined only 14 percent, less than that for any other type of accident in this age group. During the previous decade deaths from motor accidents had declined at about the same rate as that for accidental causes as a whole.

Infectious Diseases

The broad grouping "infective and parasitic diseases" in the International List covers a wide range of conditions, including, among others, measles and other so-called contagious diseases of childhood, venereal diseases, tuberculosis, and rickettsial diseases. None of the diseases or conditions in this broad group, with the exception of tuberculosis, exerted a sufficiently heavy impact on childhood mortality from 1940 on to be ranked among the five leading causes of death. Indeed, one might refer to the virtual elimination of mortality from many of these infective and parasitic diseases, in view of the very small numbers of deaths ascribed to them.

The dramatic decline of 84 percent in the death rate from infectious diseases[3] in the preschool age group within 20 years (157.1 per 100,000 in 1939–41 to 25.7 in 1959–61) attests to the spectacular progress in this area (Appendix Table III.4). However, not all the infectious diseases shared equally in the decline, and the rate of progress evident in the first half of this period was not maintained in the 1950's. For the group as a whole, the death rate declined 70 percent in the 1940's but only 45 percent in the subsequent decade. The major element in this lack of progress in recent years has been the marked slowing down in the decline of the death rate from influenza and pneumonia; the decrease was only 23 percent during the 1950's in contrast to 69 percent during the previous decade.

Also, decreases became smaller in the gastroenteritis death rate (81 percent in the 1940's and 43 percent in the 1950's), but this did not have very much of an effect on the overall picture for preschool children because of the comparatively small proportion of deaths from this type of infection. The death rate from tuberculosis, on the other hand, fell even more sharply during the 1950's (89 percent versus 53 percent during the previous decade) and the death rate from the remainder of the catch-all group of "infective and parasitic diseases" continued to decline rapidly throughout the 20-year period (66 percent in the 1940's and 65 percent in the 1950's.

Mortality from infectious diseases among children of school age

[3] Includes infective and parasitic diseases, influenza and pneumonia, and gastroenteritis.

differs to some extent from the situation among preschool children. Starting from a lower level in 1939–41 (27.6 per 100,000 in the school-age group versus 157.1 in the preschool group), the rate fell to a lesser extent in the school-age group (58 percent) than in the preschool group (70 percent) during the 1940's. In the 1950's deaths from infectious diseases continued to decline at the same rate as during the previous decade, in sharp contrast to the decided slowing down of the decline in the preschool group.

The lag in the decline in the death rate from influenza and pneumonia during the 1950's was as evident in the school-age group as in the preschool group. However, the decline in the mortality rate for the category "infective and parasitic diseases" was greater among school-age than among preschool children. The result of all these trends was an almost identical drop in the death rate from the infectious diseases among both age groups in the 20-year period from 1940 to 1960.

The sharp decline in deaths from infectious diseases since the early years of the century is attributable to a number of factors. The decline in gastroenteritis (mainly the summer diarrhea of earlier years) is undoubtedly related to improved sanitation, particularly with regard to the provision of safe milk and water. The virtual elimination of tuberculosis as a cause of death in children is partially related to the pasteurization of milk and the eradication of bovine tuberculosis and partially to the decline in tuberculosis in the adult population, for whatever reasons the latter has occurred. The long-term downward trend in mortality from the so-called contagious diseases of childhood, for which there is no adequate explanation in the early years of this century, was accelerated by the advent of immunizing agents for some diseases and the sulfonamides and antibiotics for others. The marked slowing in the decline in the death rate from influenza and pneumonia in childhood, even though the death rate has reached a very low level, is similar to what has been happening in other age groups of the population. Many of the remaining deaths may be due to viral and other pneumonias which are being identified as disease entities and which have not yet responded to specific therapies. It might be that in a substantial number of the deaths attributed to pneumonia the pneumonia is not in reality the underlying cause of death, even though the vital records so indicate.

The impact of infectious diseases on the childhood death rates by color has been explored at some length in the discussion of the leading causes of death. In the preschool-age group the decrease in the death rate from this disease among white children between 1939–41 and 1959–61 (85 percent) did not differ much from the corresponding change among the nonwhite children (82 percent). As a result, the gap between the infectious disease death rates for white and nonwhite preschool age children has not widened significantly over the years. In 1959–61 mortality due to these causes among nonwhite children was about three times the rate among white children. Furthermore, the nonwhite rate in 1959–61 was substantially higher than the figure among white children 10 years earlier. At the school ages there has been a slightly smaller relative decrease in mortality from infectious diseases over the 20-year period among white children (82 percent) as compared with nonwhite children (88 percent) and the absolute difference between white and nonwhite rates for these conditions has decreased. Nevertheless, the gap remains large, and in 1959–61 the death rate for infectious diseases was approximately 80 percent higher among the nonwhite children.

Malignant Diseases

In the preschool-age group the death rate from malignant diseases rose moderately from 9.5 per 100,000 in 1939–41 to 11.6 in the following decade, and declined slightly to 10.6 in 1959–61. With regard to the two major types of malignant disease in childhood, deaths from leukemia demonstrated the same temporal fluctuation, but deaths from malignancies of the central nervous system (mainly brain tumors) showed a progressive upward trend, from a rate of 1.3 per 100,000 in 1939–41 to 2.2 in 1959–61.

It may be supposed that the increase in the death rate from malignancy in the preschool group during the 1940's was related to better diagnosis and to the assignment of some of the deaths to malignant disease that would have been ascribed in earlier years to infectious causes. This suggestion is supported by the increase of 54 percent in the death rate for malignancies among nonwhite children in the 1940's.

The decrease during the 1950's in mortality from leukemia and other malignancies (except those of the central nervous system) is of interest despite its small magnitude. More effective care of some abdominal malignancies of early life was broadly applied during this decade. Major advances were being scored in the treatment of leukemia, although these are entirely in prolonging the life of the affected child rather than curing the disease. The small decline in the preschool leukemia death rate may be balanced against a corresponding rise in the death rate from this cause in the school-age group, suggesting that some deaths that would have occurred before the fifth birthday were being deferred beyond this age.

Among school-age children the death rate from malignancies rose from 4.8 per 100,000 in 1939–41 to 7.0 in 1959–61. The increase was evident in leukemia and in malignancies of the central nervous system. Prolongation of the lives of children with leukemia in this age group would not have a favorable effect on the death rate from this cause; leukemia is most common in the first decade of life and most deaths would occur before 10 years of age, in any event. The possible effect of survival beyond the fifth birthday has already been discussed.

The death rate from malignancies has been consistently much lower among nonwhite children than among white children in both the preschool and schoolage groups. That a large part of the difference is an artifact of unsatisfactory diagnosis and, by inference, medical care, among the nonwhite is suggested by the proportionately greater rise in the nonwhite mortality rates between 1939–41 and 1959–61. Girls have had lower malignancy mortality rates than boys throughout this period in both the preschool and school-age groups.

Congenital Malformations
The death rate from congenital malformations during childhood has shown a moderate but fairly consistent rise since the 1930's.

This increase has been proportionately greater among children of school age than among preschool children. In the younger group the death rate rose from 10.4 to 12.3 per 100,000, an increase of 18 percent, from 1939–41 to 1959–61. The corresponding increase in the older group was from 2.1 to 3.7 per 100,000, or 76 percent.

The upward trend in the death rate from congenital malformations is traceable almost entirely to the increase in the death rate from malformations of the circulatory system. In the preschool group the death rate from malformations of the circulatory system increased from 4.5 to 6.9 per 100,000 between 1939–41 and 1959–61. The increase of 2.4 per 100,000 was greater than the increase of 1.9 per 100,000 for all congenital malformations in the period. The death rate from congenital hydrocephalus and other malformations of the central nervous system actually declined from 4.7 to 3.0 per 100,000 during this time.

A similar phenomenon was observed in the school-age group. The death rate from congenital malformations of the circulatory system more than doubled between 1939–41 and 1959–61 (from 1.2 to 2.5 per 100,000). The death rate from all other congenital malformations rose only 0.3 per 100,000; among these, the death rate from hydrocephalus and other malformations of the central nervous system declined moderately during this time interval.

The rise in the reported death rate from congenital malformations of the circulatory system occurred during an era of increasingly sophisticated approaches to the diagnosis and surgical correction or amelioration of congenital heart defects. The saving of many lives, evident from clinical experience, was clearly not reflected in the recorded death rate for reasons that can only be speculated on. It does not appear likely that large numbers of children with congenital heart disease, who would have died in infancy or the preschool period, survived beyond their fifth birthday only to succumb before adolescence. More likely, rapidly developing interest in congenital heart disease, which reversed the previous professional apathy toward the problem, brought to attention many cases of congenital heart disease that would have been misdiagnosed or missed altogether. It is possible that a small part of the sharp drop in the reported death rate from rheumatic heart disease in recent years may be attributed to avoidance of missed diagnoses of congenital heart disease.

Improved techniques for the treatment of hydrocephalus and certain other central nervous system malformations would not be expected to produce a higher reported death rate, since major central nervous malformations are not easily overlooked or misdiagnosed. Studies of the vital records in upstate New York strongly suggest a major decline in the incidence of congenital hydrocephalus and other serious central nervous system malformations between 1945 and 1959 (4).

Marked differences between white and nonwhite children are evident in the trends in the death rates from congenital malformations. The death rate among nonwhite preschool children, starting from a much lower level in 1939–41 (39 percent lower than among

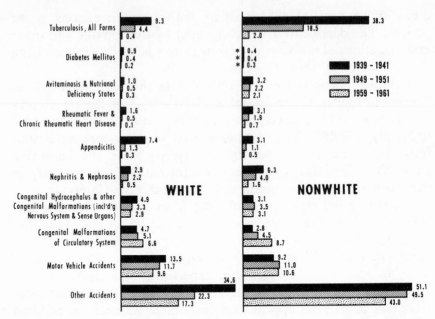

Fig. 9.17. Average annual death rates at ages 1–4 years for selected causes by color: United States, 1939–41, 1949–51, and 1959–61.

Source: National Center for Health Statistics, special tabulations and *Vital Statistics of the United States*, annual volumes.

Notes: Rates per 100,000 population. Alaska and Hawaii included for 1959–61.

*Rates based on fewer than 20 deaths.

white children), rose much more rapidly and in 1959–61 exceeded the white rate by 18 percent. The changed relation was the result mainly of the more than threefold increase in the reported death rate from congenital heart disease in the nonwhite preschool group (Fig. 9.17). The situation among the white and nonwhite children of school age was much the same as in the preschool group (Fig. 9.18). Only minor differences between the sexes were evident in the death rates or trends in the rates for congenital malformation.

Rheumatic Fever and Rheumatic Heart Disease
The long-term decline in the death rate from rheumatic fever and rheumatic heart disease in childhood has been well documented. Prior to the advent of the sulfonamides and antibiotics there were no specific factors to account for this decline. The close, but only incompletely defined, relation between rheumatic fever and hemolytic streptococcal infections suggests that the same factors respon-

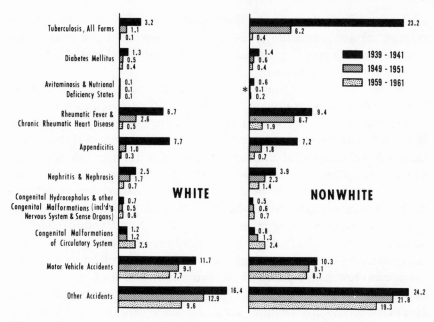

Fig. 9.18. Average annual death rates at ages 5–14 years for selected causes by color: United States, 1939–41, 1949–51, and 1959–61.

Source: National Center for Health Statistics, special tabulations and *Vital Statistics of the United States,* annual volumes.

Notes: Rates per 100,000 population. Alaska and Hawaii included for 1959–61.

*Rates based on fewer than 20 deaths.

sible for decreased mortality from streptococcal infections were also operative in relation to rheumatic fever. Possible factors have been a decrease in virulence of streptococcal infections and improved standards of living of the population, the latter being associated with better nutrition of children and less overcrowding in housing.

The drop in the mortality rate from rheumatic fever and rheumatic heart disease has been precipitous since 1940. In the preschool group the rate fell from 1.8 to 0.2 per 100,000 between 1939–41 and 1959–61. In the 5–14-year age group, the age span in which rheumatic fever is characteristically most common in the civilian population, the mortality rate fell from 7.1 to 0.7 per 100,000, a drop of 90 percent. The availability of sulfonamide and antibiotic prophylaxis of hemolytic streptococcal infections in rheumatic children and the prompt treatment of streptococcal infections with antibiotics have probably been responsible for acceleration of the decrease in the death rate. The role of steroid therapy for acute rheumatic fever in reducing the death rate is debatable, and surgery is infrequently employed for rheumatic valvular conditions in childhood.

The death rate from rheumatic fever and rheumatic heart disease is probably somewhat higher than the deaths assigned to this cause would indicate. In the school-age group in 1959–61, for example, the death rate from diseases of the circulatory system (other than deaths from congenital malformations) was 1.4 per 100,000. In other words, there was an equal number of deaths assigned to rheumatic fever or rheumatic heart disease as to other deaths related to the circulatory system (other than those of a congenital nature). There may well be some cases of myocardial and endocardial disease of unspecified nature which were of rheumatic origin. Correct assignment of these cases might at most have resulted in a minor change in the relative position of rheumatic fever and heart disease as a leading cause of death at certain times. The trends would not be altered to any great extent, since the death rates from diseases of the circulatory system not specified as rheumatic have also declined, although not as sharply as those stated to be rheumatic.

Nonwhite children have had consistently far higher death rates from rheumatic fever and rheumatic heart disease than white children, and the differences between the color groups have increased over the years. In the school-age group, for example, the death rate in 1939–41 was 6.7 per 100,000 white children and 9.4 per 100,000 nonwhite children. By 1959–61 the corresponding rates among white and nonwhite children were 0.5 and 1.9 per 100,000. The excess of 40 percent among nonwhite children in 1939–41 had increased to nearly 300 percent 20 years later (Fig. 9.18). These relative changes should not obscure the fact that very substantial progress had been achieved among nonwhite children as well, in view of the drop of 80 percent in their death rate from rheumatic fever and rheumatic heart disease within the space of 20 years. There were no remarkable differences between the sexes in the absolute death rates from rheumatic fever and rheumatic heart disease or in the trends in these rates between 1939–41 and 1959–61.

Nephritis and Nephrosis
The rubric "nephritis and nephrosis" is comprised mainly of two etiologically unrelated conditions in which the mortality rates are

affected by different factors. The first is acute glomerulonephritis, which, like acute rheumatic fever, is precipitated by hemolytic streptococcal infections; its incidence and mortality rates are presumably influenced by the same factors bearing on acute rheumatic fever. The second is the nephrotic syndrome, which has its onset most frequently between the third and fifth birthdays.

The mortality rate from nephritis and nephrosis had dropped sharply since 1940 in both the preschool and school-age groups. From a rate of 3.3 per 100,000 children in the preschool group in 1939–41, a decline of 79 percent to a rate of 0.7 per 100,000 in 1959–61 has been observed, with a greater proportional decline during the second half of this period. Improved therapy may have played some part in reducing mortality from acute glomerulonephritis, but the factors affecting hemolytic streptococcal infections were probably of greater significance. The availability of the sulfonamides and antibiotics in the 1940's made it possible to control the bacterial infections which so frequently complicated the course of the nephrotic syndrome. The subsequent development of steroid therapy further controlled the course of the illness and reduced the case fatality rate.

In the school-age group the decline in the mortality rate between 1939–41 and 1959–61 was slightly less than in the preschool group (70 percent versus 79 percent). The significance of this difference should not be exaggerated, but it may be that some of the preschool children with the nephrotic syndrome survived beyond their fifth birthday, only to succumb subsequently.

Deaths from nephritis and nephrosis have comprised about four-fifths of the total deaths during childhood from diseases and conditions of the genito-urinary tract (other than congenital malformations and malignant diseases). The decline in the death rates from all conditions of the genito-urinary tract (other than congenital malformations and malignant diseases) was very similar to that observed for nephritis and nephrosis.

Nonwhite children have shown consistently higher death rates from nephritis and nephrosis than white children, and the difference has increased somewhat since 1940. This has been more evident among the preschool children; in 1939–41 the death rate was somewhat more than twice as high in the nonwhite group (6.3 versus 2.9 per 100,000 among the nonwhite and white children, respectively) whereas it was three times as high in 1959–61 (1.6

versus 0.5 per 100,000). Among preschool children the death rate from nephritis and nephrosis has been nearly one-third higher among males than females. There were no important differences in the death rates by sex in the 5–14-year group.

Diabetes mellitus

The death rate from diabetes mellitus during childhood has dropped sharply in recent years. Among preschool children the rate declined 75 percent (from 0.8 to 0.2 per 100,000) between 1939–41 and 1959–61. Among school-age children a decline of 71 percent (1.4 to 0.4 per 100,000) occurred during the same period. There is no reason to think that the incidence of diabetes mellitus has declined during childhood. If anything, the reverse may have occurred, since more children with the disease are surviving into adult life and bearing children of their own. The reduction in mortality from this condition may therefore be ascribed to better medical care.

In the school-age group the mortality rate from diabetes in girls has been higher than in boys. The decline in mortality rates, however, has been about the same among boys and girls. No substantial difference is to be noted in the death rates from diabetes by color in the school-age group. In the preschool group the rates have been too low to permit any comparisons by sex or color.

Appendicitis

A precipitous decline in the death rate from appendicitis during childhood occurred during the two decades between 1939–41 and 1959–61. In both the preschool and school-age groups the death rate fell to about 5 percent of its previous level in the space of 20 years. The major new factor during this period was the availability of antibiotics for the control of complications of appendicitis. Another factor, probably of lesser impact on the case fatality in this condition, was the greater availability of hospital care, and by implication, earlier surgical treatment of the condition. The role of a higher level of public education regarding appendicitis, which would lead to earlier medical attention and avoidance of cathartics in the presence of abdominal pain, is debatable.

Among nonwhite children the death rate from appendicitis was lower than among white children in 1939–41 and higher in 1959–61, even though there was a marked decrease in the death rate among nonwhite children as well as the white children during this period. This suggests that the diagnosis of appendicitis was not being made in many nonwhite children in the earlier period. The death rate from appendicitis has tended to be slightly higher among boys than among girls in both the preschool and school-age periods.

Nutritional Deficiencies

The group of nutritional deficiencies includes sprue and celiac syndrome (other than cystic fibrosis), as well as the avitaminoses and other forms of malnutrition. Among preschool children the death rate declined from 1.2 to 0.6 per 100,000 between 1939–41 and 1959–61, with the bulk of the decline occurring during the first half of this period. Part of this decline may be attributed to more effective treatment of the celiac syndrome as a result of better understanding of the pathogenesis of the condition. The remainder of the decline was presumably associated in large part with higher educational and living standards and with the availability of sulfonamides and antibiotics for the control of bacterial complications of the malnutrition. The mortality rates from nutritional deficiencies among children of school age were too low by 1939–41 to permit any meaningful discussion of subsequent trends in this age group.

Nonwhite preschool children have had consistently far higher mortality rates for the nutritional deficiencies than white preschool children, and their rate of decline in mortality has been much slower. In 1939–41 the rate among nonwhite children was more than three times as high as among white children (3.2 versus 1.0 per 100,000). By 1959–61 the nonwhite rate, having practically leveled off during the 1950's, was more than twice as high as the white rate 20 years earlier. The death rates from the nutritional deficiency group were about the same in the two sexes between 1939–41 and 1959–61.

Cystic Fibrosis

Cystic fibrosis (fibrocystic disease of the pancreas) deserves specific attention in view of the widespread professional and public interest in this condition. Cystic fibrosis was not widely understood as a clinical entity until the mid-1940's, and death rates for the condition were not available for analysis until 1959–61. Deaths from cystic fibrosis for 1949–51 and 1939–41 were included under the broad rubric "diseases of the digestive system."

The death rate for cystic fibrosis in 1959–61 was 1.0 per 100,000 preschool children and 0.6 per 100,000 children of school age. This constituted just under 1 percent of the total deaths among children 1–4 years of age, and somewhat more than 1 percent of the total deaths among children 5–14 years of age. The death rate of 1.1 per 100,000 white preschool children was nearly four times as high as the rate of 0.3 per 100,000 among nonwhite children of the same age. The death rate from cystic fibrosis was 50 percent higher among preschool girls than among boys of the same age, but the rate was only slightly higher in girls of school age.

Geographic Variations

Geographic Divisions

Geographic variation in the death rate among 1–4-year-old children was fairly marked in the United States in 1959–61. Among the nine major geographic divisions, the difference between the two extremes (New England with a rate of 84.3 per 100,000 and the East South Central area with a rate of 132.0 per 100,000) was 57 percent. The three southern areas and the Mountain area, with rates above 127 per 100,000, all stood out sharply above the New England, Middle Atlantic, North Central, and Pacific areas, which had rates below 98 per 100,000 (Appendix Table III.5).

The racial characteristics of the population of the various areas is only a partial explanation of the difference evident in the preschool mortality rates. The pattern of the death rates for white preschool children alone, by geographic area, was almost the same as for the total preschool group, although the differences were not as extreme. The three southern areas and the Mountain area all had rates of 97 or more per 100,000 preschool white children, whereas the rates for the New England, Middle Atlantic, and North Central areas were all below 90 per 100,000. The death rate for white preschool children in the Pacific area was intermediate between the two groups of areas. The white preschool death rates in the three areas comprising the northeastern and north central section of the country varied from 82.4 to 89.9 per 100,000, in contrast to a range of 97.0 to 109.7 in the southern section. The highest rate for preschool white children (116.9 per 100,000) was recorded in the Mountain states. Although data are not available on this point, this is probably attributable to the relatively high proportion of the socioeconomically disadvantaged Spanish-speaking white population in this area. This may also be the case in the West South Central area, which had the second highest death rate among white preschool children (109.1 per 100,000).

The geographic pattern of the death rates for nonwhite preschool children in 1959–61 is complicated by the inclusion of children of diverse racial backgrounds as "nonwhite." In the northeastern, north central, and southern areas the nonwhite group consists mainly of Negroes. Comparison of these areas reveals more favorable rates for nonwhite preschool children in the New England, Middle Atlantic, and East North Central areas. The rates were below 160 per 100,000, whereas the rates in South Atlantic, East South Central, and West South Central areas were about 200 per 100,000. Nonwhite children in the Mountain area, predominately Indian in their background, have by far the highest mortality rate, 333 per 100,000 preschool age children. Among nonwhite children 1–4 years of age the lowest mortality rate in 1959–61 (126.1 per 100,000) was recorded in the Pacific area, where "nonwhite" consists of several racial groups other than Negro whose mortality experiences heavily influence the rate for the total nonwhite category.

Distinct geographic differences are observable in the decline in the preschool death rate between 1950 and the 1959–61 period (Appendix Table III.5). The death rates for the two color groups combined declined 30 percent or more in the West North Central, West South Central, and Mountain areas but less than 20 percent in the Middle Atlantic and South Atlantic areas. (The rates for the two periods in the Pacific area are not strictly comparable because of the inclusion of Alaska and Hawaii during the 10-year interval.) The greatest declines in the death rates among white preschool children occurred in the West South Central area (36 percent) and East South Central area (32 percent). In the nonwhite group a spectacular decline from the very high levels in 1950 occurred in the Mountain and West North Central areas, presumably among the Indian population. In the Mountain area the rate dropped 57 percent from the level of 782.5 per 100,000 in 1950; in the

West North Central area the 1950 rate of 435.1 per 100,000 dropped 58 percent within the following decade; in the other areas the percentage declines were not as marked.

Geographic differences and trends in the death rates among 5–14-year-old children generally followed the same pattern as among preschool children (Appendix Table III.5). The three southern areas and the Mountain area all had rates above 51 per 100,000 in 1959–61, whereas the other five areas all had rates below 46 per 100,000. The difference in the extremes was smaller, however, with the highest area rates (53.0 per 100,000 in the Mountain and East South Central areas) being 27 percent above the lowest area (New England, with a rate of 41.7 per 100,000).

Metropolitan-Nonmetropolitan Differences
Mortality among preschool and school-age children is higher in nonmetropolitan than in metropolitan areas (Table 9.2). There is

Table 9.2   Average annual childhood mortality rates per 100,000 population by age, color and sex in metropolitan and nonmetropolitan counties: United States, 1959–61.

Color and sex	1-4 years			5-14 years		
	All counties	Metro-politan counties	Nonmet-ropolitan counties	All counties	Metro-politan counties	Nonmet-ropolitan counties
United States	105.9	96.5	122.2	46.3	42.7	52.0
Male	115.4	106.1	131.3	55.6	51.0	62.8
Female	96.0	86.5	112.7	36.7	34.1	40.8
White	92.9	86.1	104.5	43.8	40.6	48.9
Male	101.6	94.7	113.7	52.9	48.6	59.7
Female	83.7	77.2	95.0	34.3	32.3	37.6
Nonwhite	182.6	157.1	227.5	62.5	56.5	71.7
Male	197.8	174.7	238.5	73.5	67.5	82.3
Female	167.4	139.6	216.5	51.6	45.5	60.9

Source: Special tabulations of the Division of Vital Statistics, National Center for Health Statistics, Public Health Service, Washington.

a high degree of consistency in the metropolitan-nonmetropolitan area differentials for these two age groups and the discussion that follows relates to the situation at ages 1–14 years (Appendix Table III.6). For the United States as a whole, the death rate at these ages in 1959–61 was 60.0 per 100,000 in the metropolitan counties and 73.2 in the nonmetropolitan counties, an excess of 22 percent in the latter. Both white and nonwhite children had higher mortality rates in nonmetropolitan areas, although the margin was greater for the nonwhite. Within metropolitan areas nonwhite children had a 66 percent higher mortality rate than white children; the gap between these two color groups was larger in nonmetropolitan areas (83 percent).

Excess mortality is found among male children in metropolitan and nonmetropolitan areas to almost the same relative degree. This holds for all races combined and separately for white children. Among the nonwhite children there is a higher relative risk for boys compared with girls in metropolitan counties than in nonmetropolitan.

In each of the nine geographic divisions of the country the childhood mortality rate (1–14 years) was higher in the nonmetropolitan counties. In the Middle Atlantic and North Central areas the difference was fairly small, ranging from 6 to 10 percent. Elsewhere, the nonmetropolitan areas were at a great disadvantage. The greatest difference in rates is found in the Pacific area, where the nonmetropolitan rate of 72.5 per 100,000 children (although at the midpoint in the range of area rates) is 30 percent higher than the metropolitan rate of 55.7 per 100,000. To a considerable extent these contrasts reflect the markedly different racial compositions of metropolitan and nonmetropolitan areas in various parts of the country. Among white children there is much less variation from one geographic division to another in metropolitan and nonmetropolitan mortality differentials than is found when all races are combined. Among nonwhite children the excess of mortality in nonmetropolitan areas covers a wide range; from almost double in the Pacific area to a negligible amount in the Middle Atlantic area.

Geographic Differences by Cause of Death
Some of the relationships between causes of death and geographic factors in the 1959–61 period deserve brief discussion. Reference will be made to metropolitan and nonmetropolitan counties and four major subdivisions of the country, the Northeast region, the North Central region, the South, and the West (Appendix Table III.7).

The 22 percent excess in the overall childhood (1–14 years) mortality rate in the nonmetropolitan counties over the metropolitan counties in the United States (all races) was related mainly to the higher mortality rates from accidents and infectious diseases in the nonmetropolitan counties. The 52 percent excess in the accident rate in the nonmetropolitan counties accounted for 73 percent of the difference in the rates between the two groups of counties. Of the major types of accidents, the greatest excess in the nonmetropolitan counties was in accidental deaths from fires and explosion of combustible materials (68 percent), followed by motor vehicle accidents (53 percent excess) and drownings (39 percent excess).

Most of the remaining difference in the childhood mortality rates was traceable to the higher rates for infectious diseases in the nonmetropolitan counties. The greatest difference was observed in the death rate from gastroenteritis, which was nearly twice as high (89 percent excess) in the nonmetropolitan counties. The smallest differential was in the rate for influenza and pneumonia (19 percent excess in the nonmetropolitan counties), while the differential in rates for the broad grouping in "infectious and parasitic diseases" was intermediate (44 percent excess). The nonmetropolitan counties also had a higher rate for rheumatic fever and rheumatic heart disease (75 percent excess). In contrast to the death rates from accidents and infectious diseases, the rates for congenital malformations and malignant diseases were somewhat lower in the nonmetropolitan counties.

The differentials in rates by cause of death suggest some of the reasons for the overall higher mortality outside the metropolitan counties. Adverse environmental conditions in the nonmetropolitan counties would tend to be associated with the considerably higher death rates from fires and explosion of combustible materials and from gastroenteritis and, to a lesser extent, other infectious diseases. The relative inadequacy of medical care and other health services in nonmetropolitan areas receives some confirmation from the lower recorded death rates from malignant diseases and congenital malformations in these areas; the most obvious explanation for these differences lies in the less adequate diagnosis of these conditions outside the metropolitan counties.

Except for malignant diseases and congenital malformations, the mortality rate for each major cause of death was higher among white and nonwhite children in nonmetropolitan counties than the rates in the same groups in metropolitan counties. The most striking difference was in the death rate from gastroenteritis, which was two-and-one-half times as high in nonwhite children in nonmetropolitan counties as in metropolitan counties. The corresponding excess among white children was less than two-thirds. The excess in the death rate from accidents, on the other hand, was somewhat greater (53 percent) among white nonmetropolitan versus nonmetropolitan children than among corresponding nonwhite children (44 percent).

Among the four regions of the United States, the Northeast and North Central Regions had childhood mortality rates (57.3 and 59.9 per 100,000 children 1–14 years of age, respectively) below that of the country as a whole (65.0 per 100,000). The rates by major causes of death were very similar in these two regions; the slightly higher overall rate in the North Central region was attributable to greater mortality from accidental causes, mainly from motor vehicle accidents.

The rate for the West (64.2 per 100,000), while moderately higher than in the Northeast and North Central regions, was very slightly below that for the country as a whole. Again, the higher death rate from accidental causes accounted for the difference in the overall childhood mortality rate. The highest regional mortality rate from drownings was in the West.

The mortality rate in the South was not only the highest among the four regions (75.4 per 100,000 children 1–14 years of age), but the pattern of rates by major causes also differed. The death rates from infectious diseases was about 50 percent higher than in the other regions; the greatest relative differences were evident in the rates from gastroenteritis and "infective and parasitic diseases," but a sizable difference also existed in the rates from influenza and pneumonia. The mortality rate from accidental causes was somewhat higher than in the West and about 21 percent higher than in the country as a whole. A large portion of the excess was attributable to deaths from fires and explosion of combustible substances; the death rate from this cause in the South was 79 percent higher than in any other region of the country. The death rate from motor vehicle accidents was also highest in the South, but the excess was not as marked as in the case of fires and explosions. On the other hand, the death rate from malignant diseases was lowest in the South; it is possible that some of the deaths from this cause were recorded under the other major causes of deaths, particularly under the infectious diseases. The rate for deaths from congenital malformations was at about the same level as in the other three regions.

10 / INTERNATIONAL COMPARISONS

By far the widest international differences in age-specific mortality rates are found at the preschool age level. Even the five-to-tenfold margin between countries with high and low infant mortality rates is small by comparison with the gap at ages 1–4 years. In this age group there are nations with rates 20, 30, and 40 times the rate of loss elsewhere. At no time during the twentieth century have mortality rates at ages 1–4 years in any of the low mortality countries been as high as the rates that currently prevail in the high mortality areas. The extent of the margin is staggering, and to accept its reality one has to think in terms of the differential that exist in such indices of standards of living as electrical power per unit population, housing, clothing and food consumption, and differentials in available medical manpower and hospital facilities.

As age increases beyond the fifth birthday, the relative differentials in mortality among countries decrease substantially, but the gap between areas with high and low rates remains exceedingly large. At ages 5–9 years rates are separated by factors of 5 to 9; at ages 10–14 years the high mortality countries have rates three to five times those in the low mortality countries.

Although international differentials are still large, there has been a strong downward trend in childhood mortality in many of the high mortality countries. Also, in an increasing number of countries that once might have been characterized as having moderately high childhood mortality, the rate has fallen below 2 per 1,000 at ages 1–4 and below 1 per 1,000 at ages 5–14. This brings their levels close to those in traditionally low mortality countries, such as the United States, England and Wales, the Scandinavian and other Northern European countries, and Australia and New Zealand.

Of special interest is the comparison of the United States with other low mortality nations in the mortality trend since 1950 and in the causes of death among children 1–14 years of age. The year 1950 has been selected because this preceded the slowing down in the rate of decline in the death rates in the United States. Although the data are not shown, all of the countries included in the analysis had experienced large decreases in childhood mortality over a long period of time prior to the 1950's.

Not all countries with low mortality rates at ages 1–4 and 5–14 years are covered in this discussion. The selection of countries was dictated primarily by their inclusion in the chapter on international comparisons in infant mortality. Three other countries with low childhood mortality rates have been added for illustrative purposes. These are Belgium, Czechoslovakia, and France, which are among the most recent additions to the circle of countries with comparatively low infant mortality rates.

Changes Since 1950

Trends in countries with very low death rates at 1–4 years of age in the early 1960's are first examined for two groupings of countries (Appendix Table III.8). The first group consists of nations in which the level of the mortality rates was lower than or about the same as in the United States in 1950. These include England and Wales, Denmark, Netherlands, Norway, Sweden, and Australia. The other group consists of countries in which the mortality rates in 1950 were somewhat above that in the United States, but moderately low within the context of worldwide variability in mortality. These countries include Belgium, France, Finland, and Switzerland. Although complete data are not available for Canada and Czechoslovakia for the period starting with 1950, it seems likely that they would also fall in the second category.

Most of the countries with the lowest mortality rates among 1–4-year-old children in 1950 experienced a definite slowdown during the 1950's in the rate of decline in these rates. By and large this slowdown occurred somewhat later than in the United States. Countries with moderately low rates in 1950, on the other hand, made greater relative strides in reducing mortality rates in this age group. In France, Finland, and Belgium the rates were cut approximately in half by 1960. In the following 3 years changes were minor. Switzerland, where the rate in 1950 was at the lower end of the range among the moderately low mortality countries, also showed a significant reduction in the mortality rate by 1958 but no additional gains in 1959 and 1960, the most recent years for which data were available.

The mortality situation among school-age children in other countries bears an even closer resemblance to what has been happening in the United States than is found among the 1–4-year-olds (Appendix Table III.8). In most countries the rate of decrease in the mortality rate started to level off sooner in this age group than at the younger ages. In most places the year when this occurred closely approximated the corresponding date in the United States.

Recent Status of Childhood Mortality Rates

Changes in childhood mortality rates during and since the 1950's have reduced the differentials among the countries under discussion. Mortality rates among preschool children were substantially below 90 per 100,000 in Sweden during the early 1960's (Table 10.1

Table 10.1   Average annual childhood mortality rates per 100,000 population by age and sex: Selected countries, 1961-62.

Country	1-4 years			5-14 years			5-9 years	10-14 years
	Total	Male	Female	Total	Male	Female		
Australia[1]	105.2	114.7	95.3	41.5	49.7	32.8	44.1	38.8
Belgium	100.9	112.9	88.5	43.3	50.0	36.3	47.8	38.6
Canada[2]	111.5	126.0	96.4	47.8	59.6	35.5	51.8	43.4
Czechoslovakia	112.7	128.0	96.6	43.2	53.1	32.9	49.7	36.8
Denmark	85.9	91.9	79.6	37.7	48.9	25.9	44.4	31.3
England and Wales	89.2	99.0	78.8	36.0	43.4	28.3	39.4	32.9
Finland	105.7	120.6	90.1	44.9	56.4	32.9	51.2	39.2
France	115.4	124.0	106.5	35.4	42.3	28.2	37.4	33.4
Netherlands	105.3	122.5	87.2	41.6	51.6	31.1	48.2	35.2
New Zealand[3]	127.0	136.2	117.4	44.2	51.7	36.3	44.8	43.6
Norway	96.9	111.2	81.8	40.4	51.5	28.7	47.0	33.9
Sweden	78.3	88.7	67.2	38.4	43.4	33.1	44.0	33.4
Switzerland	---	---	---	47.5	56.7	37.9	54.2	40.9
United States	99.9	107.6	91.9	43.9	52.3	35.1	45.7	42.0

Source: Files of the Statistical Office of the United Nations and annual volumes Vital Statistics of the United States, Public Health Service, Washington.

[1]Excludes full-blooded aborigines.
[2]Rates based on 1961 data.
[3]Includes Maoris. Rates for the 1-4 years age group based on 1961.

and Appendix Table III.8). In England and Wales and Denmark the rate has fluctuated around 90 per 100,000 between 1958 and 1963. The rates in three other countries (the Netherlands, Norway, and Australia) and in the United States were between 90 and 100 per 100,000 in 1963, and three countries (Belgium, Finland, and France) had rates that were moderately above 100 per 100,000 that year.

The major change in the relative position of the United States in infant mortality since the early 1950's is not repeated at the preschool level (1). Sweden, Denmark, and England and Wales, where mortality rates at ages 1–4 years were lower in the early 1960's, also tended to have slightly more favorable rates than the United States in the early 1950's. It is worth noting, however, that the differentials between the rates in these countries and the rate in the United States seem to have increased. Also, several countries that formerly had appreciably higher rates than this country have closed the gap.

There is less variability among the low mortality countries in death rates at ages 5–14 years than in the rates at preschool ages. The range among the rates was from 35 to 49 per 100,000 school-age children in the early 1960's. In four countries the rate was below 40. The United States is found among the other eight in Appendix Table III.8, with rates above 40.[1] At the start of the 1950's both absolute and relative variability were much greater, the rate in the United States falling in the middle of the range. Considering the low level of the rates and the reduction in differentials, any shift in the United States' position among low mortality countries is of little or no consequence.

In every country the minimum age-specific mortality rate occurs in the age group 10–14 years, and males have a higher death rate than females throughout childhood (Table 10.1). The magnitude of the sex differential in mortality varies, but the relative excess among males is generally greater at ages 5–14 than at 1–4 years of age. In several countries, including the United States, the margin at 1–4 years of age is 20 percent or less, whereas at the school ages males generally have rates that are at least 50 percent above the rates among girls. Although excess mortality among males at ages 1–4 years is universal among low mortality countries, higher death rates among females at these ages are common in the high mortality countries. On the other hand, it is unusual for either a high or low mortality area not to have an appreciably greater death rate among males at ages 5–14 years.

Cause of Death

Cause-of-death information is presented in Fig. 10.1 for the United States and five other countries with low childhood mortality rates (Denmark, England and Wales, the Netherlands, Norway, and

[1] Two additional countries are shown in Table 10.1 for 1961–62, Czechoslovakia and New Zealand, both of which had rates very close to that of the United States.

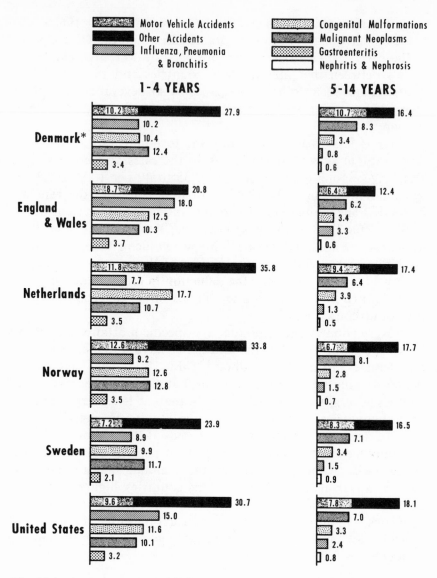

Fig. 10.1. Average annual childhood mortality for the five leading causes of death: Selected countries, 1961–62.

Source: Files of the Statistical Office of the United Nations; National Center for Health Statistics, *Vital Statistics of the United States,* annual volumes.

Notes: Rates per 100,000 population. The cause sequence conforms to sequence in the United States. Deaths coded according to the categories of the Seventh Revision of the International Classification of Diseases, 1955.

*Excluding Faeroe Islands and Greenland.

Sweden). Selection was based on the availability of data for both the 1–4-year and 5–14-year age groups. The very small proportion of deaths attributed to ill-defined and unknown conditions (3 percent or less in each age group) is reassuring about the quality of cause-of-death reporting. However, there may be some sources of incomparability in the certification and classification of causes of death that affect the precision of international comparisons of mortality rates. The latter restriction must be borne in mind in dealing with cause-of-death rates at every age level. This is undoubtedly of less importance at ages 1–14 years than in infancy, with its many ill-defined conditions, and at advanced adult ages, when many persons have multiple chronic conditions.

At ages 1–4 years the dominant cause of death is accidents, not only in the United States but in each of the low mortality countries. Accidents account for 25 to 35 percent of the deaths among preschool children in these countries. Non-motor-vehicle accidents of all types combined are more numerous as causes of death in each country than motor vehicle accidents. However, motor vehicle accidents are responsible for about 10 percent of all deaths at 1–4 years of age. The death rate for this cause varies from 7 per 100,000 to 13 per 100,000 among these countries. There is even greater variation among the countries in their death rates attributed to non-motor-vehicle accidents. The rates in the United States, Norway, and the Netherlands are far above the figure in England and Wales and appreciably higher than in Sweden and Denmark.

The next most common cause of death in the United States and England and Wales at ages 1–4 years is the respiratory diseases (influenza, pneumonia, and bronchitis). These are followed by congenital malformations and malignant neoplasms. The magnitude of the rate for each of these causes of death is similar in the two countries. In both countries, after a long period of decline in the mortality rate for influenza and pneumonia, the rate started to level off early in the 1950's. In several years between 1955 and early 1960's there were sizable increases in the rate (2).

Deaths from specific infective and parasitic diseases have become relatively rare in the United States and in England and Wales. Typhoid fever, dysentery, scarlet fever, diphtheria, whooping cough, and poliomyelitis are almost eliminated as causes of death among the 1–4-year-olds, and tuberculosis and measles are close to this point. Because of the vast reductions in mortality from these diseases, meningococcal infections have become responsible for more deaths at preschool ages in both countries than result from any of the preceding conditions. In the aggregate, infective and parasitic conditions as a group account for about 8 percent of the deaths at ages 1–4 years.

In the other low mortality countries included in Table 10.1 respiratory diseases, congenital malformations, and malignant neoplasms also predominate among the causes of death, after accidents, at ages 1–4 years. Here the similarity to the situation in the United States ends. In half of these countries, the death rate for influenza, pneumonia, and bronchitis combined is lower than the rates for congenital malformations or malignant neoplasms; in a few, malignancies cause more deaths than malformations. Exceedingly low mortality rates for infective and parasitic diseases are found in practically all of these countries.

Accidental deaths dominate the mortality picture in all six countries even more completely at ages 5–14 years than at 1–4 years of age. The most common cause of death after accidents is, uniformly, malignant neoplasms. This is followed by congenital malformations, and influenza, pneumonia, and bronchitis combined.

Comparison of cause-of-death rates for 5–14-year-olds in the United States with those of England and Wales is worth closer attention in view of the lower mortality in the latter. Greater mortality from a broad variety of conditions is found in the United States. The most important category is accidents, for which the rate is about 6 per 100,000 higher in this country. Mortality rates in the United States are also slightly higher for malignancies and for several causes of death with very low frequency, such as rheumatic fever and rheumatic heart disease, and meningitis. There are exceptions to this pattern. In England and Wales mortality from influenza, pneumonia, and bronchitis and from appendicitis, for example, are higher than in the United States. The death rate for respiratory conditions has leveled off at a higher point in both countries than in most of the others with low mortality among school-age children. In particular, the Netherlands and Denmark have death rates from influenza, pneumonia, and bronchitis that are considerably lower than the corresponding rates in the United States and in England and Wales.

Mortality rates in childhood have approached such low levels that they are no longer useful measures, in themselves, of the magnitude of existing public health problems. Nevertheless, the childhood mortality that remains is distressing, since many of the deaths appear to be avoidable through prevention of the conditions leading to death or through adequate care of the child once the condition has occurred. As discussed in Chapter 9, there are situations in which higher mortality rates point to the presence of special problems deserving intensive public health attention. In certain conditions, the deaths are only a small fraction of the total problem, the bulk of which consists of temporary or permanent disability from the same cause which results in death in a minority of the cases. Recognition of this connection has already shifted the emphasis in health services for children, to a considerable extent, from concern with mortality to the development of favorable habit patterns and health practices that will reduce morbidity.

Summary
Some major points in the trends and the recent situation in childhood mortality in the United States may be summarized as follows:

1. The trend in childhood mortality was sharply downward during the first half of the twentieth century, with a somewhat greater relative decrease in the 1–4-year age group than in the 5–14-year age group. The rate of decline in mortality in both preschool (1–4 years) and school-age (5–14 years) groups has decreased markedly since the mid-1950's.

2. The mortality level in the 5–14-year age group has been consistently lower than in the 1–4-year age group. The most favorable mortality of any age group in childhood or adult life is found among 10–14-year-old children.

3. Nonwhite children have had consistently much higher mortality rates than white children. The rates have been about twice as high in the preschool group and about 50 percent higher in the school-age group.

Boys have had consistently higher mortality rates than girls. In recent years the rates have been about 20 percent higher among boys in the 1–4-year age group and about 50 percent higher in the 5–14-year age group.

4. The nature of the leading causes of death during childhood changed markedly between 1940 and 1960. In the preschool group the infectious diseases, as represented by influenza and pneumonia, gastroenteritis, and tuberculosis, fell sharply in rank during the 20-year period. Accidents became the leading cause of death, and congenital malformations and malignant diseases became relatively more prominent. In the school-age group accidents, which were already the outstanding cause of death in 1940, remained in first place in 1960. Malignant diseases and congenital malformations have moved up immediately after accidents as causes of death, and the infectious diseases and rheumatic fever and rheumatic heart disease have decreased in importance.

5. In both the preschool and school-age groups, but more clearly in the former, the pattern of leading causes of death among the non-white children has tended to resemble the pattern among white children at least a decade earlier.

While accidents have been the cause of a greater proportion of deaths among males than among females, the nature of the leading causes of death has been similar in the two sexes.

6. Significant decreases have been recorded in the death rate from accidental causes in childhood, even though accidents have been responsible for an increasing proportion of deaths. Among the nonwhite preschool children the decline in the death rate has been far slower than among white children. The decrease in the rate among school-age children has also been less in the nonwhite group. Motor vehicle accidents have been the major cause of accidental deaths in both the preschool and school-age groups.

The recent slowing in the decline in the death rate from infectious diseases as a whole is attributable mainly to the marked slowing in the decline in the death rate from influenza and pneumonia.

The death rate from malignancies has risen slightly in the pre-school group and moderately in the school-age group. Starting from a much lower level in 1940, the death rate from malignancies among nonwhite children has shown a proportionately greater rise than among white children.

The death rate from congenital malformations during childhood has shown a moderate but fairly steady rise since 1930. This rise is traceable almost entirely to the increase in recorded mortality from congenital malformations of the circulatory system. The increase has been particularly evident among nonwhite children.

The decline in the death rate from rheumatic fever and rheumatic heart disease has been precipitous. Nonwhite children have long had far higher death rates from this cause than white children, and the difference between the two color groups has increased over the years.

The death rates from nephritis and nephrosis, diabetes mellitus, appendicitis, and nutritional deficiencies have all declined significantly during recent years.

7. Geographic differences in mortality during childhood are fairly marked in the United States, the three southern areas and the Mountain area having considerably higher rates than the New England, Middle Atlantic, and North Central areas. Regional differences are observable among both white and nonwhite children, so that the color characteristics of the various areas is only a partial explanation of these geographic differences in childhood mortality rates.

The nonmetropolitan counties as a group have moderately higher childhood mortality rates than metropolitan counties. The higher rates are concentrated in mortality from accidents and from infectious diseases, particularly gastroenteritis.

8. Comparisons between the United States and other low mortality countries in the mortality rates among preschool and school-age children show important similarities. A slowdown in the rate of decline starting in the 1950's has been a common experience; excess mortality among males is universal; accidents are the leading cause of death; and infective and parasitic diseases are uncommon causes of death. There is still a significant margin among these countries in their mortality rates at ages 1–4 years, with the rate in the United States being about in the middle. A notable difference in cause-of-death rates is found in the respiratory diseases. The United States has a higher rate for this category than the other low mortality countries, except for England and Wales.

Perspectives for Childhood Mortality

The mortality rates during childhood have fallen to such low levels in the United States that further substantial progress in reducing the absolute number of deaths occurring at 1–14 years of age appears very difficult. This seems to be reinforced by the slowdown in the rate of decline in the mortality rates among preschool age and school-age children. Nevertheless, a review of the causes of death suggests that the potential for significant reduction in mortality exists.

Accidents

Any further reduction in the mortality rate in childhood will depend to a large extent on the future trend in deaths from accidental causes, since these were responsible for 30 percent of deaths in the 1–4-year age group and 40 percent of the deaths in the 5–14-year age group in 1960. In the 5–14-year age group, progress must be made primarily against motor vehicle accidents, the principal cause of death; programs to control motor vehicle accident fatalities could also have a major impact in the preschool group. Major mortality reductions are achievable despite the anticipated continued increase in motor vehicle usage. Public concern for automotive safety and the effective organization of emergency medical services suggests that needed measures will be instituted that could affect the accident rate significantly, and more particularly, reduce the extent of injury and the number of deaths occurring as the result of motor vehicle accidents. Environmental measures, such as the development of neighborhood parks and playgrounds, would reduce the likelihood of injuries and deaths of preschool children as pedestrians.

Fires and explosion of combustible materials, which are the cause of two-thirds as many deaths as motor vehicle accidents in the preschool period, should be amenable to effective preventive measures. The marked excess of deaths from this cause among nonwhite preschool children (more than five times that of white children) suggests that correction of adverse environmental factors, such as use of dangerous methods of space-heating in non-fire-resistant housing, would have much the same effect on deaths from fires and explosions in the nonwhite group as the provision of safe milk supplies had upon infant mortality in general in earlier years. Reduction in the death rate from fires and explosions among nonwhite preschool children to the rate among white children would have decreased the total accident mortality rate among preschool children in the country as a whole by more than 8 percent in 1960. Among 5–14-year-old children the death rate from fires and explosions is much lower than among 1–4-year-old children, but the same differentials between white and nonwhite children exist.

The possibility of a major reduction in the death rate from drowning, also a leading accidental cause of death, is open to question. More leisure time, the greater availability of swimming pools, and the rapid expansion of water sports and other recreational activities involving water will greatly increase exposure to the hazard of drowning. This hazard may be offset by stricter environmental controls and by educational programs directed at recreational safety.

Reduction in other accidental causes of death can have only a minor effect on the mortality rate during childhood. Accidental poisonings caused only about 8 percent of the accidental deaths among preschool children in 1959–61 but they are particularly tragic in that they are so clearly preventable. A national educational effort to prevent accidental poisoning among preschool children has been under way since the middle 1950's. This effort may not have had maximum impact in preventing deaths from accidental poisonings because it has not placed special emphasis on the problem in the nonwhite child population, where deaths from accidental poisonings are nearly four times as frequent as among white children of the same age.

Infectious Diseases
Significant gains can still be made in the reduction of mortality among the 1–4-year age group by preventing deaths from certain of the infectious diseases. Deaths from the so-called communicable diseases of childhood and from poliomyelitis have been almost eliminated, and the residual deaths from measles are preventable through universal use of measles vaccine. The death rate from tuberculosis among preschool children has reached an extremely low level, but the remaining problem is concentrated in the nonwhite group, among whom the death rate is about five times that of white children. The death rate from gastroenteritis, which had declined to about 10 percent of its previous level in the 20 years preceding 1960, may be expected to decline further by concentration on the pockets in which the incidence of the condition remains relatively high.

Influenza and pneumonia constitutes the greater part of the remaining problem of infectious disease among 1–4-year-old children. In 1960 this group of causes was considered to be responsible for nearly 60 percent of deaths from infectious diseases in preschool children and for 14 percent of all deaths in this age group. The death rate from influenza and pneumonia has declined more slowly than for the other infectious conditions. Since many of the conditions falling under the heading of influenza and pneumonia are viral in origin and not amenable to specific therapy, it is likely that any further decline in the death rate from these causes will continue to be relatively slow unless breakthroughs in their therapy are achieved.

In the age group 5–14 years infectious diseases cause only about 10 percent of all deaths, of which about half are ascribed to influenza and pneumonia. Even if major gains were made in preventing deaths from infectious diseases in the school-age group, only a small decrease in the overall mortality would result.

Malignant Diseases
In the preschool period the death rate from malignant diseases has shown only minor fluctuations, suggesting that improved survivorship from advances in the diagnosis and treatment of some malignancies may have been counterbalanced by increased reporting of malignancies as a result of better medical care. Since leukemia is responsible for half of the deaths from malignancies in the 1–4-year age group, a major breakthrough in its prevention or treatment will probably be needed to achieve more than a minor decrease in mortality from malignant diseases as a whole in this age group.

Among children 5–14 years of age, the steady rise in the recorded death rate from malignancies suggests that an early decline in the death rate should not be anticipated in the absence of significant scientific advances.

Congenital Malformations
The moderate increase in the overall mortality rate from congenital malformations has been traced largely to the increase in deaths from congenital malformations of the circulatory system and ascribed to greater awareness and improved diagnosis of these conditions. This contrasts with the decline in the death rate from congenital malformations of the central nervous system. Only very minor fluctuations in the congenital malformation death rate may be anticipated as a result of outbreaks of rubella and the other few

known extrinsic causes of malformations in man. Improved diagnosis and treatment of certain congenital malformations is undoubtedly saving the lives of affected children. What the resultant of these factors on the future of the death rate from congenital malformations will be is problematical.

Other Causes of Death

All the remaining causes of deaths are responsible for about a quarter of the deaths during childhood, so that only large percentage decreases from these causes would have a noticeable effect on the total death rate at 1–14 years of age. The residual death rates from rheumatic fever and rheumatic heart disease, from nephritis and nephrosis, and from diabetes are very low. The death rate from cystic fibrosis in the preschool period is slightly higher than any of the three mentioned, and at about the same level as these other causes among children 5–14 years of age. Cystic fibrosis is probably being diagnosed earlier and more completely than previously. Improvements in the treatment of children with cystic fibrosis and the greater availability of special services for their care should further improve survivorship among affected children.

Part IV
Health Services and Resources

12 / HEALTH SERVICES

Historical Background

The upsurge in public concern for meeting the health needs of mothers and children through organized community health services, which has been particularly manifest since 1960, has developed on the foundation of expanding services and facilities since the turn of this century. In many instances, these new types of health services and new methods of delivering the services have set the pattern for health services to other age groups in the population.

The Shattuck Report of 1850 called attention to the need for parents and others to whom the care of infants and children is entrusted "to understand and discharge their duties so that a good foundation may be laid for vigorous manhood and old age," but this did not lead to any immediate action (1). It is ironic, however, that the recent intensive efforts to overcome poverty and to provide adequate health services in the slums of our core cities represent a return in emphasis to the first clearly identifiable public health activity in the United States specifically for infants or children. In 1879 the New York City government, in response to a mandate of the state legislature in that year, made an annual appropriation of $10,000 to employ physicians and nurses to save some of the infants dying from diarrheal diseases in the slum tenements (2). This followed 5 years after New York City's vital statistics unit, concerned about the excessive infant mortality in the tenements, first issued extensive statistical tables stressing the deaths of children under 5 years of age (3). Later in the nineteenth century, the free distribution of pasteurized milk for the children of the poor through private philanthropy, mainly in an effort to prevent diarrheal diseases, presaged the subsequent development of well-child clinics (child health conferences) for preventive health supervision of infants and young children under governmental auspices.

Much of the impetus to the development of health services for mothers and children in the United States stemmed from concern about the excessively high infant mortality rates prevailing throughout the country before and around the turn of the twentieth century. Documentation of the magnitude of the problem of infant mortality was provided about 1906, by the publication by the

223

United States Bureau of the Census of mortality statistics for 1900–1904. Disclosure of the staggering number of deaths of infants and young children aroused public concern that led to the organization of the American Association for Study and Prevention of Infant Mortality in 1909, and in that year a special session was held on the problem of infant mortality at the annual meeting of the American Medical Association. In 1917 another group of citizens, concerned about nutritional problems in school children, formed the Child Health Organization. The two organizations merged in 1922 as the American Child Health Association. The new agency conducted a number of basic studies in health problems of maternity, infancy, and childhood prior to its dissolution in 1935.

In the early years of the century concern over the poor health of school children in the large cities revolved mainly around communicable disease problems. Inspection of children for contagious diseases, supplemented in some instances by treatment services provided in the schools, gradually evolved into broader health services encompassing screening tests for visual and hearing acuity, general medical examinations, with follow-up for correction of physical defects, the provision of school lunches, and much later, in services relating to the mental and emotional health of school children.

From these small beginnings child health services expanded to include the establishment of a number of child health units within city and state departments of health prior to the First World War and to the establishment of the Children's Bureau in the federal government in 1912. The establishment of the national birth registration area by federal law in 1915 under the Bureau of the Census enabled the Public Health Service and the Children's Bureau to extend their already noteworthy studies into the causes of infant and child mortality.

The first federal grants-in-aid for any type of health service in peacetime were those for maternal and infant care under the Sheppard-Towner Act for the promotion of the welfare and hygiene of maternity and infancy, passed by Congress in 1921 (4). These grants were made available through the Children's Bureau to state departments of health, mainly for demonstration programs within the states. Before its expiration in 1929 the Sheppard-Towner program was largely responsible for the formation of maternal and child health units in all but one of the states which lacked such units previously.

The Social Security Act, passed in 1935, restored the principle of grants-in-aid to the states. Under Title V of the Act, the initial appropriation of $5,820,000 for maternal and child health services extended the scope of the program beyond maternity and newborn care to cover health services for children up to 21 years of age. Most of the funds were apportioned to the states partly on the basis of the number of live births and partly on a formula based on the financial status of the state and its rurality. The emphasis on rurality stemmed from the relative underdevelopment of health services outside of the metropolitan areas and the difficulties in financing extension of services in the rural areas without federal assistance. Part of the funds were reserved for demonstration programs of particular significance and for service programs and personnel training projects of regional and national importance. The states in which the reserve funds were to be used included these projects in their program plans required by the Children's Bureau and acted as the financial intermediaries for these special funds.

Title V of the Social Security Act also provided grants-in-aid for services for crippled children. A number of states had had programs for the rehabilitation of handicapped children, some of them for more than a decade prior to passage of the Social Security Act. However, the new type of grant-in-aid stimulated the development of crippled children's services of high quality throughout the nation. Part of the crippled children's funds were also reserved for special projects. The states have the option of determining what agency in state government shall administer the crippled children's programs; the administering agencies may be health departments, welfare departments, education departments, state universities, or special commissions.

These services were available initially mainly to children with so-called orthopedic and neuromuscular handicaps. With the passage of time, many of these programs gradually broadened in scope to cover children with heart disease, hearing handicaps, convulsive disorders, and similar partially or completely remediable conditions. More recently, an increasing number of states have included children with long-term diseases such as cystic fibrosis, nephrosis, and diabetes, and the trend is toward coverage of all long-term diseases and conditions regardless of etiology or prognosis.

The federal Emergency Maternity and Infant Care program of 1943–49, administered by the Children's Bureau through state health departments, provided prenatal, delivery, and postnatal care for wives of men in the Armed Forces, and medical care, including health supervision, of their infants under 1 year of age. During the 6 years of its existence the program financed care for 1,454,000 pregnant women and their infants, with an expenditure of $45 million in the 1945 fiscal year alone. Apart from the medical values of the program in meeting the needs of large numbers of families of military personnel, the program was broadly supported as a means of maintaining the morale of members of the Armed Forces in the lower pay grades. The program was a major force in promoting public understanding of, and demand for, a high standard of obstetric and pediatric care.

In 1956 the Dependents' Medical Care Act restored the provision of maternity and infant care for families of members of the uniformed services, this time as part of a broad program of medical care financed directly by the Department of Defense, which included diagnosis and treatment of acute medical and surgical conditions and contagious diseases. The bulk of the program, with certain specified exceptions, covered hospitalization only. However, in recognition of its special character and possibly because of precedents established under the Emergency Maternity and Infant Care program, complete maternity and infant care was covered, including care on an ambulatory basis in the physician's office or in an out-patient clinic.

In 1966 the name of the program was changed to Civilian Health and Medical Program, Uniformed Services, and the benefits were expanded to include broad out-patient services, beyond maternity and infant care, for eligible spouses and children of military personnel on active duty. In 1967, additional in-patient benefits were added for dependents of active servicemen.

Other federal legislative programs after World War II helped develop a broader base for maternal and child health services. The Hill-Burton Act of 1946 provided financial aid for the construction of general hospitals. Amendments in subsequent years extended aid to other types of hospitals and hospital-related facilities. Since the program required each state to develop a state-wide plan, with priority to be given to areas most in need of hospital beds, this had the effect of promoting the availability of hospital beds for maternity care in areas in which delivery in the home was still a common practice, thus accelerating the trend toward hospital deliveries.

Under the Social Security Act of 1935 grants-in-aid had been made available through the Public Health Service to the states for the support of general public health services. In the postwar period new legislation authorized categorical grants-in-aid to the states for services relating to specific types of health problems such as tuberculosis, venereal diseases, and mental health. Subsequently, under the Community Health Services and Facilities Act of 1961 and other legislation, special project grants were provided directly to local governmental and nongovernmental agencies for developmental projects. This was in addition to the usual formula grants to the states. These and similar projects often included the support of facilities and services for children with special health problems.

The National Institute of Mental Health, established in 1946, was the first in a series of institutes devoted to a variety of health problems. The National Institutes of Health were given increasing appropriations over the years for the provision of research grants throughout the country and abroad, and for support of their own intramural research programs. While none of the research programs were specifically related to maternal or child health, many of the disease problems studied affected children as well as adults.

These developments in governmental health services and research programs were paralleled, and often strongly influenced, by burgeoning public interest in specific health problems which led to the organization of voluntary health agencies concerned with these health problems. The two decades following the late 1930's witnessed the formation at an accelerating tempo of organizations concerned with poliomyelitis, heart disease, cancer, cerebral palsy, mental retardation, mental illness, cystic fibrosis, muscular dystrophy, and a host of other diseases and health problems. Since an important motivation in many of the voluntary health agencies has been the intensely personal experience of parents with children affected by a particular disease or condition, much of the public support for these efforts has been based on the appeal of the afflicted or handicapped child.

The resurgence of interest in the broad health problems of the pregnancy cycle and of infancy and childhood since the late 1950's may be attributed to a number of factors having a cumulative impact on national attitudes towards these issues. First in point of time was the growing realization that apparently discrete health problems, such as cerebral palsy, mental retardation, and convulsive disorders, were related to biological and socioeconomic circumstances common to all, and that a piecemeal effort would not be as effective as a coordinated approach to the study and alleviation of these factors. Almost concurrently, there emerged an awareness that the infant mortality rate for the country as a whole was not declining as rapidly as in earlier years, especially in comparison with the continued decline in a number of other countries, and that infant mortality was rising in many of the core cities in which increasing financial strains interfered with the provision of needed services of all kinds (5). Finally, there was action to implement the principle that no elements in American society should be deprived of high quality, comprehensive medical care because of poverty, race, or place of residence.

The establishment of the National Institute of Child Health and Human Development early in 1963, authorized under legislation of the previous year, as one of the National Institutes of Health was a major manifestation of interest in the health problems of the whole individual. The new institute brought together the various research projects of the other institutes which were concerned with reproductive and perinatal biology, growth and development, aging, mental retardation, congenital malformations, developmental pharmacology, and human communication, and it encouraged and supported additional research in these areas.

The initial focus on mental retardation led directly to the broadening of federal support for maternal and child health services generally. The report of the President's Panel on Mental Retardation in 1962, as might have been anticipated, called for expansion and establishment of services for the mentally retarded (6). The report went far beyond this, however, in recognizing the need for a preventive program in the field of mental retardation that would encompass adequate maternity and infant care, particularly in the areas of the core cities in which health problems of all kinds were concentrated. The amendments to the Social Security Act embodied in the Maternal and Child Health and Mental Retardation Planning Amendments of 1963 were an immediate outgrowth of the report.

Prior to the 1963 amendments the annual appropriation for formula grants to the states for maternal and child health services had reached an annual level of $25 million. The 1963 amendments authorized a gradual increase in the annual appropriation for these grants to a level of $50 million by 1970. Of greater significance, however, was the breaking of new ground by these amendments in meeting the urgent needs of deprived segments of the population. The amendments established a new program of grants for maternity and infant care for high-risk groups in low-income families, starting with $5 million in fiscal year 1964 and authorizing increasing amounts to an annual level of $30 million during 1966 through 1968. These grants, covering up to 75 percent of the costs, are made to localities for special projects either through or with the approval of state departments of health.

The 1963 amendments also authorized a new program for the support of program-oriented research aimed at the improvement of maternal and child health and crippled children's services. The research grants, for which an appropriation of $4 million was made for 1966, have covered research projects on such topics as new approaches to the provision of maternal health services, factors affecting the use of community health resources, and evaluation of the effectiveness of programs (7).

In 1964 the federal government launched a broad, multifaceted attack, in cooperation with state and local governments and non-governmental agencies, on the problems of the poor and the impact of these problems on the general welfare. This opened new avenues for the improvement of maternal and child health among the segments of the population in greatest need (8). The Economic Opportunity Act of 1964 provided the legal framework for what is popularly known as the anti-poverty program. The most novel feature of the legislation was the provision of funds directly to local governments and community agencies for community action programs in impoverished neighborhoods. Neighborhood health centers have been developed under this phase of the program. The most successful feature of this approach has been Operation Head Start, through which preschool children from disadvantaged homes are given a pre-kindergarten group experience to prepare them to enter kindergarten or the first grade on closer to an equal footing with other entering school children (9). Built into the Head Start program, with increasing effectiveness as experience has been gained, have been the important health components of health examinations and follow-up for care of adverse health conditions, dental treatment, lunches, and health education through parent participation.

A parallel approach to the problems of major geographic areas which have not fully participated in the economic advances of the country as a whole has been the encouragement of regional development embodied in the Appalachian Regional Development Act of 1965. While devoting major attention to the economic underpinnings for development, such as highways, timber development, and mining area restoration, the program does provide grants for construction of hospitals, diagnostic and treatment centers, and other health facilities. The program may also encompass medical care and health service programs on a demonstration basis.

The Social Security Act Amendments of 1965 has probably been the most significant single measure in recent years affecting health services for mothers and children and health services in general in the United States. Medicare itself, the health insurance and medical care program for the aged (Title XVIII), has lent its name to the entire bill.

Several sections of the 1965 legislation are of direct concern for maternal and child health services. The bill further strengthened the traditional grants-in-aid to states for maternal and child health and crippled children's services by authorizing larger grants for each type of grant to an annual ceiling of $60 million by fiscal year 1970, instead of the $50 million previously authorized. At the same time the states were required to show that they were extending their maternal and child health and crippled children's services to insure statewide coverage by 1975.

A new program of special project grants for comprehensive health services for children and youth was established under the 1965 legislation. Intended to reach into neighborhoods of greatest need, the projects eliminate the artificial barrier between preventive and treatment services, as well as arbitrary limitations to selected diagnostic categories. The projects provide screening, diagnosis, preventive service, treatment, and aftercare, both medical and dental, and the coordination of health care and services with other health, welfare, and education programs for children. The federal grants cover 75 percent of the costs of the projects. From an initial annual appropriation of $15 million, the bill provides increasing authorizations to a level of $50 million by 1970. The project grants may be made directly to schools of medicine and to teaching hospitals affiliated with medical schools, as well as to state and local governmental health agencies and to state crippled children's agencies (10).

Less clearly definable for health services for mothers and children, but with a greater ultimate potential, are the provisions of Title XIX of the Social Security Act. Title XIX provided a massive increase in federal aid for health services for persons who cannot pay for care either fully or in part. Under a time schedule set up in the 1965 Social Security Act Amendments a state must have a comprehensive program of health services for all such persons by 1975 if it is to receive any federal reimbursement for the costs of medical care for welfare recipients or the medically indigent. In the meantime, states may elect to provide health services only to persons in the established welfare categories of Old Age Assistance, Aid to the Disabled, Aid to the Blind, Aid to Dependent Children, and Medical Assistance for the Aged. Reimbursement to the states is increased to a range of 50 to 83 percent, depending on the states' financial condition, and no ceiling is set on either the amount expended per person or the total federal reimbursement to a state. Services for persons under 21 years of age must be of the same scope as for the other age groups, except for the provision of nursing home care. A state must not set any age requirement that would exclude any otherwise eligible person under 21 years of age.

The intent of Title XIX is to promote high quality, family-centered medical and related care for all persons who cannot meet the entire costs of such care from their own resources. The full effects of this broad program on previously established maternal and child health and crippled children's programs cannot be clearly foreseen. Crippled children's programs are most immediately affected, since Title XIX provides open-ended funds for many of the same services covered under the crippled children's programs. The use of Title XIX funds to expand and strengthen available crippled children's services, while maintaining established standards of care, depends on planning by the individual states. The impact on maternity services will be felt increasingly as states move into the provision of comprehensive health services beyond the formal categories of welfare assistance.

Health Services
Soundly conceived programs in maternal and child health are intended to ensure availability of health services for mothers and

children in all segments of the population, when and where they are needed, and to promote timely utilization of these services. Medical care alone, in its narrower sense, may not meet the full needs of the sick or handicapped child. The many hazards to which the fetus, infant, and child may be vulnerable—genetic disorders, environmental deprivation, oxygen deficiencies, hormonal and enzyme imbalances, infections, and metabolic disorders, to mention a few—call for a multidisciplinary approach to the problem of perinatal and child loss.

The application of the scientific and technical advances of recent years has been uneven. In some instances, as in the screening of the newborn infants by phenylketonuria, testing and mass application of a significant new development have proceeded almost simultaneously. In contrast, some of the highly sophisticated techniques for the evaluation of women with suspected metabolic or endocrinologic disorders can be developed initially in only a few medical centers. The application of some of these complex services to broad population groups may be deferred indefinitely. For the most part, however, the gap between the advent of new research developments and their application is probably narrower today than at any time in the past.

Changes in patterns of living in the United States, particularly transportation, have introduced an apparent contradiction in the provision of health services. The improvement in roads and the ease of movement in most rural areas have obviated the need to have a physician in every village and hamlet. This is one factor that has made possible the development of hospital centers and other facilities large enough to provide complicated services for wide geographic areas. At the same time, large segments of the population, even in the large cities, experience difficulties in making effective use of obstetric and pediatric services. This is related to a complex of economic, educational, and cultural factors, even such an obvious factor as lack of care for other children in the absence of the mother. Use of these services is further discouraged when they are provided at inconvenient times or when they are overcrowded or impersonal. It is recognized that coordinated planning is urgently required to combine the advantages of centralized regional facilities with extension of these facilities through outpatient services in outlying rural areas and in neighborhoods with special needs in cities, tied in with health services in the communities.

The level of a community's general health services, the foundation on which specialized maternal and child health services must be built, directly affects the health of mothers and children. Among the services having major impact on maternal and child health are environmental health services, community nursing and nutrition services, and health services for migrant workers.

Environmental Health Services

Over the past several decades provision of safe milk and water supplies has been the major factor in the marked reduction in mortality from diarrheal diseases in infancy. The hazards of unsafe milk and water have been reduced to such a low point in many communities that some pediatricians have advocated the use of unboiled tap water for the home preparation of infant feedings. Pasteurization of milk and control of bovine tuberculosis have made human tuberculosis of the bones and joints a rarity; this contrasts with the situation just after the turn of the century, when entire institutions were devoted to the care of children with this condition. New problems such as those of water supply and sewage disposal in suburban housing developments continue to arise. Fluoridation of water supplies is a widely applied public health procedure for the prevention of dental caries.

The presence of air pollution also has a bearing on the health of children. A recent British study has demonstrated an increased frequency and severity of lower respiratory tract infections with prolonged exposure to polluted air (11).

The potential damage from medical uses of radiation to present and future generations of infants and children has provided the chief impetus to the development of radiation control programs at the national, state, and local levels. Major areas of the country, however, still lack effective radiologic health programs.

Community Nursing Services

While public health nursing has been essentially a family service, many of the earliest activities of public health nurses were concentrated on the health problems of pregnancy and infancy. Over the years the activities of public health nurses in promoting early prenatal care and in instructing mothers in infant care have been an important factor in reducing maternal and infant mortality. The rising demands for bedside nursing care and the need to spread limited public health nursing manpower over a multitude of new health programs have resulted in decreased attention to home visiting for routine prenatal and newborn care. Nevertheless, the public health nurse remains a vital link in reaching high-risk groups of the population early in pregnancy and in ensuring care for women who have had an unfavorable outcome in a previous pregnancy.

Public health nursing responsibilities have traditionally been divided between voluntary visiting nurse services and the official nursing services of health departments. The former, found mainly in metropolitan areas, have concentrated on bedside care, while the health department nurses in these same areas have emphasized preventive and educational services. There has been a slow trend toward consolidation of the two types of services. In earlier years many agencies employed nurses for specialized services in maternal and child health, tuberculosis control, and other limited fields. While more specialized nurses are now employed as consultants, the overwhelming movement has been toward generalized public health nursing at the service level. A noteworthy exception to this trend has been nursing services in the schools, which have tended, if anything, to become even more separated from generalized community public health nursing services.

Nutrition Services
Nutrition services have traditionally been introduced into both governmental and voluntary health agencies through the medium of services to mothers and children. The rapid application of new knowledge of nutrition through child health programs was a major factor in the virtual disappearance of scurvy and rickets within a relatively few years. All professional public health workers who have close contacts with individuals are expected to include nutrition as part of the health service they provide to children and their families (12). Public health nutritionists are currently employed mainly as consultants to other public health personnel and in research settings. When they function directly with individuals, it is mainly with persons presenting unusually difficult problems or as a demonstration in the course of consultation.

Nutrition programs directed solely toward pregnant women may be relatively ineffective because they may not reach the most vulnerable groups. Women who have late or no prenatal care remain outside the scope of the programs. Also, the early age at which many first pregnancies occur suggests that any nutritional inadequacies during adolescence would carry over into pregnancy, and the limited, unbalanced diets and food fads so frequent among adolescent girls at all social levels in this country tend to carry over into adult life.

Services for Families of Migrant Workers
The families of migrant workers suffer from the general disadvantages of being at the lowest rung of the economic ladder and the manifold problems associated with their transient status. The 250,000 or more children under 14 years of age in migrant families (13) have had only rudimentary health and welfare services until recently, and these services suffered from lack of continuity. Special grants of federal funds are making possible the development of health programs aimed at following the families along the several migratory streams. In addition, funds available under the Economic Opportunity Act are being used for day care and similar projects for the children in migrant families.

Specialized Maternal and Child Health Services

Maternal Health Services
General standards for adequate obstetrical care have been developed by the American College of Obstetricians and Gynecologists (14). In assessing the adequacy of clinical features of obstetrical-gynecological care in high-risk cases, it is clear that generative tract dysfunctions, which include pregnancy inefficiency, may be the first clinical manifestation of a serious systemic disorder; and medical care designed to detect problems of this type represent an integral part of maternal and child health care. In some instances, a specific medical, anatomic, or pathologic disorder is readily discernible; but more commonly the causative factor is not obvious immediately and a subclinical defect is found only after extensive laboratory investigation.

The extent to which elaborate biochemical, endocrinologic, and other specialized studies are available throughout the country is not known. Moreover, the professional manpower available to engage in these intensive investigations of vulnerable obstetrical groups has not been specifically determined, nor has there been formulated a standard of medical audit for judging adequacy of care by region and by type of medical facility. Despite these limitations, however, some generally accepted academic guidelines have been offered on desirable clinical practices in the United States as a background for an overview of maternal health services in the country (14).

With the exception of the federal Emergency Maternity and Infant Care program of World War II, community maternal health programs have focused on the promotion of regular prenatal and postpartum care through health education and prenatal clinic services. Classes for expectant parents have been a valuable method of teaching the hygiene of pregnancy and in fostering sound parent-child relationships. When untrained midwives provided much of the obstetrical care, health department programs licensed the midwives and provided limited training and ongoing supervision through specialized maternity nurses or nurse-midwives. Medically manned clinics have also been provided mainly in the rural South for midwives' patients with suspected complications of pregnancy.

Only a few state and local programs have covered hospital care for women presenting complications of pregnancy. A survey in 1958 disclosed that only seven states included any provision for such care in their maternal and child health plans; three of these were on a statewide basis (15).

Programs in many states and large cities have developed standards and regulations for hospital maternity and newborn services. Consultation services and personnel training programs have been provided in association with these programs to assist the hospitals in meeting established standards. While originally motivated by the desire to control puerperal infections and epidemic diarrhea of the newborn infant, these supervisory services have been broadened to cover the total management of the hospital maternity and newborn units. Prepackaged infant formulas, a recent innovation, have greatly reduced the need for extensive formula room facilities in hospitals.

Studies on maternal mortality in the late 1920's and 1930's by the Children's Bureau and the New York Academy of Medicine, which disclosed that about two-thirds of maternal deaths were preventable, provoked widespread interest on the part of the medical profession. Maternal mortality committees in local medical groups and hospitals conducted ongoing reviews of maternal and, more recently, perinatal deaths. A number of states have conducted statewide maternal and perinatal mortality studies. These have become a regular practice in many parts of the country. As pointed out in the chapter on maternal mortality, other developments favorably affecting maternal care followed steadily: the availability of chemotherapeutic agents and antibiotics for the control of puerperal sepsis, the development of obstetrics as a medical specialty, the increased ease in use of blood and blood derivatives through the availability of hospital and community blood banks.

By the 1950's the majority of women delivered by private physicians were having regular prenatal care from the first trimester of pregnancy. This highly personalized type of care was probably a major factor in the decline of toxemias of pregnancy. There remained a major residue of unfavorable outcomes of pregnancy—in particular, mental retardation, cerebral palsy, and convulsive disorders—which called for intensive investigation of the responsible biological and environmental factors and for maternal health services reaching the disadvantaged segments of the population and for other high-risk groups of pregnant women.

The federal maternity and infant care grant program initiated under the Social Security Act Amendments of 1963 provided the mechanism for concentrating funds for special projects in areas of greatest need. By December 1966, 53 projects had been approved throughout the country, with more than $25 million allocated for the grants (16). Most were located in slum areas of the core cities, but some were operating in economically depressed rural areas. Basic hospital facilities and services were improved and hospital care financed under the projects, particularly for women with complicated pregnancies. Medical, nursing, social work, and nutrition staffs were expanded to provide more individual attention to mothers and infants. New clinics were organized in depressed neighborhoods; these so-called satellite clinics, staffed by personnel from the parent hospital in which delivery was scheduled, helped insure continuity of care throughout the maternity cycle, while relieving the pressures on the hospital's outpatient clinics. Imaginative use has been made of health aides from the depressed neighborhoods themselves, who assist in finding patients in need of services and who encourage them to make use of the services. In these special projects the hospital and clinic services are coordinated with public health nursing and other public health services.

During the second half of 1966, 48,300 patients were admitted to projects under the maternity and infant care program; 37,000 women were delivered; and 22,000 women were admitted for family planning services (15). While important progress has been made, very many areas with acute needs are still to be reached and the program must be viewed as still in an early stage.

Family-Planning Services

Within the space of a few years family-planning services have shifted from the realm of the highly controversial toward their acceptance as an integral and indispensable element in maternal health services. Prior to the 1960's only seven states, all in the south, were providing family-planning services, mainly in rural areas, through local health departments (17). Elsewhere in the country, such family-planning services as were available outside of an undetermined number of hospital outpatient clinics were provided through voluntary agency efforts. By 1963 only 26 counties in seven additional states, plus Puerto Rico, were providing such services. In 1965 there were 119 counties in 21 states and the District of Columbia providing family-planning services, in addition to the local health units in Puerto Rico and in the seven southern states which had provided services prior to the 1960's. Many additional state health departments had developed policy statements and were offering consultation to local health departments on the subject.

Family-planning services were included in many Maternity and Infant Care and Economic Opportunity Act projects, in programs aided by the Welfare Administration's Bureau of Family Services, and in direct services under various programs of the Public Health Service. All these services offer a choice of birth control methods in accordance with the wishes and conscience of the recipients. Family-planning services are frequently offered as part of preconceptional care to women who had difficulties in previous pregnancies.

Preconceptional Care

Increasing emphasis is being placed on having the high-risk patient, whose poor past reproductive performance may be related to underlying pathological conditions, undergo a preconceptional evaluation of the progestational development of her endometrium, as well as a general screening for primary defects which might interfere with proper ovarian function. It is clear that specific therapeutic measures are best employed prior to conception, since nutritional support of the developing embryo and placenta in the very beginnings of pregnancy is of critical importance. These measures are closely related to follow-up treatment and careful evaluations during the early gestational period, since adjustments in therapy may be necessary. For example, the insulin requirements of a diabetic patient may change dramatically. Also, biochemical, cytological and hormonal evaluation is now available for assessing the viable status of the conception.

For women who have suffered unfortunate outcomes in previous pregnancies, organized preconceptional clinics are available in a few medical centers. These services are also usually provided on a selective, consultative basis for the more difficult clinical problems; many conditions can be managed in the office of the physician or in conventional outpatient clinics. The full range of needed laboratory procedures is probably to be found almost exclusively in medical centers having a research interest in these problems.

In many centers throughout the country, specially organized facilities are available for the study of problems of infertility regardless of the specific cause. Usually multidisciplinary in character, these clinics utilize the services of a variety of health personnel and conduct sophisticated laboratory studies. Their staff may serve in a consultative capacity to the primary physician.

Care of the Newborn Infant
The dividing line between obstetrical and pediatric responsibilities for the fetus and the newborn, insofar as it can be defined at all, is artificial. In the selected examples of obstetrical practices in the discussion in Chapter 4, the potential impact on the fetus and child of events occuring during pregnancy was emphasized. This concept is cogently expressed in the description of the obstetrician as the pediatrician of the unborn. The need for the physician who is responsible for the care of the newborn infant to have an intimate knowledge of the circumstances surrounding fetal development and delivery is exemplified in the growing, but still unusual, practice of having the pediatrician in consultation during pregnancy or delivery in the presence of maternal or fetal complications, particularly when special care of the infant is desirable immediately after birth.

When this is not done, effective communication is needed between the obstetrician and pediatrician to supplement the oftentimes scanty information about the infant's background; it has been pointed out that medical intelligence in this area is often notoriously lacking. To facilitate the flow of this vital information, a short form has been devised to incorporate pertinent events of pregnancy, labor, and delivery for attachment to the infant's record (18).

The standards and recommendations for the care of newborn infants developed by the American Academy of Pediatrics in cooperation with other leading professional groups are widely accepted as authoritative in this field (19). The Academy emphasizes the need for a recovery area for the immediate postnatal care of the newborn, and for adequate nursery, observation, and isolation units. It stresses measures to minimize the possibility of cross infection, particularly to and among infants of low birth weight. Adequate laboratory services are urged, to provide round-the-clock coverage for the Coomb's test and cross-matching and for essential biochemical determinations. The desirability of further research in the area of newborn care is evident from the statement in the publication that acceptable experimental evidence bearing on many of the recommendations is not available.

Approaches to Selected Medical Problems

Genetic and Chromosomal Disorders
Research in delineating genetically determined metabolic disorders is expanding at a rapid rate. Screening in the newborn period for certain of these disorders is becoming a routine procedure. The prototype among the conditions susceptible to early detection and control is phenylketonuria (PKU), in which prolonged elevation in the blood level of phenylalanine, an essential amino acid, is associated with severe mental retardation. A widely employed screening test for this condition, which occurs in one in every 15–20,000 births, has made early diagnosis possible, followed by the prompt institution of a special diet to maintain a normal blood level of phenylalanine as a preventive measure against mental retardation (20). Screening tests are being developed for other metabolic disorders, such as galactosemia and maple syrup urine disease, which lead to death or mental retardation in the absence of adequate treatment.

In the short time since the normal number of human chromo-

somes was firmly established in 1946, many chromosomal anomalies have been identified. For example, Down's syndrome
(mongolism) and other forms of mental retardation and related
disorders have been found to be the result of an extra chromosome
or a structural abnormality of a chromosome. Chromosome
studies are of value in properly selected cases for diagnostic
purposes and as a basis for genetic counseling (21).

Genetic counseling services, staffed by medical geneticists supported by cytogenetic and biochemical laboratories, are being
financed through federal maternal and child health and other types
of grant funds in various parts of the country. Genetic counseling is
also being recognized in some areas as an operating function of
local health departments (22).

Low Birth Weight

Certain techniques, beyond those employed in the regular newborn
nursery, are applied to infants of very low birth weight. Among
these are control of temperature, humidity, nutrition, and water
balance, and the careful use of oxygen and drugs, all of which
require adequate facilities and constant supervision by specially
trained personnel (19). The precise environmental requirements for
such infants, however, still remain controversial in spite of expanding research.

Since the start of the first organized community program for the
care of premature infants in Chicago in 1934, most of the states
have provided some special measures, mostly for the very low birth-
weight infants, under their maternal and child health programs (23).
Major emphasis has been placed on the promotion and support of
special hospital nurseries or "centers" for low birth-weight infants,
to many of which infants are transported from hospitals not
prepared to provide the specially trained medical and nursing
personnel and the special facilities needed by these infants. Pay-
ment is made under the programs for transportation of the infant
under the immediate supervision of a specially trained nurse and
for care in the center. The centers often served as the focus for
training programs for professional personnel. Apart from some
city-wide programs, most of these programs have remained essentially demonstrations.

Hemolytic Disease of the Newborn.

Prenatal aspects of this condition have been discussed in relation to
obstetrical practices. Appropriate preparation is necessary prior to

delivery for care of the infant, including exchange transfusion of the affected infant soon after birth, with repetition of the procedure as needed to minimize the risks of brain damage from kernicterus, particularly in low birth-weight infants. This may require early transfer to a well-equipped hospital when the delivery takes place in a hospital not prepared to cope adequately with this problem (19).

Maternal Diabetes

Infants of diabetic mothers require special care even when their birth weight is not excessively low or excessively high (19). Indeed, such infants, when of normal birth weight, may actually be premature. Special facilities previously restricted to the care of low birth-weight infants are being used increasingly for all types of high-risk infants.

Unusual Occurrences

The thalidomide tragedy projected dramatically the need for the prompt detection of unusual events affecting infants. A system of surveillance of the incidence of congenital malformations reported on live birth certificates and other vital records (24) has been considered a first step toward a more inclusive approach to an on-going review of fetal and neonatal deaths by hospital and geographic area.

Child Health Services

While the traditional child health services after the newborn period were initiated as a result of interest in controlling disease problems in the infant, preschool, and school-age groups, the services that developed were largely of a preventive nature. Infant and preschool health supervision, through child health conferences (well-child clinics) and public health nursing services, had as its major objectives the early detection of disease and deviations from normal growth and development; the initiation of steps toward definitive diagnosis and treatment when indicated; immunization against a growing list of communicable diseases as effective immunizing agents have become available; the promotion of sound nutrition; education for the prevention of accidental injuries; and education fostering sound parent-child relationships and the child's healthy emotional development (2). Child health conferences have rarely achieved all these objectives in practice. Attendance at most child health conferences drops off sharply after the child's first birthday. In a great many child health conferences, physical examinations and immunizations have been the major points of emphasis. The pressures on maternal health services in many large cities, which have been discussed previously, have also affected preventive health services in infancy and childhood.

Health services for school-age children, or at least those offered through school health programs, have likewise stressed preventive services. While repetitive physical examinations are still common as the major element in these programs, emphasis has been placed on less frequent, but more adequate, examinations and on education of the child and his parents on sound health practices and on the proper care of adverse health conditions in the school child. Effective communication has been fostered between the school health service and the family physician and other providers of medical care for the child. The more broadly developed programs for school children are concerned with the control of communicable diseases, dietary habits and nutrition, the promotion of child safety, dental health services, and above all, the promotion of mental health. Efforts to broaden the scope and improve the quality of school health services have apparently not been more successful because efforts in the field have been fragmented and because quantity and economy have all too often been arrayed against the pursuit of medical excellence (25). Special clinics and hospital services have been developed in a number of medical centers to meet the particular needs of adolescents.

The artificial separation of preventive services from other aspects of medical care has become particularly evident in the depressed areas of large cities and in rural areas. In the latter, adequate diagnostic and treatment services are not available. In the former, the concentration of all types of health problems has overwhelmed available diagnostic and treatment resources. Even when adequate child health supervision is provided, early treatment of acute illnesses is difficult, and the pressures on available in-patient and out-patient services to provide care for acute illnesses have interfered with the provision of other essential services.

One attempt to relieve this situation has been the development of pediatric health services as an extension of the child health conference in a grossly overcrowded area in New York City (26). The treatment clinic, closely associated with, but physicially separated from, a child health conference, is staffed by a physician and public health nurse. Minor laboratory procedures and X-rays are performed in the clinic, but more definitive diagnostic services require referral to the central hospital area.

The program of special project grants for comprehensive health services for children and youth initiated under the Social Security Act Amendments of 1965 has been a federal response to the special health needs of the large urban and very rural areas. By December 1966, 28 grants had been approved for projects throughout the country (16).

Patterns of Health Care

Diversity, complexity, and change are the outstanding characteristics of the current pattern of health care in this country. The National Commission on Community Health Services has emphasized the importance of a personal physician (27). This relationship, especially in services financed directly by the individual, is undergoing critical change. An important factor has been in the growing trend toward medical specialization. The rapidly expanding fund of medical knowledge enables each specialty to offer services of greater depth within its area of competence. The public is generally eager to take advantage of these services and often directly seeks out a specialist for a particular medical problem.

Most physicians in private practice in this country are solo practitioners (28). While the number of medical groups in the United States increased by 214 percent between 1946 and 1959 (368 to 1,154), the number of physicians in group practice still constituted only 7 percent of the active practicing physicians in the country in 1959. The proportion of physicians in group practice has been higher west of the Mississippi. The trend toward group practice may have accelerated since 1959, but reliable data are not available for the subsequent years.

Group arrangements vary widely in size and in the nature and scope of the personnel in the group. Some consist of a few physicians functioning exclusively on a fee-for-service basis. Others may be a number of associated groups operating under a broad prepaid health service plan. The more highly developed groups employ nurses, social workers, technicians, and other health personnel. The National Commission on Community Health Services has recommended the stimulation and encouragement of group practice as one route towards comprehensive personal health services (27).

The services provided or financed by government proceed simultaneously under federal, state, and local auspices. To describe these as levels of service does not present a true picture of the interrelations involved, since both federal and state programs in many cases cover services to individuals in their home communities without involvement of any local governmental jurisdiction. In other instances federal or state funds, or both, may be made available to local jurisdictions as outright grants or to supplement local funds.

To complicate the picture further, voluntary agencies and private foundations have been prominent in almost every field of health, and each agency and foundation has its own policies. Some limit their activities to health education; others, to the support of research. Still others promote and support special clinical facilities and services or finance individual patient care. Coordination of these services would contribute importantly to continuity of patient care. Furthermore, it has been recommended that coordination go beyond the individual community to encompass service regions for the provision of comprehensive health care (27).

Changes in health services have been occurring on several fronts. It has been clearly brought out that further change should take place in the continued lowering of financial barriers to health care, in removing nonfinancial obstacles to the receipt of medical care, in rationalization of the system of delivery of health services, and in improving environmental conditions affecting health (29).

13 / FACILITIES, PERSONNEL, AND ECONOMICS

Hospital Facilities

Since the launching of the Hill-Burton program in 1946 the expansion of hospital facilities has proceeded at a rapid pace, the rate of increase in general hospital beds exceeding the rate of growth of the population. Between 1948 and 1962 the number of hospital beds increased from 3.2 to 3.6 per 1,000 population (Table 13.1) (1). This was the result of a net annual increase of about 7,000 beds over the increase in population (2).

The increase in the ratio of general hospital beds to population has differed regionally. The ratio in the South, starting from the lowest level of any region in 1948, increased by 27 percent to 3.3 beds per 1,000 population in 1962, equal to the ratio in the West in the same year. The number of beds in the Northeast and the West barely kept pace with the increase in population, while the North Central region increased by 18 percent in the ratio of beds to population.

The quality of hospital facilities has also improved. Whereas only 59.4 percent of the general hospital beds were considered acceptable under Hill-Burton planning in 1948, fully 80.3 percent fell into the acceptable category in 1962. However, even today there are areas without acceptable general hospital beds (2).

Emphasis in the Hill-Burton program with regard to general hospital beds has been on the needs of the smaller communities and the rural areas of the country, which had been more poorly served by hospitals than the cities. The obsolescence of hospital facilities in the major metropolitan areas, coupled with the influx of lower socioeconomic groups into the core cities and the flight of middle- and upper-income groups to the suburbs and beyond, has recently resulted in a shift in emphasis toward the large centers of population.

Information on the absolute number of obstetrical beds is not currently available. The nearest approximation is the information on hospital bassinets which is published annually in the *Journal of the American Hospital Association*. The number of bassinets per 1,000 live births increased slightly from 23.5 to 23.9 between 1948 and 1962 (Table 13.1). Actually the South was the only region to

Table 13.1   Ratio of general hospital beds to total population
and ratio of bassinets to live births: United States
and geographic regions, 1948 and 1962.

Region	General hospital beds per 1,000 population[1]		Bassinets per 1,000 live births[1]	
	1962	1948	1962	1948
Total	3.6	3.2	23.9	23.5
Northeast	4.0	3.8	26.3	29.9
North Central	3.9	3.3	25.3	26.1
South	3.3	2.6	22.3	17.6
West	3.3	3.2	21.1	22.1

Source: Hospitals, Guide Issues, J.A.H.A., (Aug. 1949 and Aug. 1963)

[1] Short-term general and special hospitals exclusive of short-term Federal hospitals and psychiatric hospitals

show an increase during this period. Even with its increase in bassinets the South in 1962 lagged behind all regions other than the West in the ratio of bassinets to live births.

Increases in the ratio of bassinets to live births, small as they are, reflect significant changes in the use made of hospitals for delivery. The proportion of deliveries that occurred in the hospital was 56 percent in 1940 (Table 13.2). It reached 88 percent in 1950, and it has exceeded 97 percent since 1962. This major shift in deliveries from the home to the hospital has been experienced by both white and nonwhite women. At present it is most unusual for a white child to be born outside the hospital (99 percent of the deliveries are in hospitals); in the nonwhite population 89 percent of the deliveries were in the hospital in 1964, as compared with 58 percent in 1950 and only 27 percent in 1940. During the period of most rapid change in the proportion of deliveries in the hospital, there were exceptionally large increases in the number of births. In 1940, 2.4 million children were born; in 1950, 3.5 million, and from 1954 to 1964 the number of births stayed above 4 million. Partially offsetting these two circumstances has been the decrease in duration of hospital stay by maternity patients.

Since 1961 the annual number of births in the United States has fallen steadily, dipping below 4 million in 1965 for the first time in

Table 13.2   Percent distribution of live births, by person in
attendance and color: United States, selected
years 1940-64.

Year and color	Total[1]	Physician in hospital[2]	Not in hospital Physician	Not in hospital Midwife
Total				
1964	100.0	97.5	0.7	1.5
1962	100.0	97.2	0.9	1.8
1960	100.0	96.6	1.2	2.0
1950	100.0	88.0	7.1	4.5
1940	100.0	55.8	35.0	8.7
White				
1964	100.0	99.1	0.4	0.3
1962[3]	100.0	99.0	0.5	0.3
1960	100.0	98.8	0.7	0.4
1950	100.0	92.8	5.9	1.1
1940	100.0	59.9	36.5	3.1
Nonwhite				
1964	100.0	89.0	2.0	8.0
1962[3]	100.0	86.9	2.7	9.9
1960	100.0	85.0	3.5	11.0
1950	100.0	57.9	14.3	26.1
1940	100.0	26.7	24.1	48.0

Source: Annual volumes Vital Statistics of the United States,
National Center for Health Statistics, Public Health Service,
Washington, and special reports.

[1]Includes other and not stated, not shown separately.

[2]It is assumed that all births in hospitals are attended by
physicians.

[3]Figures by color in 1962 exclude data for residents of New Jersey
because that State did not require reporting of the item in that year.

more than 10 years. The decline has been widespread, and in some
areas the decrease, accompanied by out-migration and a shorter
length of hospital stay after delivery, has resulted in low occupancy
of obstetrical beds. Even though there may be a new increase of
sizable proportions in the number of births by the 1970's, the
recent decline in births has reactivated interest in admitting selected
gynecological patients to the obstetrical service and in flexible

partitioning of the hospital corridor to permit contraction or expansion of the obstetrical service.

Many large cities face the more urgent and more serious problem of heavy pressure on obstetrical ward services. Municipal hospitals in a number of large cities have been forced to discharge patients within 24 to 72 hours after delivery because of overcrowding (3). Inadequacy of facilities had long been a characteristic of rural areas, but the growth of the problem in large cities has been a relatively new phenomenon.

Manpower for Health Services

Introduction

With the increasing public demand for health services and the many new health programs for delivering these services to segments of the population inadequately served in the past, the major limiting factor in the provision of health services in the future may well be the availability of enough health manpower of all kinds properly distributed throughout the country. The appointment of a National Advisory Committee on Health Manpower by the President in May 1966 is an indication of the widespread recognition of this situation. Further, the Public Health Service has a major unit devoted to the health manpower problem. A brief examination of the manpower available for health services for mothers and children follows.

Physicians

Obstetrical and pediatric care in the United States is characteristically rendered through arrangements between the individual patient and the practicing physician. Outside the larger cities, in areas where outpatient hospital, prenatal, postnatal, and pediatric care is not available, or where special programs of maternal and child care are nonexistent, indigent and medically indigent patients generally receive their care from individually practicing physicians under the sponsorship of a public welfare or other official agency.

Any assessment of the trends in obstetrical and pediatric care services must first consider the quantity and training of medical manpower available for all types of medical care. The overall ratio of physicians to total population—about 138 per 100,000 population—remained essentially unchanged between 1949 and 1962 (Table 13.3) (4). However, the ratio of physicians in private practice to population has declined from 101 to 90 per 100,000. About half of this decline is accounted for by an increase in the ratio of physicians in full-time practice other than private practice, from 15 to 21 per 100,000 population; the other half is related to an increase in the number of physicians still in graduate training.

Table 13.3 Ratio of physicians to total population and percent distribution, by type of practice: United States, 1949 and 1962.

Type of practice	Ratios per 100,000 population		Percent distribution	
	1962[1]	1949[2]	1962[1]	1949[2]
Total	136.9	138.3	100.0	100.0
Private practice	89.8	100.9	65.6	72.9
Full-time specialists	52.6	36.8	38.4	26.6
Part-time specialists	6.7	15.4	4.9	11.1
General practitioners	30.5	48.7	22.3	35.2
Other full-time practice[3]	20.6	15.2	15.1	11.0
Training programs[3]	20.0	15.7	14.6	11.4
Retired, not in practice	6.5	6.5	4.7	4.7

Source: Adapted from Division of Public Health Methods: Medical specialists, by P. Q. Peterson and M. Y. Pennell. Health Manpower Source Book, Section 14. PHS Pub. No. 263, Public Health Service, Washington, 1962.

Note: Population includes Armed Forces overseas.

[1]Includes 50 States, District of Columbia, and Puerto Rico and outlying areas.

[2]Includes the 48 States and the District of Columbia.

[3]Includes Federal and non-Federal physicians and all interns and residents.

Between 1949 and 1962 the number of privately practicing general practitioners and part-time specialists declined from 64 to 37 per 100,000 population. This decline has been offset only in part by the increase in full-time specialists in private practice from 37 to 53 per 100,000 population during this 13-year span.

The decline in the number of general practitioners and part-time specialists in private practice is reflected in wide variations in the distribution of physicians in metropolitan versus rural areas. In

1962 there were 195 physicians per 100,000 population in the greater metropolitan counties,[1] and 145 physicians per 100,000 in the lesser metropolitan counties (5). This was in marked contrast to 94 physicians per 100,000 in isolated semirural counties and only 53 per 100,000 in isolated rural counties, where limited manpower is spread over wider geographic areas.

Of more direct pertinence to obstetrical and pediatric care are the ratios of general practitioners and of specialists in obstetrics-gynecology and pediatrics to the specific segments of the population served (Table 13.4). Between 1949 and 1962 the number of full-

Table 13.4 Ratio per 100,000 population of general practitioners and full-time specialists in obstetrics-gynecology and in pediatrics to specified population and birth groups: United States, 1949 and 1962.

Population group	1962[1]	1949[2]
General practitioners		
Total population	30.5	48.7
Fetal deaths[3] and live births	1,340.0	1,998.6
Children under 15 years	97.7	179.5
Specialists in obstetrics-gynecology		
Total population	6.2	3.4
Fetal deaths[3] and live births	270.8	139.8
Specialists in pediatrics		
Total population	5.6	2.9
Children under 15 years	17.8	10.7

Source: Adapted from Division of Public Health Methods: Medical Specialists, by P. Q. Peterson and M. Y. Pennell. Health Manpower Source Book, Section 14, PHS Pub. Nc. 263. Public Health Service, Washington, 1962.

Note: Data for specialists include those in private practice, hospital service (other than interns and residents), teaching, administration, research, and preventive medicine; data for general practitioners refer to those in private practice. Population includes Armed Forces overseas.

[1]Includes 50 States, District of Columbia, and Puerto Rico and outlying areas.

[2]Includes the 48 States and the District of Columbia.

[3]Fetal deaths of 20 weeks or more gestation or gestation not stated.

[1] Greater metropolitan counties are those with populations of 1 million or more; lesser metropolitan, between 50,000 and 1 million; isolated semirural, not adjacent to greater or lesser metropolitan counties and having less than 50,000 population but with at least one incorporated place of 2,500 or more persons; isolated rural, same as isolated semirural but not having at least one incorporated place of 2,500 or more persons.

time obstetrician-gynecologists per 100,000 deliveries almost doubled, from 140 to 271. This figure would be more meaningful if the trend in the proportion of obstetrician-gynecologists not in private practice could be determined, but this information is not available. In any event, the increase in the availability of specialist manpower has been more than offset by the decrease in the number of general practitioners per 100,000 deliveries from 1,999 to 1,340, and in the ratio of part-time specialists in obstetrics-gynecology from 137 to 44 (Table 13.5).

Definitive assessment of the actual amount of physicians' time devoted to obstetrical care would require information on the proportion of their time that general practitioners devote to obstetrics, and similarly, the proportion of time that obstetrical-gynecologists devote to the obstetrical aspects of their specialty. In the absence

Table 13.5   Part-time specialists in obstetrics-gynecology and in pediatrics per 100,000 in specified population and birth groups: United States, 1949 and 1962.

Population group	1962^1	1949^2
Part-time specialists in obstetrics-gynecology		
Total population	1.0	3.3
Fetal deaths[3] and live births	44.2	137.0
Part-time specialists in pediatrics		
Total population	0.5	1.2
Children under 15 years	1.5	4.4

Source: Adapted from Division of Public Health Methods: Medical Specialists, by P.Q. Peterson and M.Y. Pennell. Health Manpower Source Book, Section 14, PHS Pub. No. 263, Public Health Service, Washington, 1962.

Note: Data for specialists include those in private practice, hospital service (other than interns and residents), teaching, administration, research, and preventive medicine. Population includes Armed Forces overseas.

[1]Includes 50 States, District of Columbia, and Puerto Rico and outlying areas.

[2]Includes the 48 States and the District of Columbia.

[3]Fetal deaths of 20 weeks or more gestation or gestation not stated.

of specific information, broad assumptions may be made on these points, namely, that general practitioners, in the aggregate, devote about 10 percent of their time to obstetrical care, that full-time obstetrician-gynecologists devote 60 percent of their time to obstetrics, and that part-time obstetrician-gynecologists devote 30 percent of their time to obstetrics. On these assumptions, the ratio of physician time to the number of deliveries decreased from the equivalent of 325 full-time obstetricians per 100,000 deliveries in 1949 to 310 in 1962.

Other factors which cannot be adequately quantified suggest that the decline in available obstetrical manpower may actually have been greater. It is likely that physicians in general practice have reduced the proportion of their time devoted to obstetrical care, particularly in those localities in which the concentration of specialists has increased most rapidly. Part of the impact of this factor is undoubtedly offset by the increase in the proportion of physicians still in training, but the care given by interns and residents must still be supervised by other physicians. Also, the broadening concept of obstetrics and gynecology, especially with respect to endocrinologic problems and to the meticulous and time-consuming diagnostic and therapeutic services required by women with a history of relative infertility or previously complicated deliveries, makes increased inroads on the time of specialists in obstetrics-gynecology at the expense of general obstetrical care.

In the mid-1940's the goal was suggested that "in the United States all maternity patients should have advice and treatment throughout the maternity cycle by or under the immediate supervision of a doctor of medicine recognized as a specialist in obstetrics" (6). Recent estimates throw some light on the extent to which this goal is being achieved (7). Using a generous figure of an annual average of 200 deliveries for all diplomates of the American Board of Obstetrics and Gynecology, whether in private practice, academic medicine, or administration, it has been estimated that 17 percent of the births during the 1950–54 period were attended by diplomates, with an increase to 27 percent of the births in the 1960–64 period, and only a slight further increase thereafter.[2] Unless something unforeseen occurs, this will be accompanied by a contin-

[2]Other data indicate that in 1963 in about 50 percent of the deliveries the attending physician was either a diplomate in obstetrics and gynecology or had reported obstetrics and gynecology as his primary or secondary specialty (8). About a third of the women with eight grades of school education or less were delivered by such specialists; the proportion was 3 out of 5 among women with some college education.

ued decrease in the proportion of general practitioners and part-time specialists providing obstetrical care. This points to the need to make full use of the skills of qualified obstetricians at the highest level of medical care; with the use of other, and perhaps new types of health personnel to assume responsibilities for which they receive special training.

The ratio of full-time pediatric specialists to the population under 15 years of age has increased sharply in recent years (11 per 100,000 in 1949 to 18 per 100,000 in 1962—Table 13.4). This is only a part of the picture of the availability of medical manpower for pediatric care, since the medical care of infants and children is still provided to a major extent by general practitioners. Between 1949 and 1962 the ratio of general practitioners declined from 180 to 98 per 100,000 child population, and the ratio of part-time pediatric specialists dropped from 4.4 to 1.5 per 100,000 (Table 13.5).

It may be estimated that general practitioners devote at least 20 percent of their professional time to the care of children under 15 years of age, and that part-time pediatric specialists devote 40 percent of their time to the care of this age group. If these conservative estimates are accepted, it follows that medical manpower for this age group, consisting of the total time of the pediatric specialists plus the percentage of time devoted to pediatric care by general practitioners and part-time specialists, declined from 48 to 38 physicians per 100,000 infants and children under 15 years of age between 1949 and 1962. The actual decline has probably been even greater, since general practitioners in areas with a high proportion of pediatric specialists tend to devote a smaller fraction of their time to the care of children than do general practitioners elsewhere. Furthermore, pediatrics is moving increasingly in the direction of subspecialization, removing a corresponding proportion of pediatricians from the role of primary physicians to children. The American Academy of Pediatrics, in an official policy statement (9), has recognized the progressive difficulty in delivering high quality, private pediatric care in view of the unparalleled growth in child population, and to an even greater degree, in affording proper health services for the nation's underprivileged children.

One index of the quality of medical care available is the proportion of physicians in a specialty who are diplomates of their respective specialty boards (Table 13.6). Of the full-time specialists in obstetrics-gynecology in clinical practice, about half (49 percent)

Table 13.6   Diplomate status of full-time specialists in
obstetrics-gynecology and in pediatrics, exclusive
of those in training: United States, 1961.

Type of specialist	Percent diplomates		
	Total	Among those in clinical practice	Among those in other full-time practice
Obstetrics-gynecology	48.1	48.8	36.7
Pediatrics	62.7	62.8	62.3

Source: Adapted from Division of Public Health Methods: Medical Specialists, by P. Q. Peterson and M. Y. Pennell. Health Manpower Source Book, Section 14. PHS Pub. No. 263. Public Health Service, Washington, 1962.

are diplomates of the American Board of Obstetrics and Gynecology. Full-time pediatricians as a group have a higher proportion of diplomates (licentiates) of the American Board of Pediatrics. Among those in clinical practice, fully 63 percent fall in this group. With nearly 2,000 physicians in residency programs in obstetrics-gynecology in 1961, and nearly 1,400 in residency programs in pediatrics in the same year, it may be anticipated that the proportion of diplomates in both these specialties will continue to rise.

The distribution of obstetricians and pediatricians is highly variable in different regions of the United States (Table 13.7) (4). The number of specialists in obstetrics-gynecology per 100,000 deliveries ranged from a high of 398 in the Northeast to a low of 234 in the South during 1961. The North Central region had only a slightly higher ratio of specialists in obstetrics-gynecology than the South, with the West in an intermediate position. The Northeast had the highest level of pediatricians, with 26 pediatric specialists per 100,000 children under 15 years. However, the North Central region, with 15 pediatricians per 100,000 child population, had a slightly lower ratio than the South, where the ratio was 16 per 100,000 children under 15.

The supply of physicians for maternal and child health programs does not appear to be keeping pace with the increasing needs in this field. An annual average of about 14 physicians were majoring in maternal and child health in schools of public health during the decade starting with the 1951–52 academic year (10). There were 76

Table 13.7   Ratio per 100,000 population of full-time specialists
in obstetrics-gynecology and in pediatrics to specified
population and birth groups: United States and
geographic regions, 1961.

Population group	United States	North-east	North Central	South	West
Specialists in obstetrics-gynecology					
Total population	6.7	8.7	5.7	5.8	7.3
Fetal deaths[1] and live births	283.9	397.8	238.9	234.2	300.6
Specialists in pediatrics					
Total population	5.8	7.5	4.6	5.2	6.6
Children under 15 years	18.5	26.0	14.6	15.6	20.6

Source: Adapted from Division of Public Health Methods: Medical Specialists,
by P. Q. Peterson and M. Y. Pennell. Health Manpower Source Book, Section 14. PHS Pub.
No. 263. Public Health Service, Washington, 1962.

Note: Data for specialists include non-Federal physicians and interns and residents.
Population is 1961 estimated population exclusive of Armed Forces abroad. Data from
the 1960 census used for the population under 15 years of age.

[1]Fetal deaths of 20 weeks or more gestation or gestation not stated.

majors during the second half of this period and 68 during the first half (11).

In January 1962, 17 percent of the positions of directors of state maternal and child health programs were unfilled (10). Of those filled, 27 percent were certified by the American Board of Preventive Medicine, 9 percent by the Board of Pediatrics, and 5 percent by the Board of Obstetrics and Gynecology.

Nurses

It is generally agreed that there is a continuing shortage in nursing personnel at all levels of training even though the ratio of nursing personnel to total population has increased during the past decade (Table 13.8). The shortage of nurses, as evidenced by a high proportion of vacancies in nursing positions, may in large measure be traced to a decrease in the proportion of women entering the nursing field, an increasing demand for nursing services, and a decline in the work week of nursing personnel toward a national standard of 40 hours. Professional nurses, that is, registered nurses or nurses with a bachelor's degree or higher, have increased from 249 to 298 per 100,000 population, a rise of 20 percent, between 1950 and 1962

Table 13.8   Nursing personnel per 100,000 population, by type of nurse: United States, 1950 and 1962.

Type of nurse	1962	1950
Total	642	487
Professional	298	249
Practical	122	91
Aides, orderlies, and attendants	222	147

Source: Adapted from Division of Public Health Methods: Manpower in the 1960's. Health Manpower Source Book. Section 18. PHS Pub. No. 263. Public Health Service, Washington, 1964.

(11). During this period, the ratio of practical nurses has increased by one-third, from 91 to 122 per 100,000 population; the proportionate increase in nurses' aides, orderlies, and other attendants— 147 to 222 per 100,000 population—has been even greater than that of practical nurses.

Marked regional variations are found in the ratios of professional nurses to population (Table 13.9). The ratio of professional nurses to population was nearly twice as high in the Northeast as

Table 13.9   Professional and practical nurses in practice per 100,000 population: United States and geographic regions, 1960 and 1962.

Region	Professional nurse 1962	Practical nurse 1960
Total	298	114
Northeast	396	115
North Central	290	111
South	209	113
West	321	122

Sources: Division of Public Health Methods: Manpower in the 1960's. Health Manpower Source Book, Section 18. PHS Pub. No. 263 (1964), and Surgeon General's Consultant Group on Nursing: Toward Quality in Nursing, Needs and Goals. PHS Pub. No. 992 (1963); Public Health Service, Washington.

in the South, with the other regions of the country at a level about half way between these two extremes. The distribution of practical nurses, however, was practically the same throughout the country, the variation being within the very narrow limits of a low of 111 per 100,000 population in the North Central states to a high of 122 per 100,000 in the West. There is an even greater variation in the ratio of active registered nurses to population in metropolitan versus nonmetropolitan areas (5). From a high of 340 and 328 nurses per 100,000 population in lesser and greater metropolitan areas, respectively, in 1962, the ratio dropped to 243 and 126 in the isolated semirural and isolated rural areas.

The total number of public health nurses, if nurses employed by boards of education are included, has exceeded the growth of the population. The absolute increase in numbers from 25,800 to 34,700 between 1954 and 1962 represents an increase from about 16 to 19 in the number of nurses employed for such public health work per 100,000 population (11). A major part of the increase resulted from the increased numbers of nurses employed by boards of education (12). As a result the slight increase in the number of public health nurses during this period, other than those employed by boards of education, did not appear to be sufficient to maintain the earlier ratio of public health nurses to population. There are indications that referrals to public health nurses for services in the area of maternal and child health care are decreasing. At the same time, the increasing demands for home bedside nursing care may build up even more rapidly as a result of new medical care programs which place emphasis on health services in the home. These developments suggest the need for more flexible use of qualified public health nurses and for greater use of nurses with lesser educational attainments for less demanding tasks.

Midwives

As previously indicated, the untrained midwife is rapidly disappearing from the American scene. In 1964 midwives were in attendance at only 1.5 percent of live births in the United States, in contrast to 8.7 percent in 1940 and 4.5 percent in 1950 (Table 13.2). In 1964 midwife deliveries constituted 8 percent of the total among nonwhite and 0.3 percent among white persons.

Well-qualified nurse-midwives are employed to only a very limited extent in the actual conduct of deliveries in the United

States (13). A survey in 1963 disclosed that not more than 95 nurse-midwives, and possibly as few as 34, were engaged in direct nurse-midwifery practice in the entire country. Most of the nurse-midwives were functioning in teaching and consultant positions or as nursing supervisors on hospital obstetrical services. The gross overcrowding of large municipal hospital obstetrical services and the depletion of medical manpower in the extreme rural areas have led to the development of a number of demonstration programs using nurse-midwives as members of maternity-care teams. In 1968, there were nine schools providing academic training of nurse-midwives in the United States.

Other Health Personnel

Growing pressures on all types of professional personnel in the health field dictate their use at their highest levels of competence if newly authorized programs are to be staffed adequately. To do this requires a flexible approach to the legally and ethically acceptable functions to be performed by physicians, nurses, therapists, and other types of personnel in the health professions. Functions that require lesser degrees of training are increasingly being delegated to technicians and health aides of many kinds. For some of these, as in the case of X-ray and laboratory technicians, a formal post-high-school course of 2 years is being recognized as a minimal requirement, and the tendency is in the same direction for other types of health personnel.

The American Academy of Pediatrics has pointed out that, if pediatric care is to be adequate in the future, much that is now done by physicians must be accomplished by allied health personnel. It suggests that nurses and a new type of health worker called a "pediatric assistant" can assume many of the traditional responsibilities of physicians (14). The National Commission on Community Health Services has recommended that governmental, private, and voluntary agencies, together with the professional associations, encourage and give financial support to innovations in ways of providing health services that will increase the productivity of highly skilled personnel and improve the range and quality of services (15).

In more recent programs aimed at the health problems of the poor as part of a broad attack on poverty, an effort is being made to use neighborhood workers recruited from the population groups served (16). With a limited degree of highly directed training, these neighborhood workers search out persons with health problems, inform them of available services, and encourage them to make use of the services. They also serve in limited capacities, under close supervision, in the provision of services.

Financing Health Services

Expenditures for Health Purposes
Expenditures for health purposes more than doubled in the 1950 decade alone, rising from $12.9 billion to $26.9 billion between 1950 and 1960 (Table 13.10) (17). This represented an increase

Table 13.10   Private and governmental expenditures for all health purposes: United States, 1950, 1960 and 1964.

Type of expenditure	1964	1960	1950
Total, millions	$36,763	$26,892	$12,867
Total, percent	100.0	100.0	100.0
Private expenditures	74.1	75.5	72.2
Public expenditures	25.9	24.5	27.8
State and local government	13.0	13.1	14.5
Federal government	12.9	11.4	13.3

Source: Reed, L.S., and Hanft, R.S., National Health Expenditures, 1950-64, Social Security Bulletin, January 1966.

from 4.5 to 5.3 percent in the proportion of the gross national product devoted to health and medical care expenditures. Between 1960 and 1964 there was another large increase, and expenditures totaled $36.8 billion, or 5.8 percent of the gross national product.

Mounting expenditures for all types of health purposes from both private and public sources have been a reflection of the higher costs of hospital care and other health services, increased utilization of services, and a rise in public expenditures for facilities and research. A survey of private expenditures for personal health services indicated that the prices of the services had increased 42 percent between 1953 and 1963 and that the use of the services increased 20 percent during the same period (18). Changes in public and private expenditures for health purposes have just about kept pace since 1950. In both cases there has been almost a tripling in expenditures between 1950 and 1964. Nevertheless, slight changes have taken place in the proportion of health expenditures accounted for by each source. The proportion represented by public expenditures went from 28 percent in 1950 to 25 percent in 1960. This was partially reversed during the early 1960's, and the proportion of health expenditures that came from public funds was 26 percent in 1964. The potential effect of the new federal health programs in the mid-1960's on the proportion of public versus private health expenditures is debatable. While the rise in public expenditures may be expected to accelerate, private expenditures may be affected simultaneously as a result of heightened public interest in medical care and increased costs of services.

State and local governments have contributed a slowly declining proportion of the total expenditures for health purposes. The proportion spent by the federal government has fluctuated moderately but by 1964 it was practically equal to that of state and local governments (Table 13.10) (17). The level of health expenditures by the federal government may be expected to surpass that of state and local governments as a result of new and broadened federal health programs.

Changes in the proportions of governmental expenditures for different health purposes have varied markedly (Table 13.11). Expenditures for health research have increased the most sharply; the proportion of governmental expenditures for health research rose from 2.3 to 12.3 percent of the total such expenditures between 1950 and 1964, almost all at the federal level. On the other hand, the proportion of expenditures for construction of health facilities had declined markedly, particularly at the state and local level. Also noteworthy has been the moderate decline in expenditures for general public health activities by state and local governments.

Of the somewhat more than $2 billion spent for health services under identifiable government health service programs in 1964, 56 percent went for public assistance medical care and related purposes (Table 13.12) (17). About one-quarter of the expenditures was devoted to health services under workmen's compensation pro-

Table 13.11 Governmental expenditures for health purposes: 1950, 1960 and 1964.

Type of expenditure	1964	1960	1950
Total, millions	$9,531	$6,579	$3,578
Total, percent	100.0	100.0	100.0
Health services and supplies	80.2	83.3	82.4
Hospital care	51.1	53.7	48.8
Physicians' services	5.3	5.6	4.2
Dentists' services	0.3	0.2	0.4
Medical activities in Federal units other than hospitals	7.4	9.6	15.3
Public health activities	8.4	8.6	11.2
School health services	1.4	1.6	1.0
Other	6.3	3.9	1.6
Research	12.3	8.2	2.3
Construction	7.5	8.6	15.3
Federal			
Total, millions	$4,756	$3,067	$1,706
Total, percent	49.9	46.6	47.7
Health services and supplies	34.4	34.6	39.1
Hospital care	19.6	20.5	20.5
Physicians' services	1.2	1.1	0.4
Dentists' services	0.2	0.1	0.3
Medical activities in Federal units other than hospitals	7.4	9.6	15.3
Public health activities	2.9	1.7	2.4
Other	3.1	1.6	0.1
Research	11.7	7.8	2.2
Construction	3.8	4.3	6.4
State and local			
Total, millions	$4,775	$3,512	$1,872
Total, percent	50.1	53.4	52.3
Health services and supplies	45.8	48.7	43.3
Hospital care	31.5	33.2	28.3
Physicians' services	4.1	4.5	3.8
Dentists' services	0.1	0.1	0.1
Public health activities	5.5	6.9	8.8
School health services	1.4	1.6	1.0
Other	3.2	2.3	1.5
Research	0.5	0.4	0.1
Construction	3.7	4.3	8.9

Source: Reed and Hanft. See Table 13.10.

Table 13.12   Government payments for health services[1] under specified
                government programs, by source of funds: 1964.

Program	Total	Federal	State and local
Total, millions	$2,184.3	$848.7	$1,335.6
Total, percent	100.0	100.0	100.0
Maternal and child health[2]	10.1	7.5	11.8
Public assistance	56.1	75.1	44.0
Workmen's compensation	25.5	1.3	40.9
Medical vocational rehabilitation	1.6	2.6	1.0
Military dependents	3.5	9.1	-
Other	3.1	4.5	2.2

Source: Reed and Hanft. See Table 13.10.

[1]Includes hospital care, physicians' and dentists' services, other
professional services, drugs, eyeglasses and appliances, nursing home
care, and public health services.

[2]Services for crippled children and maternal and child health
services.

grams, almost entirely by state and local governments. Identifiable
expenditures for maternal and child health services comprised
about 10 percent of the total under the specified governmental
health services, with a greater proportion spent at state and local
levels than by the federal government. These are only a fraction of
the total public expenditures for maternal and child health purposes, since they do not include the large but indefinable segments
of other governmental programs devoted to the care of mothers
and children, especially under public assistance and the health care
of military dependents.

Health-care expenditures are being met increasingly through
third-party payments. From slightly over one-third in 1950, third-
party payments (health insurance, government, and philanthropy)
covered nearly half of all health-care expenditures in 1964 (Table
13.13) (17). Payments through health insurance accounted for the
entire increase; the proportion covered under health insurance rose

Table 13.13   Amount and percent of expenditures for personal health care met by third parties: United States, 1950, 1960 and 1964.

Year	Total health care expenditures* (in millions)	Health care expenditures by third parties		Third party payment (percent)		
		Amount (in millions)	Percent	Health insurance	Government	Philanthropy and others
1964	$31,201	$15,318	49.1	25.0	22.0	2.1
1960	23,515	10,445	44.4	21.2	20.9	2.3
1950	11,069	3,860	34.9	9.0	23.0	2.9

Source: Reed and Hanft. See Table 13.10.

*All expenditures for health services and supplies other than (1) net cost of insurance, (2) government public health activities, and (3) expenditures of private voluntary health agencies.

from 9 percent in 1950 to 25 percent in 1964. The proportion covered through governmental programs fluctuated slightly but did not change significantly, while the small proportion covered by philanthropy and other sources shrank even further.

Despite the greater availability of governmental funds for the support of health services, the economic burden of health services remains especially heavy in families with low income (Table 13.14) (18). Families with annual incomes of less than $2,000 spent $228 for health services in 1963 in comparison to an outlay of $480 in families with incomes of $7,500 or more. The former represented 15.7 percent of family income in the poorest families in contrast to 3.8 percent in the higher-income group. These are the extremes in the inverse relation between family income and percentage of family outlay devoted to health services. Similar inverse relations were evident in 1953 and 1958. In interpreting these relations, it should be borne in mind that low-income families are more heavily weighted with units of one or two persons and that there tend to be more elderly and chronically ill persons among them.

Personal expenditures for health services increase progressively with age (Table 13.15) (19). In 1963 the average individual expenditure was $47 for children under 6 years of age and $56 for children 6–17 years of age, in contrast to average expenditures of $124 for persons 18–34 years of age and $185 for those 65 and over. Average expenditures were substantially higher than in 1953 at every age. Among children under 6, expenditures increased by about two-

Table 13.14   Personal health services - mean charges incurred and
               family outlay by family income group: United States, 1953,
               1958 and 1963.

Family income (dollars)	Mean gross charge per family (dollars)			Aggregate family outlay as percent of family income		
	1963	1958	1953	1963	1958	1953
Total	370	294	207	5.0	5.5	4.8
0-1,999	228	165	130	15.7	13.0	11.8
2,000-3,499	245	226	152	8.5	8.4	6.1
3,500-4,999	289	287	207	6.8	6.4	5.4
5,000-7,499	409	336	259	5.6	5.4	4.7
7,500 or more	480	411	353	3.8	3.9	3.0

Source: Anderson, O.W., Collette, P. and Feldman, J.J.: Family
expenditure patterns for personal health service, 1953 and 1958:
nationwide surveys. HIF Research Series, No. 14, New York, Health
Information Foundation, 1960, and personal communication from O. W.
Anderson.

Table 13.15   Average individual expenditures for
               health services by age category:
               United States, 1953, 1958 and 1963.

Age (years)	1963	1958	1953
Under 6	$ 47	$ 48	$ 28
6-17	56	49	38
18-34	124	98	70
35-54	151	108	80
55-64	165	129	96
65 and over	185	177	102

Source: Anderson, O.W., Collette, P., and Feldman, J.J.:
Trends in personal health spending. Progress in Health Services,
Health Information Foundation, University of Chicago, Vol. 14,
No. 5: November-December 1965.

thirds. This was not an unusual rise. In fact, at all adult ages, the increase was proportionately at least as large.

Expenditures for Maternity Care

Personal expenditures for maternity care, from which free care has been excluded, rose 64 percent in the decade from 1953 to 1963. Average expenditures per confinement increased from $193 in 1953 to $272 in 1958 and to $316 in 1963 (Table 13.16) (20). The cost of

Table 13.16   Average expenditures per live birth by type of services: United States, 1953, 1958 and 1963.

Type of service	1963		1958		1953	
	Amount	Percent of all services	Amount	Percent of all services	Amount	Percent of all services
All services	$316	100	$272	100	$193	100
Hospital	162	51	128	47	82	42
Physician	133	42	118	43	91	47
Drugs and medicines	16	5	17	6	10	5
Laboratory fees	3	1	2	1	3	1
Other medical care	2	1	6	2	7	4

Source: Andersen, R. and Anderson, O.W., Maternity care and costs: A ten-year trend. Progress in Health Services, Health Information Foundation, University of Chicago, Vol. 15, No. 2:1-6, March-April 1966.

hospital care nearly doubled between 1953 and 1963, and the percentage of the costs of all maternity services devoted to hospital care rose from 42 to 51 percent during the 10-year interval. Expenditures for physician services increased by almost 50 percent during this period, going from $91 per capita in 1953 to $133 in 1963. In 1953 expenditures for doctors averaged more than hospital costs; by 1958 the situation was reversed, and by 1963 hospital costs for maternity cases exceeded physician costs by an appreciable margin. Other types of services accounted for only a minor proportion of the total costs.

The total costs of maternity care rose despite a decreased average length of hospital stay for maternity care. In the Health Information Foundation survey of 1953, the median number of days per hospitalized delivery was 4.7 (20). Succeeding surveys by HIF showed that this dropped to 4.4 days in 1958 and to 3.7 days in 1963.[3] Over this 10-year period, there was a decrease from 28 to 12 percent in the number of women who remained in the hospital for 6 or more days for delivery. Average length of hospital stay was at all times greater at higher income levels, but the differences among income levels became less pronounced as the average length of stay decreased for the middle- and high-income groups.

Personal expenditures for maternity care have increased relatively more in low-income families than in higher-income families (Table 13.17). The average expenditure per live birth in families in the lowest third in income rose from $112 in 1953 to $194 in 1963,

Table 13.17   Average expenditures per live birth by family income group: United States, 1953, 1958 and 1963.

Family income group[1]	1963	1958	1953
Low	$194	$172	$112
Medium	327	283	208
High	393	348	276

Source: See Table 13.16.

[1]In 1953 family incomes were classifed as follows: low, under $3,000 annually; middle, $3,000-$4,999; and high, $5,000 and over. In 1958 the corresponding groups were: under $3,500; $3,500-$5,999; and $6,000 and over. In 1963 the groups were: low, under $3,999; middle, $4,000-$6,999; and high, $7,000 or more. In each survey these class intervals divided the families of the sample as a whole into three approximately equal-sized groups.

[3] It should be noted that national data on hospital discharges in July 1963–June 1964 released by the National Center for Health Statistics show an average duration of hospital stay for deliveries of 4.2 days (21).

an increase of 73 percent. Among the highest third in income, the corresponding figures were $276 and $393, an increase of 42 percent. These dollar figures refer to payments (or unpaid bills) for services and exclude the value of free care. Increasing coverage by health insurance may have shifted some of the medical service for low-income families out of the free-care category and thereby contributed to the sharp increase in personal expenditures by these families for maternity care.

In 1953, 45 percent of all the families with a child born during the year had health insurance benefits for maternity care. This figure increased to 55 percent in 1958 and to 58 percent in 1963 (20). The average benefits for maternity care in the covered families rose from $129 in 1953 to $187 in 1958 and to $236 in 1963, and the proportion of expenditures met by health insurance in covered families rose from 53 to 63 percent from 1953 to 1963. The proportion of all uninsured and insured family expenditures for maternity care covered by health insurance rose from 30 percent of the total of all such expenditures in 1953 to 43 percent of the total in 1963 (22).

Conclusion

This review of specific changes in medical facilities, manpower, and economics covers the period that ends just prior to the start of governmental support for new maternity and infant care programs. From the preceding discussion, it is clear that these programs arrived on the scene following a period of diminishing supply of obstetrical and pediatric manpower. Also, all major components of health expenditures, including costs per maternity case, had increased markedly, with low-income families experiencing the largest relative increase. The recent maternal and infant care legislation injects a new element into the picture. Its impact on patterns of medical care and on infant and perinatal mortality remains to be documented, but there is a strong potential for an important, positive effect.

APPENDIX TABLES

APPENDIX TABLES

Table I.la   **Infant mortality rates per 1,000 live births by age at death:**
United States, 1935-64.

Year	Under 1 Year	Under 1 day	1-6 days	Under 7 days	7-27 days	Under[1] 28 days	28 days[1] - 5 months	6-11 months	28 days[1] - 11 months
TOTAL									
1964[2]	24.8	10.2	5.9	16.1	1.8	17.9	5.1	1.8	6.9
1963[2]	25.2	10.4	6.0	16.4	1.8	18.2	5.2	1.8	7.0
1962[2]	25.3	10.4	6.1	16.5	1.9	18.3	5.2	1.8	7.0
1961[2]	25.3	10.3	6.2	16.5	1.9	18.4	5.2	1.8	6.9
1960[2]	26.0	10.3	6.4	16.7	2.0	18.7	5.4	1.9	7.3
1959[2]	26.4	10.3	6.6	16.9	2.1	19.0	5.4	1.9	7.3
1958	27.1	10.2	6.9	17.1	2.3	19.5	5.6	2.0	7.6
1957	26.3	9.9	6.8	16.7	2.4	19.1	5.3	2.0	7.3
1956	26.0	9.9	6.7	16.6	2.2	18.9	5.1	2.0	7.1
1955	26.4	10.0	7.0	17.0	2.2	19.1	5.2	2.1	7.3
1954	26.6	9.6	7.1	16.8	2.3	19.1	5.3	2.2	7.5
1953	27.8	9.7	7.5	17.1	2.4	19.6	5.8	2.4	8.2
1952	28.4	9.7	7.5	17.3	2.6	19.8	6.0	2.6	8.6
1951	28.4	9.8	7.7	17.5	2.6	20.0	5.9	2.5	8.4
1950	29.2	10.2	7.7	17.8	2.7	20.5	6.0	2.7	8.7
1949	31.3	10.5	7.8	18.3	3.1	21.4	7.0	2.9	9.9
1948	32.0	10.7	8.2	18.9	3.3	22.2	6.9	3.0	9.8
1947	32.2	10.7	8.5	19.3	3.5	22.8	6.7	2.7	9.4
1946	33.8	11.4	8.6	20.0	4.0	24.0	6.8	2.9	9.7
1945	38.3	11.2	8.5	19.7	4.6	24.3	9.6	4.4	13.9
1944	39.8	11.5	8.5	19.9	4.7	24.7	10.1	4.9	15.1
1943	40.4	11.6	8.4	20.0	4.8	24.7	10.5	5.2	15.6
1942	40.4	12.3	8.5	20.9	4.8	25.7	9.9	4.8	14.7
1941	45.3	13.2	9.0	22.2	5.4	27.7	11.8	5.9	17.7
1940	47.0	13.9	9.4	23.3	5.5	28.8	12.2	6.0	18.3
1939	48.0	14.1	9.6	23.8	5.5	29.3	12.2	6.6	18.7
1938	51.0	14.1	9.6	23.7	5.9	29.6	13.8	7.7	21.4
1937	54.4	14.7	10.0	24.7	6.5	31.3	15.0	8.2	23.2
1936	57.1	15.1	10.7	25.7	6.8	32.6	15.8	8.7	24.6
1935	55.7	15.0	10.5	25.5	6.9	32.4	15.0	8.3	23.3

Source: Annual volumes <u>Vital Statistics of the United States</u>, National Center for Health Statistics, Public Health Service, Washington, and special tabulations.

[1]From 1935 to 1948 these categories refer to deaths at ages "under 1 month," "1 to 5 months" and "1 to 11 months" respectively.

[2]Includes Alaska and Hawaii.

Table I.1b   Infant mortality rates per 1,000 live births by age at death and sex:
United States, 1935-64 - continued.

Year	Under 1 Year	Under 1 day	1-6 days	Under 7 days	7-27 days	Under[1] 28 days	28 days[1] - 5 months	6-11 months	28 days[1] - 11 months
MALE									
1964[2]	27.8	11.5	6.8	18.3	1.9	20.3	5.7	1.9	7.6
1963[2]	28.4	11.7	7.0	18.7	2.0	20.7	5.8	1.9	7.7
1962[2]	28.6	11.7	7.1	18.8	2.0	20.9	5.8	1.9	7.7
1961[2]	28.4	11.5	7.2	18.7	2.1	20.8	5.7	1.9	7.6
1960[2]	29.3	11.6	7.4	19.0	2.2	21.2	6.0	2.1	8.1
1959[2]	29.6	11.6	7.7	19.2	2.3	21.6	6.0	2.0	8.0
1958	30.2	11.4	7.9	19.3	2.6	21.9	6.2	2.1	8.3
1957	29.5	11.1	7.8	19.0	2.6	21.6	5.9	2.1	7.9
1956	29.2	11.3	7.8	19.0	2.5	21.5	5.7	2.1	7.7
1955	29.6	11.2	8.1	19.3	2.4	21.7	5.7	2.2	7.9
1954	29.8	10.8	8.3	19.1	2.6	21.7	5.8	2.3	8.1
1953	31.2	10.9	8.7	19.6	2.7	22.3	6.3	2.6	8.9
1952	31.8	11.0	8.8	19.7	2.8	22.5	6.5	2.8	9.3
1951	32.0	11.1	9.0	20.0	2.8	22.9	6.4	2.7	9.1
1950	32.8	11.5	8.9	20.4	2.9	23.3	6.6	2.8	9.4
1949	35.1	11.9	9.1	21.0	3.5	24.5	7.6	3.0	10.7
1948	35.9	12.1	9.5	21.6	3.6	25.2	7.6	3.1	10.7
1947	36.1	12.1	9.9	22.0	3.9	25.9	7.4	2.9	10.3
1946	37.8	12.9	10.0	22.9	4.3	27.2	7.5	3.0	10.6
1945	42.7	12.6	9.9	22.5	5.1	27.6	10.5	4.6	15.1
1944	44.1	12.8	9.8	22.5	5.2	27.7	11.2	5.2	16.3
1943	45.1	13.1	9.7	22.8	5.2	28.1	11.5	5.5	17.0
1942	44.9	13.9	9.9	23.8	5.3	29.1	10.8	5.1	15.8
1941	50.4	14.9	10.4	25.3	5.9	31.2	12.9	6.3	19.2
1940	52.5	15.7	10.9	26.6	6.0	32.6	13.4	6.5	19.9
1939	53.3	15.8	11.0	26.8	6.1	32.9	13.3	7.1	20.4
1938	56.7	16.0	11.0	27.0	6.4	33.4	15.1	8.2	23.3
1937	60.3	16.5	11.5	27.9	7.1	35.1	16.4	8.8	25.2
1936	63.4	17.1	12.3	29.3	7.4	36.8	17.4	9.3	26.7
1935	62.2	17.0	12.1	29.1	7.6	36.7	16.6	9.0	25.6

Note: See table for TOTAL births for footnotes and source.

Table I.1c   Infant mortality rates per 1,000 live births by age at death and sex: United States, 1935-64 - continued.

Year	Under 1 Year	Under 1 day	1-6 days	Under 7 days	7-27 days	Under[1] 28 days	28 days[1] - 5 months	6-11 months	28 days[1] - 11 months
FEMALE									
1964[2]	21.6	8.9	4.8	13.7	1.7	15.4	4.5	1.7	6.2
1963[2]	21.9	9.0	5.0	14.0	1.6	15.6	4.6	1.7	6.3
1962[2]	21.9	8.9	5.0	14.0	1.7	15.7	4.5	1.7	6.2
1961[2]	22.0	9.0	5.1	14.1	1.7	15.8	4.6	1.6	6.2
1960[2]	22.6	9.0	5.3	14.3	1.8	16.1	4.7	1.8	6.5
1959[2]	23.0	9.0	5.5	14.4	1.9	16.3	4.9	1.8	6.7
1958	23.7	9.0	5.9	14.8	2.0	16.8	5.0	1.9	6.9
1957	23.0	8.7	5.6	14.3	2.1	16.4	4.7	1.9	6.6
1956	22.6	8.5	5.6	14.?	2.0	16.2	4.5	1.9	6.4
1955	23.0	8.8	5.8	14.5	1.9	16.4	4.7	2.0	6.6
1954	23.2	8.4	5.9	14.2	2.1	16.3	4.8	2.1	6.9
1953	24.2	8.3	6.2	14.5	2.2	16.7	5.2	2.3	7.5
1952	24.9	8.4	6.2	14.7	2.3	17.0	5.4	2.5	7.9
1951	24.7	8.4	6.4	14.8	2.3	17.1	5.2	2.4	7.7
1950	25.5	8.8	6.4	15.1	2.4	17.5	5.4	2.6	8.0
1949	27.3	9.0	6.5	15.5	2.8	18.3	6.3	2.7	9.1
1948	27.9	9.1	6.9	16.0	3.0	19.0	6.1	2.8	8.9
1947	28.1	9.3	7.1	16.4	3.2	19.5	6.0	2.6	8.5
1946	29.5	9.9	7.2	17.1	3.6	20.7	6.1	2.8	8.8
1945	33.6	9.7	7.1	16.8	4.1	20.9	8.6	4.1	12.7
1944	35.2	10.1	7.1	17.2	4.3	21.5	9.0	4.7	13.7
1943	35.4	9.9	7.0	16.9	4.3	21.2	9.3	4.8	14.2
1942	35.7	10.6	7.1	17.7	4.3	22.1	9.1	4.5	13.6
1941	40.0	11.4	7.6	19.1	4.9	23.9	10.7	5.4	16.1
1940	41.3	12.1	7.7	19.8	4.9	24.7	11.0	5.5	16.5
1939	42.5	12.4	8.2	20.5	4.9	25.5	10.9	6.1	17.0
1938	45.1	12.2	8.1	20.3	5.4	25.6	12.4	7.1	19.4
1937	48.3	12.8	8.5	21.3	5.9	27.3	13.4	7.5	21.0
1936	50.5	13.0	9.0	22.0	6.2	28.2	14.2	8.1	22.3
1935	48.9	12.8	8.8	21.6	6.3	27.9	13.4	7.6	21.0

Note: See table for TOTAL births for footnotes and source.

Table I.1d   Infant mortality rates per 1,000 live births by age at death and color: United States, 1935-64 - continued.

Year	Under 1 Year	Under 1 day	1-6 days	Under 7 days	7-27 days	Under 28 days[1]	28 days - 5 months[1]	6-11 months	28 days - 11 months[1]
WHITE									
1964[2]	21.6	9.3	5.4	14.7	1.5	16.2	4.0	1.4	5.4
1963[2]	22.2	9.5	5.6	15.2	1.5	16.7	4.1	1.4	5.5
1962[2]	22.3	9.6	5.7	15.3	1.5	16.9	4.0	1.4	5.5
1961[2]	22.4	9.5	5.8	15.4	1.6	16.9	4.1	1.4	5.5
1960[2]	22.9	9.6	6.0	15.6	1.7	17.2	4.2	1.5	5.7
1959[2]	23.2	9.5	6.2	15.7	1.7	17.5	4.2	1.5	5.7
1958	23.8	9.5	6.4	15.9	1.9	17.8	4.4	1.6	6.0
1957	23.3	9.3	6.3	15.6	2.0	17.5	4.2	1.6	5.8
1956	23.2	9.3	6.3	15.6	1.9	17.5	4.1	1.6	5.7
1955	23.6	9.3	6.6	15.9	1.8	17.7	4.2	1.7	5.9
1954	23.9	9.0	6.8	15.8	2.0	17.8	4.3	1.8	6.1
1953	25.0	9.1	7.1	16.2	2.1	18.3	4.7	2.0	6.7
1952	25.5	9.2	7.1	16.3	2.2	18.5	4.8	2.1	7.0
1951	25.8	9.3	7.3	16.6	2.3	18.9	4.8	2.1	6.9
1950	26.8	9.7	7.4	17.1	2.3	19.4	5.1	2.3	7.4
1949	28.9	10.1	7.5	17.6	2.7	20.3	6.0	2.5	8.5
1948	29.9	10.3	7.9	18.2	2.9	21.2	6.1	2.7	8.7
1947	30.1	10.4	8.2	18.5	3.2	21.7	5.9	2.4	8.4
1946	31.8	11.2	8.4	19.5	3.6	23.1	6.1	2.6	8.7
1945	35.6	11.0	8.1	19.1	4.1	23.3	8.5	3.9	12.3
1944	36.9	11.2	8.1	19.3	4.3	23.6	9.0	4.3	13.3
1943	37.5	11.4	7.9	19.3	4.4	23.7	9.3	4.5	13.8
1942	37.3	12.1	8.1	20.1	4.4	24.5	8.7	4.1	12.7
1941	41.2	12.9	8.4	21.3	4.8	26.1	10.2	4.9	15.1
1940	43.2	13.6	8.8	22.4	4.8	27.2	10.8	5.2	16.0
1939	44.3	13.8	9.1	22.9	4.9	27.8	10.7	5.7	16.5
1938	47.1	13.9	9.0	23.0	5.3	28.3	12.2	6.6	18.8
1937	50.3	14.5	9.4	23.9	5.9	29.7	13.4	7.2	20.6
1936	52.9	14.9	10.0	24.9	6.1	31.0	14.1	7.7	21.9
1935	51.9	14.8	9.9	24.7	6.3	31.0	13.5	7.4	20.9

Note: See table for TOTAL births for source.

[1]From 1935 to 1948 these categories refer to deaths at ages "under 1 month," "1 to 5 months" and "1 to 11 months" respectively.

[2]Includes Alaska and Hawaii. New Jersey excluded from data for 1962 and 1963; color not reported on vital record.

Table I.1e   Infant mortality rates per 1,000 live births by age at death and color: United States, 1935-64 - continued.

Year	Under 1 Year	Under 1 day	1-6 days	Under 7 days	7-27 days	Under[1] 28 days	28 days[1] - 5 months	6-11 months	28 days[1] - 11 months
NONWHITE									
1964[2]	41.1	15.0	8.0	23.0	3.5	26.5	11.1	3.5	14.6
1963[2]	41.5	14.6	8.2	22.7	3.4	26.1	11.5	3.9	15.4
1962[2]	41.4	14.3	8.1	22.4	3.6	26.1	11.5	3.8	15.3
1961[2]	40.7	14.2	8.3	22.4	3.8	26.2	11.0	3.5	14.5
1960[2]	43.2	14.4	8.5	22.9	4.0	26.9	12.1	4.2	16.3
1959[2]	43.7	14.5	8.8	23.3	4.2	27.5	12.1	4.1	16.2
1958	45.7	14.3	10.0	24.3	4.7	29.0	12.4	4.3	16.7
1957	43.7	13.9	9.3	23.2	4.6	27.8	11.6	4.3	15.9
1956	42.1	13.7	8.9	22.6	4.4	27.0	10.9	4.1	15.0
1955	42.8	13.9	9.1	22.9	4.2	27.2	11.3	4.3	15.6
1954	42.9	13.3	9.4	22.6	4.4	27.0	11.3	4.6	15.9
1953	44.7	12.9	9.8	22.7	4.7	27.4	12.3	5.0	17.3
1952	47.0	12.8	10.2	23.0	5.0	28.0	13.3	5.7	19.0
1951	44.8	12.7	10.0	22.7	4.6	27.3	12.2	5.3	17.5
1950	44.5	13.0	9.8	22.8	4.8	27.5	11.7	5.2	16.9
1949	47.3	12.8	10.1	22.9	5.7	28.6	13.5	5.3	18.8
1948	46.5	12.9	10.4	23.4	5.7	29.1	12.3	5.0	17.3
1947	48.5	13.5	11.2	24.7	6.2	31.0	12.4	5.1	17.5
1946	49.5	13.4	11.0	24.4	7.2	31.5	12.5	5.4	17.9
1945	57.0	12.7	11.3	24.0	8.0	32.0	17.3	7.8	25.0
1944	60.3	13.2	11.3	24.5	8.0	32.5	18.4	9.4	27.8
1943	62.5	13.2	11.7	24.9	8.0	32.9	19.2	10.3	29.6
1942	64.6	14.4	12.0	26.4	8.3	34.6	19.7	10.2	30.0
1941	74.8	15.7	13.5	29.2	9.8	39.0	23.0	12.8	35.8
1940	73.8	16.0	13.7	29.7	10.0	39.7	22.5	11.5	34.1
1939	74.2	16.2	13.5	29.7	9.8	39.6	22.2	12.5	34.7
1938	79.1	15.8	13.4	29.2	9.9	39.1	24.9	15.1	40.0
1937	83.2	16.1	14.7	30.8	11.3	42.1	26.0	15.1	41.1
1936	87.6	16.4	15.6	32.0	11.9	43.9	27.9	15.9	43.7
1935	83.2	16.2	14.8	31.0	11.6	42.7	25.8	14.7	40.6

Note: See table for WHITE births for footnotes and source.

Table I.1f   Infant mortality rates per 1,000 live births by age at death, color and sex: United States, 1935-64 - continued.

Year	Male				Female			
	Under 1 Year	Under 7 days	Under[1] 28 days	28 days[1,2] - 11 months	Under 1 year	Under 7 days	Under[1] 28 days	28 days[1,2] - 11 months
WHITE								
1964[3]	24.4	16.9	18.5	5.9	18.6	12.5	13.8	4.8
1963[3]	25.1	17.4	19.1	6.1	19.0	12.8	14.1	4.9
1962[3]	25.4	17.6	19.4	6.1	19.1	12.9	14.2	4.8
1961[3]	25.4	17.6	19.3	6.1	19.3	13.0	14.4	4.9
1960[3]	26.0	17.8	19.7	6.3	19.6	13.2	14.7	4.9
1959[3]	26.3	18.0	20.0	6.3	20.0	13.3	14.8	5.1
1958	26.7	18.0	20.2	6.6	20.6	13.6	15.2	5.4
1957	26.4	17.8	20.0	6.4	20.1	13.2	14.9	5.2
1956	26.2	17.9	20.0	6.3	20.0	13.2	14.8	5.1
1955	26.7	18.2	20.3	6.5	20.3	13.5	15.1	5.3
1954	27.0	18.1	20.4	6.6	20.6	13.3	15.1	5.5
1953	28.4	18.7	21.0	7.4	21.5	13.6	15.4	6.0
1952	28.7	18.7	21.1	7.5	22.1	13.8	15.8	6.4
1951	29.2	19.1	21.6	7.6	22.4	14.0	16.0	6.3
1950	30.2	19.6	22.2	8.0	23.1	14.4	16.4	6.7
1949	32.5	20.2	23.3	9.2	25.0	14.8	17.2	7.8
1948	33.7	21.0	24.2	9.5	25.9	15.3	18.0	7.9
1947	33.9	21.3	24.8	9.2	26.0	15.7	18.5	7.5
1946	35.8	22.3	26.3	9.5	27.5	16.5	19.7	7.8
1945	39.9	21.9	26.5	13.4	31.1	16.3	19.9	11.2
1944	41.2	21.9	26.6	14.6	32.4	16.6	20.4	12.0
1943	42.0	22.1	26.9	15.1	32.7	16.3	20.2	12.5
1942	41.6	23.0	27.8	13.8	31.3	16.3	20.1	11.2
1941	46.0	24.2	29.5	16.5	36.1	18.2	22.5	13.7
1940	48.3	25.6	30.9	17.5	37.8	19.0	23.3	14.5
1939	49.2	25.9	31.3	17.9	39.1	19.8	24.2	14.9
1938	52.5	26.2	32.0	20.5	41.4	19.6	24.4	17.0
1937	56.0	27.0	33.4	22.6	44.4	20.6	25.8	18.6
1936	58.9	28.3	35.1	23.8	46.5	21.2	26.7	19.8
1935	58.1	28.3	35.2	22.9	45.2	20.8	26.5	18.8

Note: See table for TOTAL births for source.

[1]From 1935 to 1948 these categories refer to deaths at ages "under 1 month" and "1 to 11 months" respectively.

[2]From 1935 to 1948, "28 days to 11 months" rates computed by subtracting "Under 28 days" rates from "Under 1 year" rates for respective year.

[3]Includes Alaska and Hawaii. New Jersey excluded from data for 1962 and 1963; color not reported on vital record.

Table I.1g   Infant mortality rates per 1,000 live births by age at death, color and sex: United States, 1935-64 - continued.

	Male				Female			
Year	Under 1 year	Under 7 days	Under[1] 28 days	28 days[1,2] - 11 months	Under 1 year	Under 7 days	Under[1] 28 days	28 days[1,2] - 11 months
NONWHITE								
1964[3]	45.5	25.8	29.6	15.9	36.6	20.1	23.3	13.3
1963[3]	46.0	25.5	29.2	16.7	36.9	19.8	22.9	14.0
1962[3]	45.7	25.1	28.9	16.7	36.9	19.8	23.1	13.8
1961[3]	44.8	25.0	29.1	15.7	36.5	19.7	23.2	13.3
1960[3]	47.9	25.8	30.0	17.8	38.5	19.9	23.6	14.8
1959[3]	47.8	25.9	30.5	17.3	39.5	20.6	24.4	15.1
1958	50.3	26.9	32.0	18.3	41.0	21.7	25.9	15.1
1957	47.8	25.8	30.7	17.0	39.6	20.5	24.7	14.8
1956	46.7	25.6	30.4	16.3	37.3	19.6	23.6	13.7
1955	46.9	25.5	30.2	16.7	38.6	20.3	24.1	14.5
1954	47.1	25.4	30.1	16.9	38.6	19.8	23.7	14.8
1953	48.4	25.0	30.1	18.3	40.8	20.3	24.6	16.3
1952	52.3	26.0	31.6	20.7	41.7	19.9	24.4	17.3
1951	50.0	25.8	31.0	18.9	39.6	19.5	23.6	16.0
1950	48.9	25.6	30.8	18.1	39.9	19.8	24.2	15.7
1949	52.5	25.9	32.1	20.4	42.0	19.7	25.0	17.1
1948	51.4	26.2	32.4	19.0	41.4	20.5	25.8	15.6
1947	53.2	27.9	34.6	18.6	43.7	21.5	27.4	16.4
1946	54.0	27.4	35.0	19.0	44.8	21.3	28.0	16.8
1945	63.2	27.3	36.0	27.2	50.8	20.6	28.0	22.8
1944	65.5	27.3	36.0	29.5	55.0	21.6	29.0	26.1
1943	68.9	28.4	36.9	32.0	55.9	21.3	28.8	27.1
1942	70.7	29.7	38.6	32.1	58.3	23.0	30.6	27.7
1941	82.1	33.2	43.5	38.6	67.3	25.0	34.4	32.9
1940	82.2	34.0	44.9	37.3	65.2	25.4	34.5	30.7
1939	82.3	33.6	44.5	37.8	66.0	25.7	34.5	31.5
1938	87.0	32.9	43.5	43.6	70.9	25.3	34.5	36.4
1937	91.0	34.7	46.6	44.3	75.2	26.8	37.5	37.7
1936	96.3	36.5	49.0	47.3	78.6	27.4	38.6	40.1
1935	91.7	35.0	47.3	44.4	74.6	26.9	37.9	36.6

Note: See table for TOTAL births for source.

[1]From 1935 to 1948 these categories refer to deaths at ages "under 1 month" and "1 to 11 months" respectively.

[2]From 1935 to 1948, "28 days to 11 months" rates computed by subtracting "Under 28 days" rates from "Under 1 year" rates for respective year.

[3]Includes Alaska and Hawaii. New Jersey excluded from data for 1962 and 1963; color not reported on vital record.

Table I.2a   Average annual infant mortality rates per 10,000 live births for selected causes of death by age at death: United States, selected decennium periods.

Cause of death	1959-61			1949-51			1939-41		
	Under 1 year	Under 28 days	28 days -11 months	Under 1 year	Under 28 days	28 days -11 months	Under 1 year	Under 1 month	1-1 mont♦
Total									
All causes	259.0	187.1	71.9	296.4	206.5	89.9	467.5	285.5	182.♦
Infective and parasitic diseases (001-138)	3.4	0.5	2.9	8.2	1.2	7.0	26.6	4.5	22.♦
Influenza and pneumonia, including pneumonia of newborn (480-493,763)	31.0	8.6	22.4	31.7	8.1	23.6	70.6	12.5	58.♦
All other diseases of respiratory system (470-475,500-527)	6.2	0.7	5.5	3.9	0.6	3.3	5.1	1.1	4.♦
Gastritis and duodenitis, etc.[1] (543,571,572,764)	6.9	1.1	5.8	14.7	2.3	12.3	37.2	4.7	32.♦
All other diseases of digestive system (530-542,544-570,573-587)	3.8	2.4	1.4	4.3	2.0	2.2	7.1	1.5	5.♦
Congenital malformations (750-759)	36.4	23.9	12.5	39.9	25.7	14.2	46.5	32.0	14.♦
Birth injuries (760,761)	23.9	23.9	0.0	33.1	32.8	0.4	44.2	43.3	0.♦
Intracranial and spinal injury at birth (760)	7.5	7.5	0.0*	14.3	14.1	0.2	---	---	--♦
Other birth injury (761)	16.4	16.4	0.0	18.8	18.7	0.1	---	---	--♦
Postnatal asphyxia and atelectasis (762)	45.7	45.0	0.7	38.3	37.4	0.8	---	---	--♦
Hemolytic disease of newborn (770)	5.0	5.0	0.0	7.1	6.9	0.2	---	---	--♦
Immaturity unqualified (776)	45.4	45.1	0.3	63.6	62.7	0.8	137.2	133.0	4.♦
Nutritional maladjustment and ill-defined diseases peculiar to early infancy (772,773)	18.9	17.1	1.9	11.1	8.4	2.7	11.9	7.2	4.♦
Neonatal disorders arising from certain diseases of mother during pregnancy, etc.[2] (765-769,771,774)	8.6	7.9	0.7	9.9	8.4	1.5	---	---	--♦
Symptoms and ill-defined conditions (780-793,795)	5.8	2.4	3.4	10.0	5.4	4.5	23.7	13.8	9.♦
Accidents (E800-E962)	8.8	1.4	7.4	10.2	1.9	8.2	11.1	2.5	8.♦
Residual (140-468,590-749,E963-E985)	9.2	2.5	6.7	10.8	2.7	8.1	---	---	--♦
Certain diseases of early infancy (760-776)	157.1	153.5	3.6	173.2	166.7	6.5	234.1	222.3	11.♦

Source: Annual volumes Vital Statistics of the United States, National Center for Health Statistics, Public Health Service, Washington, and special tabulations.

[1]Includes gastritis and duodenitis; gastroenteritis and colitis, except ulcerative, age 4 weeks and over; chronic enteritis and ulcerative colitis; diarrhea of newborn.

[2]Includes neonatal disorders arising from certain diseases of the mother during pregnancy; immaturity with mention of other subsidiary condition; and other diseases peculiar to early infancy not already mentioned.

Note: Alaska and Hawaii included in 1959-61 deaths. Numbers after causes of death are category numbers of the Seventh Revision of the International Classification of Diseases, 1955. Deaths are classified according to the Sixth Revision, 1948, for 1949-1951 and Fifth Revision, 1938, for 1939-1941. A major source of incomparability between rates for the 1939-41 period and rates for later decennium periods is the classification of causes of death with mention of "immaturity" or "prematurity". In the Fifth Revision, "prematurity" was given priority over other diseases of early infancy, except injury at birth. In later revisions, prematurity or immaturity was made a secondary axis of classification. The effect of this change is to understate rates for the following categories of disease in the period 1939-41 as compared with rates for succeeding decennium periods (rubrics are Seventh Revision): 762, 763, 764, 768-774. Similarly, 1939-41 rates shown in the table on the line for "immaturity, unqualified" are about 80 per cent above the rates that would have been obtained under the classification rules of the Sixth and Seventh Revisions.

* Rates based on less than 20 deaths.

Table I.2b   Average annual infant mortality rates per 10,000 live births
for selected causes of death by age at death and sex:
United States, selected decennium periods - continued.

Cause of death	1959-61			1949-51			1939-41		
	Under 1 year	Under 28 days	28 days -11 months	Under 1 year	Under 28 days	28 days -11 months	Under 1 year	Under 1 month	1-11 months
Male									
All causes	291.0	212.2	78.8	332.6	235.4	97.2	520.0	322.0	198.0
Infective and parasitic diseases	3.8	0.6	3.2	8.7	1.4	7.3	27.8	4.9	22.9
Influenza and pneumonia, including pneumonia of newborn	34.6	9.9	24.7	34.6	9.1	25.5	77.7	14.0	63.7
All other diseases of respiratory system	7.1	0.8	6.3	4.4	0.7	3.6	5.7	1.2	4.5
Gastritis and duodenitis, etc.[1]	7.5	1.2	6.3	16.1	2.6	13.4	40.9	5.3	35.6
All other diseases of digestive system	4.4	2.7	1.7	5.0	2.4	2.7	8.6	1.8	6.8
Congenital malformations	39.2	26.1	13.1	42.4	27.8	14.6	49.8	34.4	15.4
Birth injuries	28.1	28.0	0.0	39.7	39.3	0.4	52.9	51.8	1.1
Intracranial and spinal injury at birth	9.4	9.4	-	17.9	17.6	0.3	---	---	---
Other birth injury	18.7	18.7	0.0	21.8	21.6	0.1	---	---	---
Postnatal asphyxia and atelectasis	53.0	52.2	0.7	45.0	44.1	0.9	---	---	---
Hemolytic disease of newborn	5.2	5.1	0.0	8.1	7.9	0.2	---	---	---
Immaturity unqualified	50.0	49.7	0.3	70.4	69.5	0.9	151.7	147.6	4.1
Nutritional maladjustment and ill-defined diseases peculiar to early infancy	22.1	19.9	2.2	12.5	9.5	3.0	13.5	8.3	5.2
Neonatal disorders arising from certain diseases of mother during pregnancy, etc.[2]	9.9	9.2	0.7	11.2	9.7	1.5	---	---	---
Symptoms and ill-defined conditions	6.3	2.6	3.7	11.1	6.3	4.8	26.0	15.5	10.5
Accidents	9.7	1.5	8.1	11.3	2.2	9.1	12.2	2.7	9.5
Residual	10.3	2.9	7.4	12.1	3.0	9.1	---	---	---
Certain diseases of early infancy	179.2	175.1	4.0	198.4	191.5	7.0	264.7	252.2	12.5

Note: For sources and footnotes see table for TOTAL.

Table I.2c

Average annual infant mortality rates per 10,000 live births
for selected causes of death by age at death and sex:
United States, selected decennium periods - continued.

Cause of death	1959-61			1949-51			1939-41		
	Under 1 year	Under 28 days	28 days -11 months	Under 1 year	Under 28 days	28 days -11 months	Under 1 year	Under 1 month	1- mor
Female									
All causes	225.4	160.8	64.6	258.3	176.1	82.3	412.2	246.9	165
Infective and parasitic diseases	3.0	0.4	2.6	7.6	1.0	6.6	25.3	4.0	21
Influenza and pneumonia, including pneumonia of newborn	27.3	7.3	20.0	28.7	7.0	21.6	63.1	10.9	52
All other diseases of respiratory system	5.2	0.6	4.6	3.4	0.4	3.0	4.4	1.0	3
Gastritis and duodenitis, etc.[1]	6.3	0.9	5.3	13.2	2.0	11.2	33.3	4.0	29
All other diseases of digestive system	3.2	2.1	1.1	3.5	1.7	1.7	5.6	1.2	4
Congenital malformations	33.5	21.5	12.0	37.2	23.5	13.7	43.1	29.4	13
Birth injuries	19.6	19.5	0.0	26.2	25.9	0.3	35.0	34.2	0
Intracranial and spinal injury at birth	5.6	5.6	0.0*	10.5	10.3	0.2	---	---	-
Other birth injury	14.0	13.9	0.0	15.7	15.6	0.1	---	---	-
Postnatal asphyxia and atelectasis	38.0	37.4	0.6	31.2	30.5	0.8	---	---	-
Hemolytic disease of newborn	4.9	4.9	0.0	5.9	5.8	0.1	---	---	-
Immaturity unqualified	40.5	40.2	0.3	56.3	55.5	0.8	121.9	117.7	4
Nutritional maladjustment and ill-defined diseases peculiar to early infancy	15.7	14.1	1.5	9.6	7.2	2.4	10.3	6.0	4
Neonatal disorders arising from certain diseases of mother during pregnancy, etc.[2]	7.2	6.5	0.7	8.5	7.0	1.5	---	---	-
Symptoms and ill-defined conditions	5.2	2.1	3.1	8.7	4.5	4.2	21.3	12.0	9
Accidents	7.9	1.3	6.6	9.0	1.7	7.2	9.9	2.2	7
Residual	8.0	2.0	5.9	9.4	2.3	7.1	---	---	-
Certain diseases of early infancy	134.0	130.8	3.2	146.6	140.7	5.9	201.7	190.8	10

Note: For sources and footnotes see table for TOTAL.

Table I.2d   Average annual infant mortality rates per 10,000 live births
for selected causes of death, by age at death and color:
United States, selected decennium periods - continued.

Cause of death	1959-61			1949-51			1939-41		
	Under 1 year	Under 28 days	28 days -11 months	Under 1 year	Under 28 days	28 days -11 months	Under 1 year	Under 1 month	1-11 months
White									
All causes	228.5	172.2	56.3	271.4	195.2	76.2	428.6	270.1	158.5
Infective and parasitic diseases	2.6	0.3	2.3	6.5	0.8	5.8	20.6	2.8	17.8
Influenza and pneumonia, including pneumonia of newborn	22.9	6.6	16.3	25.3	6.8	18.5	61.1	11.3	49.8
All other diseases of respiratory system	5.3	0.6	4.6	3.4	0.5	2.9	4.4	0.8	3.5
Gastritis and duodenitis, etc.[1]	4.0	0.6	3.4	12.0	1.9	10.1	33.4	4.3	29.0
All other diseases of digestive system	3.6	2.4	1.2	4.0	2.1	2.0	6.7	1.4	5.3
Congenital malformations	37.5	25.0	12.5	41.8	27.2	14.7	49.9	34.4	15.5
Birth injuries	23.4	23.3	0.0	32.9	32.6	0.3	45.4	44.5	0.9
Intracranial and spinal injury at birth	6.9	6.9	-	13.7	13.5	0.2	---	---	---
Other birth injury	16.5	16.5	0.0	19.2	19.1	0.1	---	---	---
Postnatal asphyxia and atelectasis	42.2	41.6	0.5	37.4	36.7	0.8	---	---	---
Hemolytic disease of newborn	5.6	5.5	0.0	7.6	7.4	0.2	---	---	---
Immaturity unqualified	39.4	39.2	0.2	58.1	57.5	0.6	131.7	128.2	3.5
Nutritional maladjustment and ill-defined diseases peculiar to early infancy	16.6	15.7	0.9	9.3	7.3	2.0	8.9	5.0	3.9
Neonatal disorders arising from certain diseases of mother during pregnancy, etc.[2]	7.4	6.9	0.5	8.9	7.7	1.2	---	---	---
Symptoms and ill-defined conditions	2.7	1.1	1.6	5.3	2.6	2.6	12.5	6.9	5.6
Accidents	7.3	1.1	6.2	8.8	1.6	7.2	9.9	2.1	7.8
Residual	8.1	2.3	5.8	10.0	2.6	7.4	---	---	---
Certain diseases of early infancy	141.7	139.5	2.2	162.9	157.8	5.1	224.3	214.3	10.0

Note: For sources and footnotes see table for TOTAL.

Table I.2e   Average annual infant mortality rates per 10,000 live births
for selected causes of death by age at death and color:
United States, selected decennium periods - continued.

Cause of death	1959-61			1949-51			1939-41		
	Under 1 year	Under 28 days	28 days -11 months	Under 1 year	Under 28 days	28 days -11 months	Under 1 year	Under 1 month	1- mon
Nonwhite									
All causes	425.3	268.6	156.7	455.1	278.0	177.1	742.8	394.1	348
Infective and parasitic diseases	7.9	1.5	6.4	18.8	4.2	14.6	69.2	16.5	52
Influenza and pneumonia, including pneumonia of newborn	75.2	19.2	56.1	72.3	16.1	56.2	138.0	21.3	116
All other diseases of respiratory system	11.3	1.2	10.1	7.1	1.3	5.8	10.2	3.0	7
Gastritis and duodenitis, etc.[1]	23.0	3.9	19.1	31.4	5.0	26.4	64.0	6.9	57
All other diseases of digestive system	4.7	2.3	2.5	5.7	2.0	3.7	10.5	2.5	8
Congenital malformations	30.4	17.8	12.6	27.4	16.2	11.2	22.7	14.6	8
Birth injuries	26.9	26.8	0.1*	34.3	33.8	0.5	35.7	34.8	0
Intracranial and spinal injury at birth	11.2	11.2	0.0*	18.1	17.8	0.4	---	---	-
Other birth injury	15.7	15.6	0.1*	16.2	16.0	0.2	---	---	-
Postnatal asphyxia and atelectasis	64.8	63.5	1.3	43.7	42.4	1.3	---	---	-
Hemolytic disease of newborn	2.2	2.2	0.1*	3.4	3.2	0.2	---	---	-
Immaturity unqualified	77.8	76.9	0.9	97.9	95.5	2.4	176.3	167.8	8
Nutritional maladjustment and ill-defined diseases peculiar to early infancy	31.5	24.6	6.9	22.5	15.2	7.3	33.6	22.5	11
Neonatal disorders arising from certain diseases of mother during pregnancy, etc.[2]	15.3	13.4	1.9	16.2	12.8	3.3	---	---	-
Symptoms and ill-defined conditions	22.2	9.2	13.1	39.9	23.3	16.5	102.9	62.3	40
Accidents	17.0	3.1	14.0	18.9	4.0	14.9	19.7	5.5	14
Residual	15.0	3.6	11.3	15.7	3.0	12.8	---	---	-
Certain diseases of early infancy	241.1	230.0	11.2	238.4	223.3	15.1	302.9	279.0	23

Note: For sources and footnotes see table for TOTAL.

able I.3   Infant mortality rates per 100,000 live births
by detailed age, color, and sex: United States, 1964.

(Data refer only to deaths occurring within the United States. Excludes fetal deaths.)

Age	Total			White			Nonwhite		
	Both Sexes	Male	Female	Both Sexes	Male	Female	Both Sexes	Male	Female
Under 1 year	2,477.5	2,783.7	2,157.0	2,158.6	2,443.6	1,858.8	4,109.6	4,549.1	3,660.5
nder 28 days	1,788.4	2,028.6	1,536.8	1,620.4	1,848.6	1,380.2	2,648.1	2,962.9	2,326.3
nder 1 day	1,022.6	1,151.2	887.9	929.3	1,051.3	800.9	1,500.0	1,669.7	1,326.5
Under 1 hour	196.1	206.7	184.9	181.8	188.7	174.5	269.2	300.2	237.4
1-23 hours	826.5	944.5	702.9	747.5	862.6	626.3	1,230.8	1,369.5	1,089.1
day	263.2	307.6	216.8	244.9	286.6	201.1	357.0	416.5	296.1
days	160.2	188.2	130.9	152.4	180.7	122.7	200.2	227.2	172.6
days	72.2	85.2	58.6	66.8	79.5	53.4	99.8	114.5	84.8
days	40.0	44.9	34.9	36.3	40.5	31.8	59.4	67.9	50.7
days	28.4	31.7	24.9	24.8	28.1	21.4	46.6	50.8	42.4
days	21.4	25.4	17.2	19.0	23.4	14.3	33.9	35.8	31.9
-13 days	85.5	93.4	77.3	72.8	80.0	65.2	150.5	162.9	137.9
4-20 days	51.3	54.7	47.7	41.2	44.1	38.2	102.7	109.7	95.5.
1-27 days	43.5	46.2	40.6	32.8	34.3	31.2	98.0	107.9	87.8
8-59 days	165.4	186.3	143.5	130.6	150.3	109.8	343.6	373.0	313.6
months	128.7	141.9	114.9	99.4	111.8	86.2	278.9	298.1	259.2
months	95.9	107.5	83.7	74.8	83.1	66.0	204.0	234.1	173.2
months	69.7	75.1	64.1	52.3	57.5	46.8	158.9	166.2	151.4
months	53.4	58.4	48.2	40.2	43.9	36.2	121.4	133.4	109.0
months	43.4	46.4	40.3	33.8	36.8	30.8	92.2	96.2	88.1
months	34.9	36.6	33.1	27.8	27.5	28.1	71.1	83.8	58.0
months	29.1	30.1	28.1	22.8	23.1	22.5	61.5	66.4	56.5
months	26.1	27.7	24.4	21.7	22.7	20.6	48.9	53.8	43.9
0 months	21.9	24.1	19.6	17.8	20.1	15.4	42.8	44.8	40.8
1 months	20.6	21.0	20.2	17.2	18.1	16.2	38.3	36.4	40.2

Source: Annual volume <u>Vital Statistics of the United States</u>, National Center for Health Statistics, Public Health
ervice, Washington,

Table I.4a   Average annual infant mortality rates per 10,000 live births
for selected causes of death, by age at death, color and sex: United States, 1959-61.

Cause of Death	Under 1 year	Under 1 day	1-6 days	Under 7 days	7-27 days	Under 28 days	28 days -5 months	6-11 months	28 days -11 months
Total All Causes	259.0	103.1	63.9	166.9	20.2	187.1	53.3	18.6	71.9
Infective and parasitic diseases (001-138)	3.4	0.0	0.1	0.2	0.3	0.5	1.9	1.1	2.9
Dysentery, All Forms (045-048)	0.3	-	0.0*	0.0*	0.0	0.0	0.2	0.1	0.3
Tuberculosis, septicemia and pyemia, meningococcal infections and measles (001-019,053,057,085)	1.7	0.0*	0.0*	0.0*	0.0	0.0	1.0	0.6	1.6
All other infective and parasitic diseases (020-044, 049-052,054-056,058-064,086-138)	1.5	0.0	0.1	0.1	0.3	0.4	0.7	0.4	1.1
Diseases of nervous system and sense organs (330-398)	4.2	0.1	0.3	0.4	0.4	0.9	2.0	1.3	3.3
Diseases of respiratory system (470-527)	28.7	0.2	0.3	0.4	0.4	0.8	21.9	6.1	28.0
Acute upper respiratory infections (470-475)	1.0	0.0*	0.0	0.0	0.1	0.1	0.7	0.2	0.9
Influenza and pneumonia, except pneumonia of the newborn (480-493)	22.5	0.0*	0.0	0.0	0.1	0.1	17.4	5.0	22.4
Bronchitis and other diseases of the respiratory system (500-502,510-522,525-527)	5.2	0.2	0.2	0.4	0.2	0.6	3.8	0.9	4.7
Diseases of digestive system (530-587)	9.6	0.8	0.9	1.7	0.7	2.4	4.9	2.4	7.3
Hernia and intestinal obstruction (without mention of hernia) (560,561,570)	2.2	0.8	0.5	1.3	0.3	1.6	0.5	0.2	0.7
Gastritis, duodenitis, enteritis, and colitis, except diarrhea of newborn (543,571,572)	5.8	-	0.0*	0.0*	0.0*	0.0	3.8	2.0	5.8
All other diseases of digestive system (530-542, 544-553,573-587)	1.6	0.1	0.4	0.5	0.3	0.8	0.6	0.2	0.8
Congenital malformations (750-759)	36.4	9.5	8.9	18.4	5.5	23.9	9.4	3.1	12.5
Congenital malformations of nervous system and sense organs (750-753)	9.0	3.6	1.4	5.0	1.0	6.0	2.1	0.9	3.0
Congenital malformations of circulatory system (754)	17.8	2.4	5.3	7.7	2.8	10.5	5.6	1.7	7.3
All other congenital malformations (755-759)	9.6	3.5	2.2	5.7	1.7	7.4	1.7	0.5	2.2
Birth injuries (760-761)	23.9	15.9	7.4	23.3	0.6	23.9	0.0*	0.0*	0.0*
Intracranial and spinal injury at birth (760)	12.5	3.1	4.0	7.1	0.5	7.5	0.0*	-	0.0*
Other birth injury (761)	16.4	12.8	3.4	16.2	0.2	16.4	0.0*	0.0*	0.0*
Postnatal asphyxia and atelectasis (762)	45.7	27.4	16.4	43.8	1.2	45.0	0.6	0.1	0.7
Pneumonia of newborn (763)	8.5	1.1	3.4	4.4	4.1	8.5	0.0*	...	...*
Diarrhea of newborn (764)	1.1	0.0*	0.1	0.1	1.0	1.1	0.0*	...*	0.0*
Other infections of newborn (765-768)	1.8	0.2	0.8	0.9	0.9	1.8	0.0	0.0*	0.0
Neonatal disorders arising from certain diseases of the mother during pregnancy (769)	2.2	1.3	0.8	2.1	0.1	2.2	0.0	0.0*	0.0
Hemolytic disease of newborn (erythroblastosis) (770)	5.0	3.3	1.5	4.8	0.2	5.0	0.0	0.0*	0.0
Hemorrhagic disease of newborn (771)	1.5	0.5	0.8	1.3	0.2	1.4	0.0*	0.0*	0.0*
Nutritional maladjustment and ill-defined diseases peculiar to early infancy (772,773)	18.9	8.6	7.6	16.1	1.0	17.1	1.6	0.3	1.9
Immaturity with mention of any other subsidiary condition (774)	3.1	1.2	1.0	2.2	0.3	2.5	0.6	0.0	0.6
Immaturity, unqualified (776)	45.4	31.3	12.2	43.5	1.6	45.1	0.3	0.0*	0.3
Accidents (E800-E962)	8.8	0.2	0.5	0.6	0.8	1.4	5.1	2.3	7.4
Residual (140-326,400-468,590-749,780-793,795,E963-E999)	10.8	1.6	1.3	2.9	1.1	4.0	4.8	2.0	6.8

Source: Special tabulations of the Division of Vital Statistics, National Center for Health Statistics, Public Health Service, Washington.

for selected causes of death, by age at death, color and sex: United States, 1959-61 - Continued.

Cause of Death	Under 1 year	Under 1 day	1 - 6 days	Under 7 days	7 - 27 days	Under 28 days	28 days -5 months	6 - 11 months	28 days -11 months
Male									
All Causes	291.0	115.7	74.2	189.9	22.3	212.2	59.2	19.6	78.8
Infective and parasitic diseases	3.8	0.0	0.1	0.2	0.4	0.6	2.1	1.2	3.2
Dysentery, All Forms	0.3	-	0.0*	0.0*	0.0*	0.0	0.2	0.1	0.3
Tuberculosis, septicemia and pyemia, meningococcal infections and measles	1.9	0.0*	0.0*	0.0*	0.0*	0.0	1.2	0.7	1.9
All other infective and parasitic diseases	1.6	0.0	0.1	0.2	0.3	0.5	0.7	0.4	1.1
Diseases of nervous system and sense organs	4.7	0.1	0.4	0.5	0.5	1.0	2.3	1.4	3.7
Diseases of respiratory system	32.0	0.2	0.3	0.5	0.4	0.9	24.7	6.4	31.1
Acute upper respiratory infections	1.1	0.0*	0.0	0.0	0.1	0.1	0.8	0.2	1.0
Influenza and pneumonia, except pneumonia of the newborn	24.8	0.2	0.0*	0.2	0.1	0.1	19.5	5.2	24.7
Bronchitis and other diseases of the respiratory system	6.0	0.2	0.2	0.4	0.2	0.7	4.4	0.9	5.3
Diseases of digestive system	10.7	0.9	1.1	2.0	0.8	2.7	5.4	2.6	8.0
Hernia and intestinal obstruction (without mention of hernia)	2.6	0.8	0.6	1.4	0.4	1.8	0.6	0.2	0.8
Gastritis, duodenitis, enteritis, and colitis, except diarrhea of newborn	6.3	-	0.0*	0.0*	0.0*	0.0*	4.1	2.2	6.3
All other diseases of digestive system	1.8	0.1	0.5	0.6	0.4	0.9	0.7	0.2	0.9
Congenital malformations	39.2	9.8	10.3	20.1	6.0	26.1	10.0	3.0	13.1
Congenital malformations of nervous system and sense organs	8.1	3.0	1.4	4.4	0.9	5.3	2.0	0.9	2.9
Congenital malformations of circulatory system	19.9	2.7	6.5	9.1	3.2	12.3	6.0	1.6	7.6
All other congenital malformations	11.2	4.1	2.5	6.6	2.0	8.6	2.1	0.5	2.6
Birth Injuries	28.1	18.4	8.9	27.3	0.7	28.0	0.0	0.0*	0.0
Intracranial and spinal injury at birth	9.4	3.8	5.1	8.8	0.5	9.4	-	-	-
Other birth injury	18.7	14.7	3.8	18.5	0.2	18.7	0.0*	-	0.0*
Postnatal asphyxia and atelectasis	53.0	31.6	19.4	51.0	1.3	52.2	0.7	0.1	0.7
Pneumonia of newborn	9.7	1.2	3.9	5.1	4.6	9.7	...	...	...
Diarrhea of newborn	1.2	0.0*	0.1	0.1	1.1	1.2	0.0*	0.0*	0.0*
Other infections of newborn	2.1	0.2	0.9	1.1	1.0	2.1	0.0*	0.0*	0.0*
Neonatal disorders arising from certain diseases of the mother during pregnancy	2.5	1.5	0.9	2.4	0.1	2.5	0.0*	0.0*	0.0*
Hemolytic disease of newborn (erythroblastosis)	5.2	3.1	1.7	4.9	0.3	5.1	0.0	0.0*	0.0
Hemorrhagic disease of newborn	1.8	0.6	1.0	1.6	0.2	1.8	0.0	0.0*	0.0
Nutritional maladjustment and ill-defined diseases peculiar to early infancy	22.1	9.9	8.9	18.8	1.1	19.9	1.9	0.3	2.2
Immaturity with mention of any other subsidiary condition	3.5	1.4	1.1	2.5	0.4	2.9	0.6	0.0*	0.6
Immaturity, unqualified	50.0	35.0	13.1	48.1	1.6	49.7	0.3	0.0*	0.3
Accidents	9.7	0.2	0.6	0.7	0.8	1.5	5.6	2.5	8.1
Residual	11.9	1.7	1.6	3.3	1.2	4.5	5.3	2.2	7.4

Note: See table for TOTAL deaths for footnote and source.

Table I.4c
Average annual infant mortality rates per 10,000 live births
for selected causes of death, by age at death, color and sex: United States, 1959-61 - Continued.

Cause of Death	Under 1 year	Under 1 day	1-6 days	Under 7 days	7-27 days	Under 28 days	28 days -5 months	6-11 months	28 days -11 months
Female									
All Causes	225.4	89.7	53.0	142.8	18.0	160.8	47.1	17.5	64.6
Infective and parasitic diseases	3.0	0.0	0.1	0.1	0.3	0.4	1.6	1.0	2.6
Dysentery, All Forms	0.3	-	0.0*	0.0*	0.0*	0.0*	0.2	0.1	0.3
Tuberculosis, septicemia and pyemia, meningococcal infections and measles	1.4	0.0*	0.0*	0.0*	0.0*	0.0	0.8	0.6	1.4
All other infective and parasitic diseases	1.3	0.0	0.1	0.1	0.2	0.3	0.6	0.3	0.9
Diseases of nervous system and sense organs	3.6	0.1	0.3	0.4	0.4	0.7	1.8	1.1	2.9
Diseases of respiratory system	25.3	0.2	0.2	0.4	0.3	0.7	18.9	5.8	24.7
Acute upper respiratory infections	0.9	-	0.0*	0.0*	0.1	0.1	0.6	0.2	0.8
Influenza and pneumonia, except pneumonia of the newborn	20.1	-	0.0*	0.0*	0.1	0.1	15.2	4.8	20.0
Bronchitis and other diseases of the respiratory system	4.3	0.2	0.2	0.4	0.2	0.5	3.1	0.8	3.8
Diseases of digestive system	8.5	0.8	0.8	1.5	0.5	2.1	4.3	2.1	6.4
Hernia and intestinal obstruction (without mention of hernia)	1.8	0.7	0.4	1.2	0.3	1.4	0.3	0.1	0.4
Gastritis, duodenitis, enteritis, and colitis, except diarrhea of newborn	5.3	-	0.0*	0.0*	0.0*	0.0*	3.6	1.8	5.3
All other diseases of digestive system	1.4	0.3	0.3	0.4	0.3	0.7	0.5	0.2	0.7
Congenital malformations	33.5	9.2	7.4	16.6	4.9	21.5	8.7	3.2	12.0
Congenital malformations of nervous system and sense organs	9.9	4.2	1.4	5.6	1.2	6.8	2.2	1.0	3.2
Congenital malformations of circulatory system	15.6	2.1	4.1	6.2	2.5	8.6	5.2	1.8	7.0
All other congenital malformations	7.9	2.9	1.9	4.8	1.3	6.1	1.4	0.4	1.8
Birth Injuries	19.6	13.2	5.8	19.0	0.5	19.5	0.0*	0.0*	0.0
Intracranial and spinal injury at birth	5.6	2.3	2.9	5.2	0.4	5.6	0.0*	-	0.0*
Other birth injury	14.0	10.9	2.9	13.8	0.1	13.9	0.0*	0.0*	0.0
Postnatal asphyxia and atelectasis	38.0	23.0	13.3	36.3	1.1	37.4	0.5	0.1	0.6
Pneumonia of newborn	7.2	0.9	2.8	3.6	3.5	7.2	...	...	...
Diarrhea of newborn	0.9	0.0*	0.1	0.1	0.5	0.9	0.0*	0.0*	0.0*
Other infections of newborn	1.5	0.2	0.6	0.8	0.7	1.5	0.0*	-	0.0*
Neonatal disorders arising from certain diseases of the mother during pregnancy	1.9	1.2	0.6	1.8	0.1	1.8	0.0*	-	0.0*
Hemolytic disease of newborn (erythroblastosis)	4.9	3.5	1.2	4.7	0.2	4.9	0.0	0.0*	0.0
Hemorrhagic disease of newborn	1.1	0.4	0.5	1.0	0.2	1.1	0.0*	-	0.0*
Nutritional maladjustment and ill-defined diseases peculiar to early infancy	15.7	7.2	6.1	13.3	0.9	14.1	1.3	0.3	1.5
Immaturity with mention of any other subsidiary condition	2.7	1.0	0.8	1.8	0.3	2.1	0.6	0.0*	0.6
Immaturity, unqualified	40.5	27.3	11.3	38.6	1.6	40.2	0.3	0.0*	0.3
Accidents	7.9	0.2	0.4	0.5	0.8	1.3	4.5	2.1	6.6
Residual	9.5	1.4	1.1	2.5	1.0	3.4	4.3	1.8	6.1

for selected causes of death, by age at death, color and sex: United States, 1959-61 - Continued.

Cause of Death	Under 1 year	Under 1 day	1 - 6 days	Under 7 days	7 - 27 days	Under 28 days	28 days -5 months	6 - 11 months	28 days -11 months
White									
All Causes	228.5	95.6	60.0	155.6	16.6	172.2	41.5	14.8	56.3
Infective and parasitic diseases	2.6	0.0	0.1	0.1	0.2	0.3	1.4	0.9	2.3
Dysentery, All Forms	0.2	-	0.0*	0.0*	0.0*	0.0*	0.1	0.1	0.2
Tuberculosis, septicemia and pyemia, meningococcal infections and measles	1.4	0.0*	0.0*	0.0*	0.0	0.0	0.8	0.5	1.3
All other infective and parasitic diseases	1.0	0.1	0.1	0.1	0.2	0.3	0.5	0.3	0.8
Diseases of nervous system and sense organs	3.5	0.1	0.3	0.4	0.4	0.8	1.7	1.0	2.7
Diseases of respiratory system	21.6	0.2	0.2	0.4	0.3	0.7	16.6	4.3	20.9
Acute upper respiratory infections	0.8	0.0*	0.0	0.0	0.1	0.1	0.5	0.2	0.7
Influenza and pneumonia, except pneumonia of the newborn	16.3	0.0*	0.0*	0.0*	0.0	0.0	12.8	3.4	16.3
Bronchitis and other diseases of the respiratory system	4.5	0.2	0.2	0.4	0.0	0.5	3.2	0.7	3.9
Diseases of digestive system	7.0	0.9	0.9	1.8	0.6	2.4	2.9	1.7	4.6
Hernia and intestinal obstruction (without mention of hernia)	2.2	0.9	0.5	1.4	0.3	1.7	0.4	0.1	0.5
Gastritis, duodenitis, enteritis, and colitis, except diarrhea of newborn	3.4	-	0.0*	0.0*	0.0*	0.0*	2.0	1.4	3.4
All other diseases of digestive system	1.4	0.1	0.4	0.4	0.3	0.7	0.5	0.2	0.7
Congenital malformations	37.5	10.1	9.3	19.3	5.7	25.0	9.4	3.1	12.5
Congenital malformations of nervous system and sense organs	9.7	3.9	1.5	5.4	1.1	6.5	2.2	1.0	3.2
Congenital malformations of circulatory system	18.3	2.4	5.6	8.0	3.0	11.0	5.6	1.6	7.2
All other congenital malformations	9.6	3.7	2.2	5.9	1.6	7.5	1.6	0.5	2.1
Birth Injuries	23.4	15.7	7.1	22.8	0.5	23.3	0.0	0.0*	0.0
Intracranial and spinal injury at birth	6.9	2.7	3.7	6.5	0.4	6.9	-	-	-
Other birth injury	16.5	12.9	3.4	16.3	0.1	16.5	0.0	0.0*	0.0
Postnatal asphyxia and atelectasis	42.2	24.9	15.8	40.6	1.0	41.6	0.5	0.1	0.5
Pneumonia of newborn	6.6	0.8	2.8	3.6	3.0	6.6	...	...	...
Diarrhea of newborn	0.6	0.0*	0.1	0.1	0.5	0.6	-	-	...
Other infections of newborn	1.5	0.2	0.6	0.8	0.7	1.4	0.0*	0.0*	0.0*
Neonatal disorders arising from certain diseases of the mother during pregnancy	2.0	1.2	0.7	2.0	0.1	2.0	0.0	0.0*	0.0
Hemolytic disease of newborn (erythroblastosis)	5.6	3.8	1.6	5.3	0.2	5.5	0.0	0.0*	0.0
Hemorrhagic disease of newborn	1.2	0.4	0.7	1.1	0.1	1.2	0.0*	0.0*	0.0*
Nutritional maladjustment and ill-defined diseases peculiar to early infancy	16.6	7.7	7.4	15.0	0.6	15.7	0.8	0.2	0.9
Immaturity with mention of any other subsidiary condition	2.7	1.1	0.9	2.0	0.3	2.3	0.4	0.0*	0.4
Immaturity, unqualified	39.4	27.5	10.6	38.2	1.1	39.2	0.2	0.0*	0.2
Accidents	7.3	0.1	0.3	0.5	0.6	1.1	4.2	2.0	6.2
Residual	7.3	1.0	0.9	1.9	0.7	2.6	3.2	1.5	4.7

Note: See table for TOTAL deaths for footnote and source.

Table I.4e   Average annual infant mortality rates per 10,000 live births for selected causes of death, by age at death, color and sex: United States, 1959-61 - Continued.

Cause of Death	Under 1 year	Under 1 day	1 - 6 days	Under 7 days	7 - 27 days	Under 28 days	28 days -5 months	6 - 11 months	28 days -11 months
Nonwhite									
All Causes	425.3	143.3	85.3	228.5	40.1	268.6	117.3	39.4	156.7
Infective and parasitic diseases	7.9	0.1	0.3	0.4	1.1	1.5	4.2	2.2	6.4
Dysentery, All Forms	1.1	-	0.0*	0.0*	0.1	0.1	0.6	0.4	1.0
Tuberculosis, septicemia and pyemia, meningococcal infections and measles	3.1	0.0*	0.0*	0.0*	0.1*	0.1*	2.0	1.0	3.0
All other infective and parasitic diseases	3.8	0.1	0.3	0.4	0.9	1.3	1.7	0.8	2.5
Diseases of nervous system and sense organs	7.8	0.2	0.5	0.7	0.7	1.4	3.7	2.6	6.3
Diseases of respiratory system	67.8	0.3	0.4	0.7	0.8	1.6	50.5	15.7	66.2
Acute upper respiratory infections	2.2	-	0.1*	0.1*	0.3	0.3	1.5	0.4	1.9
Influenza and pneumonia, except pneumonia of the newborn	56.4	0.0*	0.1	0.1	0.2	0.3	42.3	13.8	56.1
Bronchitis and other diseases of the respiratory system	9.1	0.3	0.3	0.5	0.4	0.9	6.7	1.5	8.2
Diseases of digestive system	23.9	0.4	1.1	1.5	0.8	2.3	15.7	5.9	21.6
Hernia and intestinal obstruction (without mention of hernia)	2.3	0.3	0.4	0.8	0.4	1.1	1.0	0.3	1.2
Gastritis, duodenitis, enteritis, and colitis, except diarrhea of newborn	19.1	-	0.0*	0.0*	0.0*	0.0*	13.8	5.3	19.1
All other diseases of digestive system	2.4	0.0*	0.7	0.7	0.4	1.1	1.0	0.3	1.3
Congenital malformations	30.4	6.4	6.8	13.2	4.6	17.8	9.2	3.5	12.6
Congenital malformations of nervous system and sense organs	5.6	1.8	0.8	2.6	0.7	3.3	1.5	0.8	2.3
Congenital malformations of circulatory system	15.4	2.0	3.8	5.8	2.1	7.9	5.4	2.1	7.5
All other congenital malformations	9.4	2.6	2.2	4.7	1.9	6.6	2.2	0.6	2.8
Birth injuries	26.9	16.9	8.9	25.8	1.0	26.8	0.1*	0.0*	0.1*
Intracranial and spinal injury at birth	11.2	4.8	5.6	10.4	0.8	11.2	0.0*	-	0.0*
Other birth injury	15.7	12.0	3.4	15.4	0.2	15.6	0.1*	0.0*	0.1*
Postnatal asphyxia and atelectasis	64.8	41.2	20.0	61.2	2.3	63.5	1.1	0.2	1.3
Pneumonia of newborn	18.8	2.2	6.4	8.7	10.2	18.8	...	...	...
Diarrhea of newborn	3.9	0.0*	0.2	0.3	3.6	3.8	0.0*	...	0.0*
Other infections of newborn	3.9	0.4	1.6	2.0	1.9	3.8	0.1*	0.0*	0.1*
Neonatal disorders arising from certain diseases of the mother during pregnancy	3.0	1.9	0.9	2.8	0.1	3.0	0.0*	0.0*	0.0*
Hemolytic disease of newborn (erythroblastosis)	2.2	0.9	1.0	1.9	0.3	2.2	0.1*	-	0.1*
Hemorrhagic disease of newborn	2.8	0.9	1.5	2.3	0.4	2.8	0.0*	-	0.0*
Nutritional maladjustment and ill-defined diseases peculiar to early infancy	31.5	13.3	8.6	21.9	2.7	24.6	6.0	0.9	6.9
Immaturity with mention of any other subsidiary condition	5.6	1.7	1.4	3.1	0.7	3.8	1.7	0.1*	1.8
Immaturity, unqualified	77.8	51.6	21.0	72.6	4.3	76.9	0.9	0.0*	0.9
Accidents	17.0	0.4	1.1	1.5	1.5	3.1	10.1	3.9	13.9
Residual	29.5	4.7	3.8	8.4	3.0	11.4	13.6	4.5	18.1

Table I.5

Average annual infant mortality rates per 1,000 live births by age at death and color; United States and each geographic division, selected decennium periods.

Age, color and decennium	United States	Geographic division								
		New England	Middle Atlantic	East North Central	West North Central	South Atlantic	East South Central	West South Central	Mountain	Pacific
Under 1 year										
Total										
1959-61[1]	25.9	22.5	24.2	24.1	22.8	30.4	31.7	28.3	27.4	23.6
1949-51	29.6	24.3	25.8	26.6	26.1	34.0	37.4	36.2	37.1	25.3
1939-41	46.8	38.6	39.3	39.1	39.5	58.6	56.1	58.3	60.6	37.8
White										
1959-61[1]	22.8	21.9	21.8	22.3	21.6	23.7	25.3	24.2	25.7	22.7
1949-51	27.1	24.0	24.3	25.6	25.2	28.4	33.4	33.7	33.9	24.7
1939-41	42.9	38.3	37.8	38.2	38.1	49.4	50.9	54.1	56.7	37.1
Nonwhite										
1959-61[1]	42.5	37.5	41.9	38.2	41.4	46.5	46.9	43.5	48.7	30.4
1949-51	45.5	41.2	42.2	39.4	47.6	46.9	46.8	46.3	94.4	34.5
1939-41	74.3	59.2	62.8	58.3	80.5	79.7	69.7	76.1	160.1	55.1
Under 28 days[2]										
Total										
1959-61[1]	18.7	17.1	18.5	18.0	17.1	20.7	21.2	19.5	19.2	17.4
1949-51	20.7	18.6	19.6	19.4	19.3	22.4	24.1	22.6	23.3	18.7
1939-41	28.5	26.0	26.2	25.7	25.9	33.5	32.2	32.0	31.5	24.9
White										
1959-61[1]	17.2	16.7	16.8	16.9	16.5	17.9	18.7	17.6	18.9	16.8
1949-51	19.5	18.4	18.5	18.7	19.0	20.2	22.5	21.4	22.7	18.3
1939-41	27.0	25.8	25.5	25.2	25.5	30.0	30.4	29.8	30.7	24.8
Nonwhite										
1959-61[1]	26.9	27.2	30.7	26.8	26.6	27.3	27.1	26.4	23.5	21.2
1949-51	27.8	31.0	30.5	26.8	27.7	27.6	27.9	27.4	34.2	23.2
1939-41	39.4	37.0	37.6	34.8	39.2	41.6	36.9	41.0	52.4	28.1
28 days-11 months[2]										
Total										
1959-61[1]	7.2	5.4	5.7	6.0	5.7	9.7	10.6	8.8	8.2	6.3
1949-51	9.0	5.7	6.3	7.3	6.8	11.6	13.3	13.6	13.8	6.7
1939-41	18.2	12.6	13.1	13.4	13.6	25.1	23.9	26.4	29.1	12.9
White										
1959-61[1]	5.6	5.2	5.0	5.4	5.1	5.7	6.7	6.6	6.8	5.9
1949-51	7.6	5.6	5.7	6.8	6.2	8.2	10.9	12.3	11.2	6.3
1939-41	15.8	12.5	12.3	13.0	12.6	19.4	20.5	24.3	26.0	12.3
Nonwhite										
1959-61[1]	15.7	10.3	11.2	11.4	14.9	19.2	19.8	17.1	25.3	9.2
1949-51	17.7	10.2	11.7	12.6	19.8	19.2	18.9	18.8	60.2	11.3
1939-41	34.9	22.3	25.3	23.5	41.3	38.1	32.8	35.0	107.7	27.0

Source: Annual volumes Vital Statistics of the United States, National Center for Health Statistics, Public Health Service, Washington.

[1]Includes Alaska and Hawaii.

[2]1939-41 age categories are "under 1 month" and "1-11 months," respectively.

Table I.6   Infant mortality rates per 1,000 live births by age at death and color
for urban and rural areas and population-size groups:
United States, 1940, 1950 and 1960.

Area	1960			1950			1940		
	Total	White	Nonwhite	Total	White	Nonwhite	Total	White	Nonwhite
Under 1 year	26.0	22.9	43.2	29.2	26.8	44.5	47.0	43.2	73.8
Urban	26.3	23.2	40.9	28.4	26.3	42.6	44.4	41.1	74.4
100,000 or more	27.9	23.9	39.3	27.1	24.6	39.0	39.3	36.1	64.0
50,000-100,000	24.4	22.6	37.7	27.8	25.8	43.3 }			
25,000-50,000	23.9	21.8	44.3	28.2	26.5	43.4 }	46.5[1]	42.9[1]	86.2
10,000-25,000	24.5	22.3	47.7	29.0	27.0	51.0 }			
2,500-10,000	26.6	24.3	48.8	32.2	30.0	54.4	53.4	50.2	90.0
Rural	25.7	22.4	48.5	30.4	27.6	47.0	50.1	45.9	73.4
Under 28 days	18.7	17.2	26.9	20.5	19.4	27.5	28.8	27.2	39.7
Urban	19.5	17.9	27.6	21.2	20.0	29.0	28.9	27.4	42.8
100,000 or more	20.7	18.3	27.7	20.7	19.1	28.3 }			
50,000-100,000	18.5	17.7	24.7	20.7	19.7	28.6 }	28.0[1]	26.4[1]	42.3[1]
25,000-50,000	17.9	16.9	28.0	21.1	20.3	28.1 }			
10,000-25,000	18.4	17.3	29.6	21.2	20.2	32.2 }			
2,500-10,000	19.4	18.5	27.5	22.8	21.9	31.6	32.8	31.7	45.3
Rural	17.4	16.3	25.1	19.5	18.4	25.5	28.6	27.0	37.5
28 days - 11 months	7.3	5.7	16.3	8.7	7.4	16.9	18.3	16.0	34.1
Urban	6.7	5.4	13.3	7.2	6.3	13.6	15.5	13.7	31.6
100,000 or more	7.2	5.6	11.6	6.4	5.5	10.7 }			
50,000-100,000	5.9	4.9	13.0	7.0	6.0	14.7 }	14.3[1]	12.6[1]	29.2[1]
25,000-50,000	6.0	5.0	16.3	7.1	6.2	15.3 }			
10,000-25,000	6.2	5.0	18.1	7.8	6.8	18.8 }			
2,500-10,000	7.2	5.7	21.3	9.4	8.1	22.7	20.6	18.5	44.7
Rural	8.3	6.1	23.3	11.0	9.2	21.5	21.5	18.9	35.9

Source: Annual volumes Vital Statistics of the United States, National Center for Health Statistics, Public Health Service, Washington.

Note: In general, urban includes incorporated places with 2,500 inhabitants or more; all remaining places are classified as rural. Cities are classified by size as of the particular census period for which the rates have been computed.

[1]Data available only for cities of 10,000-100,000 combined for "under 1 year"; and only for cities of 10,000 or more combined for "under 28 days" and for "28 days-11 months."

Average annual infant mortality rates per 1,000 live births, as by age at death and race, for urban and rural areas, and population-size groups in metropolitan and nonmetropolitan counties: United States, 1950 and 1960-61.

Area	Total						White						Nonwhite					
	Under 1 year		Under 28 days		28 days-11 months		Under 1 year		Under 28 days		28 days-11 months		Under 1 year		Under 28 days		28 days-11 months	
	1960-61	1950	1960-61	1950	1960-61	1950	1960-61	1950	1960-61	1950	1960-61	1950	1960-61	1950	1960-61	1950	1960-61	1950
United States	25.7	29.2	18.6	20.5	7.1	8.7	22.7	26.8	17.1	19.4	5.6	7.4	42.0	44.5	26.5	27.5	15.4	16.9
Urban[1,2]																		
Places of 1,000,000 or more	25.9	28.4	19.3	21.2	6.5	7.2	22.9	26.3	17.7	20.0	5.3	6.3	40.0	42.6	27.3	29.0	12.6	13.6
Places of 250,000-1,000,000	27.1	26.0	20.1	21.2	7.0	6.1	22.5	23.3	17.0	18.0	5.5	5.3	38.4	38.3	27.7	28.6	10.7	9.7
Places of 100,000-250,000	27.9	27.4	20.9	21.1	7.0	6.3	24.2	25.2	18.6	19.8	5.6	5.4	37.7	37.4	26.9	27.1	10.7	10.4
Places of 50,000-100,000	26.5	28.2	19.8	21.2	6.7	6.9	23.3	25.8	18.0	19.7	5.3	5.8	39.8	43.7	27.5	30.2	12.3	13.5
Places of 25,000-50,000	24.3	27.8	18.4	20.7	5.9	7.0	22.3	25.8	17.4	19.7	5.0	6.0	38.9	43.3	26.3	28.6	12.6	14.7
Places of 10,000-25,000	23.8	28.2	17.9	21.1	5.9	7.1	21.9	26.5	16.9	20.3	4.9	6.2	42.5	43.4	27.4	28.1	15.0	15.3
Places of 2,500-10,000	26.1	29.0	18.2	21.1	6.1	7.8	22.2	27.0	17.2	20.2	5.1	6.8	45.8	51.0	28.6	32.2	17.2	18.8
	26.1	32.2	19.1	22.8	7.0	9.4	23.8	30.0	18.3	21.9	5.5	8.1	48.0	54.4	27.5	31.6	20.6	22.7
Rural[1]	25.3	30.4	17.3	19.5	8.0	11.0	22.3	27.6	16.2	18.4	6.1	9.2	46.5	47.0	24.7	25.5	21.8	21.5
Metropolitan Counties	24.7	26.4	18.4	19.8	6.2	6.7	22.0	24.5	16.9	18.6	5.2	5.9	38.6	40.0	26.8	28.1	11.8	11.9
Urban[1,2]																		
Places of 1,000,000 or more	25.4	26.5	19.1	20.2	6.3	6.3	22.4	24.4	17.3	18.9	5.1	5.5	38.3	39.5	27.1	28.2	11.3	11.3
Places of 250,000-1,000,000	27.1	26.0	20.1	19.9	7.0	6.1	22.5	23.3	17.0	18.0	5.5	5.3	38.4	38.3	27.7	28.6	10.7	9.7
Places of 100,000-250,000	27.9	27.4	20.9	21.1	7.0	6.3	24.2	25.2	18.6	19.8	5.6	5.4	37.7	37.4	26.9	27.1	10.7	10.4
Places of 50,000-100,000	26.5	28.2	19.8	21.2	6.7	6.9	23.3	25.8	18.0	19.7	5.3	5.8	39.8	43.7	27.5	30.2	12.3	13.5
Places of 25,000-50,000	24.4	27.8	18.5	20.7	5.9	7.0	22.3	25.8	17.4	19.7	5.0	6.0	38.9	43.3	26.3	28.6	12.6	14.7
Places of 10,000-25,000	21.4	25.0	16.5	19.2	4.9	5.8	20.4	24.2	15.9	18.8	4.4	5.3	36.2	37.0	26.8	25.3	13.1	13.1
Places of 2,500-10,000	21.5	22.6	16.6	17.3	4.9	5.3	21.0	21.9	16.0	16.8	4.9	5.0	39.8	44.1	26.6	26.2	14.3	10.8
	21.8	23.4	16.5	17.9	5.3	5.6	20.4	22.6	16.2	17.4	5.5	5.2	36.7	44.1	22.4	29.9	14.3	14.2
Rural[1]	22.3	26.4	16.3	18.2	6.0	8.2	20.8	24.9	15.6	17.4	5.2	7.5	40.6	44.0	24.5	27.6	16.1	16.3
Nonmetropolitan Counties	27.5	32.6	18.8	21.4	8.7	11.2	23.8	29.7	17.5	20.4	6.3	9.3	48.4	49.0	26.1	26.9	22.3	22.1
Urban[1,2]																		
Places of 25,000-50,000	27.6	33.8	20.1	24.0	7.5	9.8	24.5	31.3	18.8	22.9	5.7	8.4	48.3	52.9	28.7	31.8	19.6	21.1
Places of 10,000-25,000	26.6	30.4	19.6	22.3	7.0	8.0	23.5	28.7	18.2	21.4	5.3	6.9	45.5	45.0	28.2	29.0	17.3	16.0
Places of 2,500-10,000	27.2	33.3	19.8	23.8	7.4	9.5	24.2	30.7	18.4	22.6	5.8	8.1	48.4	55.5	29.5	34.2	18.9	21.3
	28.6	36.0	20.7	24.9	7.9	11.1	25.5	33.5	19.5	24.1	6.0	9.4	50.4	55.8	28.5	31.9	21.9	23.9
Rural[1]	27.4	32.0	17.9	20.0	9.5	12.0	23.3	28.7	16.6	18.9	6.7	9.8	48.4	47.5	24.8	25.1	23.7	22.4

Source: Annual volumes Vital Statistics of the United States, National Center for Health Statistics, Public Health Service, Washington, and special tabulations.

[1] In general, urban includes incorporated places with 2,500 inhabitants or more; all remaining places are classified as rural.

[2] Cities are classified by their size size as of the particular census period for which the rates have been computed.

Table I.8   Average annual infant mortality rates per 1,000 live
births by age at death for Negroes and other races:
United States and each geographic division, 1959-61.

Area and race	Under 1 year	Under 28 days	Under 1 day	1-6 days	7-27 days	28 days - 11 months
United States[1]	25.9	18.7	10.3	6.4	2.0	7.2
Negro	43.7	27.8	14.8	8.8	4.2	15.9
Other	30.0	16.7	9.2	5.3	2.2	13.4
New England[1]	22.5	17.1	9.9	5.6	1.6	5.4
Negro	39.7	28.8	18.4	7.6	2.9	10.9
Other	13.7†	10.2†	*	*	*	*
Middle Atlantic[1]	24.2	18.5	10.7	6.1	1.7	5.7
Negro	42.6	31.2	19.2	9.0	3.0	11.4
Other	20.5	16.1	9.8	5.3†	*	4.3†
East North Central[1]	24.1	18.0	10.5	5.8	1.7	6.0
Negro	38.6	27.2	16.3	8.0	2.9	11.4
Other	24.6	14.0	8.9	3.3†	*	10.6
West North Central[1]	22.8	17.1	9.6	5.8	1.8	5.7
Negro	41.3	28.1	15.3	8.8	3.9	13.2
Other	41.9	18.8	10.0	5.2	3.5†	23.1
South Atlantic[1]	30.4	20.7	10.7	7.4	2.7	9.7
Negro	46.8	27.5	13.6	9.2	4.7	19.3
Other	26.7	15.6	8.9	4.1†	2.6†	11.0
East South Central[1]	31.7	21.2	10.5	7.6	3.0	10.6
Negro	47.0	27.2	12.5	9.2	5.4	19.9
Other	25.1†	*	*	*	*	*
West South Central[1]	28.3	19.5	9.7	7.3	2.6	8.8
Negro	44.1	26.8	12.7	9.1	5.0	17.3
Other	26.9	14.9	7.8	5.1†	2.1†	12.0
Mountain[1]	27.4	19.2	10.2	7.0	2.0	8.2
Negro	46.1	30.8	17.1	8.9	4.8	15.3
Other	50.0	19.9	9.1	6.9	3.9	30.2
Pacific[1]	23.6	17.4	10.0	5.8	1.6	6.3
Negro	35.5	25.7	15.7	7.4	2.6	9.8
Other	24.6	16.2	9.4	5.2	1.6	8.5

Source: Annual volumes Vital Statistics of the United States,
National Center for Health Statistics, Public Health Service, Washington, and
special tabulations.

[1]Includes all races. (See Table I.9).
*Rates not computed, based on less than 20 deaths.
†Rates based on between 20 and 49 deaths.

Table I.9a   Average annual infant mortality rates per 1,000 live births by age at death and color: United States, each geographic division and State, 1959-61.

Area and color	Under 1 year	Under 28 days	Under 1 day	1-6 days	7-27 days	28 days - 11 months
United States	25.9	18.7	10.3	6.4	2.0	7.2
White	22.8	17.2	9.6	6.0	1.7	5.6
Nonwhite	42.5	26.9	14.3	8.6	4.0	15.7
New England	22.5	17.1	9.9	5.6	1.6	5.4
White	21.9	16.7	9.6	5.6	1.6	5.2
Nonwhite	37.5	27.2	17.5	7.1	2.6	10.3
Maine	25.6	18.8	10.8	6.0	2.0	6.8
White	25.7	18.9	10.8	6.0	2.0	6.8
Nonwhite	*	*	*	*	-	*
New Hampshire	23.4	17.6	10.0	5.8	1.7	5.8
White	23.4	17.6	10.1	5.8	1.7	5.8
Nonwhite	*	*	-	*	*	*
Vermont	25.0	18.6	11.6	5.3	1.7†	6.4
White	25.0	18.7	11.6	5.4	1.7†	6.4
Nonwhite	-	-	-	-	-	-
Massachusetts	21.8	16.6	9.3	5.8	1.6	5.2
White	21.3	16.3	9.1	5.7	1.5	5.0
Nonwhite	34.3	24.0	14.5	6.8	2.7†	10.3
Rhode Island	23.3	17.1	10.2	5.5	1.4	6.1
White	22.8	16.9	10.1	5.5	1.3	5.9
Nonwhite	34.2	22.3	13.1†	*	*	11.8†
Connecticut	21.9	17.1	10.5	5.2	1.5	4.8
White	20.4	16.0	9.6	5.0	1.4	4.4
Nonwhite	43.9	33.5	23.1	7.8	2.7†	10.4

Area and color	Under 1 year	Under 28 days	Under 1 day	1-6 days	7-27 days	28 days - 11 months
East North Central—continued						
Illinois	24.8	18.0	10.7	5.6	1.7	6.8
White	22.1	16.6	9.8	5.3	1.5	5.5
Nonwhite	38.5	25.1	15.3	7.0	2.7	13.4
Michigan	24.1	18.3	10.7	5.8	1.7	5.8
White	22.5	17.2	10.0	5.6	1.6	5.4
Nonwhite	36.9	27.2	16.4	7.9	2.9	9.7
Wisconsin	22.6	17.1	10.1	5.5	1.5	5.5
White	22.0	16.8	9.9	5.4	1.4	5.3
Nonwhite	37.4	25.6	15.9	6.9	2.3†	11.8
West North Central	22.8	17.1	9.6	5.8	1.8	5.7
White	21.6	16.5	9.2	5.6	1.7	5.1
Nonwhite	41.4	26.5	14.4	8.2	3.9	14.9
Minnesota	21.6	16.1	9.5	5.1	1.5	5.5
White	21.4	16.1	9.4	5.1	1.5	5.3
Nonwhite	30.4	17.6	11.2	5.0†	*	12.3
Iowa	21.3	16.3	9.3	5.4	1.6	5.0
White	21.1	16.2	9.2	5.4	1.6	4.9
Nonwhite	35.9	23.7	16.5	*	*	12.2†
Missouri	24.6	18.1	9.8	6.1	2.2	6.5
White	21.6	16.3	8.8	5.6	1.9	5.3
Nonwhite	43.5	29.2	15.9	9.2	4.1	14.3

Middle Atlantic	24.2	18.5	10.7	6.1	1.7	5.7
White	21.8	16.3	9.6	5.8	1.5	5.0
Nonwhite	41.9	30.7	18.9	8.9	3.0	11.2
New York	24.2	18.4	10.8	5.9	1.6	5.8
White	21.6	16.5	9.5	5.6	1.4	5.1
Nonwhite	41.5	30.6	19.4	8.5	2.7	10.9
New Jersey	24.2	18.5	10.0	6.6	1.9	5.7
White	21.4	16.6	9.0	6.0	1.6	4.8
Nonwhite	42.3	30.4	16.0	10.4	3.9	12.0
Pennsylvania	24.3	18.7	11.0	6.1	1.7	5.6
White	22.2	17.3	9.9	5.8	1.6	4.9
Nonwhite	42.3	31.1	19.9	8.5	2.7	11.2
East North Central	24.1	18.0	10.5	5.8	1.7	6.0
White	22.3	16.9	9.8	5.6	1.5	5.4
Nonwhite	38.2	26.8	16.1	7.9	2.8	11.4
Ohio	24.1	18.5	10.6	6.3	1.6	5.5
White	22.3	17.2	9.8	5.9	1.5	5.1
Nonwhite	38.7	29.4	17.7	9.0	2.7	9.3
Indiana	23.7	17.4	10.0	5.6	1.8	6.4
White	22.4	16.6	9.6	5.4	1.6	5.3
Nonwhite	38.8	26.6	14.8	8.3	3.5	12.2

North Dakota	23.9	18.3	9.9	6.6	1.8	5.6
White	23.1	18.1	9.9	6.6	1.6	5.0
Nonwhite	43.8	23.5†	10.9†	*	*	20.3†
South Dakota	25.4	17.7	9.7	5.7	2.4	7.6
White	22.3	17.0	9.5	5.4	2.1	5.4
Nonwhite	63.5	27.3	12.7	9.1†	5.6†	36.2
Nebraska	22.7	17.5	9.6	6.2	1.6	5.2
White	22.0	17.2	9.4	6.2	1.6	4.9
Nonwhite	36.7	24.2	14.1	7.0†	*	12.5
Kansas	22.3	17.0	9.4	5.9	1.7	5.3
White	21.5	16.6	9.3	5.8	1.6	4.9
Nonwhite	33.1	22.5	11.2	8.0	3.3†	10.6
South Atlantic	30.4	20.7	10.7	7.4	2.7	9.7
White	23.7	17.9	9.5	6.6	1.8	5.7
Nonwhite	46.5	27.3	13.5	9.1	4.7	19.2
Delaware	24.9	18.2	10.2	6.2	1.8	6.8
White	19.8	15.5	8.7	5.5	1.3†	4.3
Nonwhite	47.0	29.7	16.6	9.4	3.7†	17.3
Maryland	27.2	20.0	10.9	6.8	2.3	7.1
White	22.1	17.2	9.5	5.9	1.7	5.0
Nonwhite	44.4	29.7	15.5	9.7	4.5	14.6
District of Columbia	36.2	27.4	17.6	7.7	2.1	8.8
White	29.4	23.4	13.8	7.7	1.9†	6.0
Nonwhite	39.4	29.3	19.4	7.6	2.2	10.1

Source: Annual volumes Vital Statistics of the United States, National Center for Health Statistics, Public Health Service, Washington, and special tabulations.

*Rates not computed, based on less than 20 deaths.

†Rates based on between 20 and 49 deaths.

Table I.9b Average annual infant mortality rates per 1,000 live births by age at death and color: United States, each geographic division and State, 1959-61 - continued.

Area and color	Under 1 year	Under 28 days	Under 1 day	1-6 days	7-27 days	28 days - 11 months
South Atlantic - continued						
Virginia	29.6	20.9	10.9	7.5	2.5	8.7
White	24.2	18.2	9.6	6.8	1.8	6.0
Nonwhite	45.9	29.0	14.6	9.6	4.7	17.0
West Virginia	26.5	18.7	8.9	7.4	2.4	7.7
White	26.0	18.7	9.0	7.4	2.4	7.3
Nonwhite	34.6	19.6	8.2	8.2	*	15.0
North Carolina	31.7	20.6	10.2	7.5	2.9	11.1
White	23.1	17.4	9.0	6.6	1.8	5.7
Nonwhite	50.3	27.5	12.7	9.5	5.2	22.8
South Carolina	33.9	20.0	9.1	7.5	3.4	13.8
White	23.4	17.0	8.5	6.8	1.7	6.5
Nonwhite	48.1	24.2	9.3	8.6	5.8	23.9
Georgia	31.6	20.8	10.6	7.3	2.9	10.8
White	23.5	17.9	9.5	6.7	1.7	5.6
Nonwhite	46.3	26.0	12.7	8.3	5.0	20.3
Florida	30.1	21.1	11.2	7.4	2.5	9.0
White	24.0	18.6	10.2	6.5	1.8	5.4
Nonwhite	46.5	27.7	13.7	9.8	4.3	18.8
East South Central	31.7	21.2	10.5	7.6	3.0	10.6
White	25.3	18.7	9.7	7.0	2.0	6.7
Nonwhite	46.9	27.1	12.5	9.2	5.4	19.8

Area and color	Under 1 year	Under 28 days	Under 1 day	1-6 days	7-27 days	28 days - 11 months
West South Central - continued						
Texas	28.0	19.3	9.6	7.3	2.4	8.3
White	25.5	18.1	9.1	6.9	2.0	7.4
Nonwhite	42.6	26.0	12.3	9.2	4.4	16.5
Mountain	27.4	19.2	10.2	7.0	2.0	8.2
White	25.7	18.9	10.1	6.9	1.9	6.8
Nonwhite	48.7	23.5	11.7	7.6	4.2	25.3
Montana	25.0	17.4	9.3	6.3	1.9	7.6
White	23.5	17.1	9.1	6.2	1.8	6.4
Nonwhite	44.1	21.3	10.8†	7.4†	*	22.9
Idaho	22.7	17.1	9.2	6.3	1.7	5.6
White	22.5	17.1	9.2	6.4	1.6	5.4
Nonwhite	35.2†	*	*	*	*	*
Wyoming	27.4	20.8	11.4	7.4	2.1	6.6
White	26.6	20.5	11.2	7.3	2.0†	6.1
Nonwhite	50.9†	29.6†	*	*	*	*
Colorado	27.5	20.9	12.0	7.1	1.8	6.6
White	27.0	20.6	11.3	7.0	1.8	6.4
Nonwhite	40.9	29.3	17.9	8.2†	*	11.6
New Mexico	31.9	20.6	10.0	8.0	2.6	11.3
White	30.1	20.4	10.3	8.0	2.4	9.7
Nonwhite	46.8	21.8	9.8	7.6	4.5†	24.9

Kentucky	27.7	19.7	10.2	7.0	2.5	8.0
White	26.1	18.8	9.8	6.7	2.3	7.3
Nonwhite	44.0	28.6	13.8	9.5	5.4	15.4
Tennessee	29.5	20.6	10.6	7.4	2.6	9.1
White	25.7	19.0	9.7	7.2	2.1	6.8
Nonwhite	43.1	26.1	13.5	8.2	4.4	17.0
Alabama	31.7	20.8	10.1	7.7	3.1	10.9
White	24.0	17.9	9.3	6.8	1.7	6.2
Nonwhite	44.6	25.8	11.3	9.2	5.3	18.9
Mississippi	39.4	24.3	11.5	8.6	4.2	15.2
White	24.9	19.2	10.2	7.2	1.8	5.7
Nonwhite	51.8	28.6	12.7	9.7	6.2	23.2
West South Central	28.3	19.5	9.7	7.3	2.6	8.8
White	24.2	17.6	8.9	6.8	1.9	6.6
Nonwhite	43.5	26.4	12.5	9.0	4.9	17.1
Arkansas	27.1	17.4	7.9	6.9	2.6	9.7
White	22.2	16.2	7.7	6.8	1.8	6.0
Nonwhite	38.6	20.1	8.3	7.4	4.5	18.5
Louisiana	31.8	22.0	11.1	7.6	3.4	9.7
White	22.0	17.2	9.0	6.4	1.8	4.8
Nonwhite	46.9	29.5	14.3	9.5	5.8	17.4
Oklahoma	24.5	17.6	9.1	6.5	2.1	6.9
White	22.1	16.6	8.6	6.3	1.8	5.4
Nonwhite	39.6	23.8	12.2	7.6	4.0	15.8
Arizona	31.9	20.1	10.8	6.8	2.5	11.7
White	27.5	19.5	10.7	6.6	2.1	8.0
Nonwhite	55.3	23.6	11.4	7.7	4.5	31.7
Utah	20.0	15.0	7.2	6.5	1.3	5.0
White	19.4	14.9	7.1	6.5	1.2	4.6
Nonwhite	43.1	20.5†	11.1†	*	*	22.7†
Nevada	30.2	21.5	11.0	8.2	2.3	8.7
White	28.3	21.3	11.0	8.4	1.9†	6.9
Nonwhite	43.6	22.9	10.7†	*	*	20.7
Pacific	23.6	17.4	10.0	5.8	1.6	6.3
White	22.7	16.8	9.6	5.7	1.5	5.9
Nonwhite	30.4	21.2	12.7	6.3	2.2	9.2
Washington	23.4	17.0	9.7	5.8	1.5	6.3
White	22.5	16.7	9.5	5.7	1.5	5.8
Nonwhite	37.8	22.6	13.2	7.3	2.2†	15.2
Oregon	23.7	16.8	9.6	5.8	1.4	6.9
White	23.4	16.8	9.5	5.9	1.4	6.6
Nonwhite	32.0	17.6	11.5†	*	*	14.4
California	23.4	17.3	10.0	5.7	1.6	6.1
White	22.6	16.8	9.6	5.7	1.6	5.8
Nonwhite	29.7	21.6	13.1	6.4	2.1	8.1
Alaska	40.0	23.3	12.0	7.6	3.7	16.7
White	26.8	20.0	11.5	6.7	1.9†	6.8
Nonwhite	66.9	30.0	13.1	9.4	7.5	36.8
Hawaii	22.9	18.0	11.0	5.8	1.1	4.9
White	22.1	17.6	10.6	6.3	*	4.5
Nonwhite	23.3	18.2	11.2	5.7	1.3†	5.1

Table I.10a   Average annual infant mortality rates per 10,000 live births for selected causes of death by age at death and color, in metropolitan and nonmetropolitan counties: United States and each geographic region, 1959-61.

Cause of Death (7th Revision-International Classification of Diseases)	Total			White			Nonwhite		
	Under 1 year	Under 28 days	28 days - 11 months	Under 1 year	Under 28 days	28 days - 11 months	Under 1 year	Under 28 days	28 days - 11 months
United States[1]									
All causes	259.0	187.1	71.9	228.5	172.2	56.3	425.3	268.6	156.7
Infective and parasitic diseases (001-138)	3.4	0.5	2.9	2.6	0.3	2.3	7.9	1.5	6.4
Influenza and pneumonia, including pneumonia of newborn (480-493,763)	31.0	8.6	22.4	22.9	6.6	16.3	75.2	19.2	56.1
All other diseases of respiratory system (470-475, 500-527)	6.2	0.7	5.5	5.3	0.6	4.6	11.3	1.2	10.1
Gastritis, duodenitis, enteritis and colitis, including diarrhea of newborn[2] (543, 571, 572, 764)	6.9	1.1	5.8	4.0	0.6	3.4	23.0	3.9	19.1
All other diseases of digestive system (530-542, 544-570, 573-587)	3.8	2.4	1.4	3.6	2.4	1.2	4.7	2.3	2.5
Congenital malformations (750-759)	36.4	23.9	12.5	37.5	25.0	12.5	30.4	17.8	12.6
Birth injuries (760, 761)	23.9	23.9	0.0	23.4	23.3	0.0	26.9	26.8	0.1*
Intracranial and spinal injury at birth (760)	7.5	7.5	0.0*	6.9	6.9	-	11.2	11.2	0.0*
Other birth injury (761)	16.4	16.4	0.0	16.5	16.5	0.0	15.7	15.6	0.1*
Postnatal asphyxia and atelectasis (762)	45.7	45.0	0.7	42.2	41.6	0.5	64.8	63.5	1.3
Hemolytic disease of newborn (770)	5.0	5.0	0.0	5.6	5.5	0.0	2.2	2.2	0.1*
Immaturity unqualified (776)	45.4	45.1	0.3	39.4	39.2	0.2	77.8	76.9	0.9
Neonatal disorders arising from certain diseases of mother, etc.[3] (769, 771-774)	25.7	23.2	2.5	22.6	21.2	1.4	42.8	34.1	8.7
Accidents (E800-E962)	8.8	1.4	7.4	7.3	1.1	6.2	17.0	3.1	14.0
Residual (140-468, 590-749, 765-768, 780-793, 795, E963-E999)	16.8	6.7	10.1	12.3	4.8	7.5	41.1	16.7	24.5
Metropolitan Counties									
All causes	249.1	186.5	62.6	222.0	170.4	51.7	392.6	272.0	120.6
Infective and parasitic diseases (001-138)	2.4	0.3	2.1	2.0	0.2	1.8	4.5	0.6	3.9
Influenza and pneumonia, including pneumonia of newborn (480-493, 763)	28.2	8.2	20.0	21.6	6.5	15.1	63.1	17.4	45.7
All other diseases of respiratory system (470-475, 500-527)	6.5	0.7	5.9	5.6	0.6	5.0	11.5	1.0	10.5
Gastritis, duodenitis, enteritis and colitis, including diarrhea of newborn[2] (543, 571, 572, 764)	4.5	0.7	3.8	2.9	0.4	2.5	12.7	2.0	10.7
All other diseases of digestive system (530-542, 544-570, 573-587)	3.7	2.4	1.3	3.5	2.4	1.1	4.5	2.5	2.1

Congenital malformations (750-759)	36.1	23.7	12.4	37.0	24.7	12.3	31.4	18.5	12.9
Birth injuries (760, 761)	23.2	23.1	0.0	22.5	22.5	0.0	26.9	26.8	0.1*
Intracranial and spinal injury at birth (760)	7.7	7.7	-	6.9	6.9	-	12.0	12.0	-
Other birth injury (761)	15.5	15.4	0.0	15.5	15.5	0.6	14.8	14.8	0.1*
Postnatal asphyxia and atelectasis (762)	49.5	48.8	0.7	44.5	44.0	0.6	76.0	74.6	1.4
Hemolytic disease of newborn (770)	5.2	5.1	0.0	5.7	5.7	0.0	2.3	2.2	0.1*
Immaturity unqualified (776)	44.8	44.5	0.2	38.2	38.1	0.2	79.5	78.9	0.6
Neonatal disorders arising from certain diseases of mother, etc.[3] (769, 771-774)	24.3	22.5	1.7	21.2	20.2	1.0	40.7	35.2	5.5
Accidents (E800-E962)	7.0	1.0	6.0	6.0	0.8	5.2	12.5	2.0	10.5
Residual (140-468, 590-749, 765-768, 780-793, 795, E963-E999)	13.8	5.4	8.4	11.4	4.5	6.9	26.9	10.3	16.6
Nonmetropolitan Counties									
All causes	276.5	188.8	87.7	239.8	175.8	64.0	486.8	263.3	223.6
Infective and parasitic diseases(001-138)	5.2	0.8	4.4	3.6	0.4	3.2	14.2	3.2	11.1
Influenza and pneumonia, including pneumonia of newborn (480-493, 763)	36.1	9.3	26.8	25.2	7.0	18.3	98.2	22.6	75.6
All other diseases of respiratory system (470-475, 500-527)	5.6	0.8	4.8	4.7	0.7	4.0	11.0	1.6	9.4
Gastritis, duodenitis, enteritis, and colitis, including diarrhea of newborn[2] (543, 571, 572, 764)	11.3	1.8	9.5	5.8	0.8	5.0	42.3	7.4	35.0
All other diseases of digestive system (530-542, 544-570, 573-587)	4.0	2.3	1.7	3.8	2.4	1.4	5.1	1.9	3.2
Congenital malformations (750-759)	36.9	24.2	12.7	38.4	25.5	12.8	28.4	16.4	12.1
Birth injuries (760, 761)	25.2	25.2	0.1	24.9	24.9	0.0*	27.0	26.9	0.2*
Intracranial and spinal injury at birth (760)	7.2	7.2	0.0*	6.8	6.8	-	9.7	9.7	0.0*
Other birth injury (761)	18.1	18.0	0.1	18.2	18.1	0.0*	17.4	17.3	0.1*
Postnatal asphyxia and atelectasis (762)	38.9	38.3	0.6	38.1	37.5	0.5	43.6	42.5	1.1
Hemolytic disease of newborn (770)	4.8	4.8	0.1	5.3	5.3	0.1*	2.1	2.0	0.1*
Immaturity unqualified (776)	46.5	46.1	0.4	41.5	41.3	0.2	74.5	73.0	1.5
Neonatal disorders arising from certain diseases of mother, etc.[3] (769, 771-774)	28.3	24.3	3.9	25.0	23.0	2.0	46.9	32.1	14.8
Accidents (E800-E962)	12.0	2.1	9.8	9.6	1.6	8.0	25.4	5.0	20.4
Residual (140-468, 590-749, 765-768, 780-793, 795, E963-E999)	21.9	8.9	13.1	13.9	5.4	8.5	67.9	28.7	39.3

Source: Special tabulations of the Division of Vital Statistics, National Center for Health Statistics, Public Health Service, Washington.

[1] Includes Alaska and Hawaii.

[2] Rates for cause 764 (Diarrhea of newborn) for geographic regions estimated on basis of number of deaths from this cause reported for United States by age at death and color in metropolitan and nonmetropolitan regions. Deaths from this cause not tabulated by geographic region.

[3] Includes neonatal disorders arising from certain diseases of the mother during pregnancy, hemorrhagic disease of newborn; illdefined diseases peculiar to early infancy, including nutritional maladjustment; immaturity with mention of any other subsidiary condition.

*Rates based on less than 20 deaths.

Table I.10b Average annual infant mortality rates per 10,000 live births for selected causes of death by age at death and color, in metropolitan and nonmetropolitan counties: United States and each geographic region, 1959-61 - continued.

Cause of Death (7th Revision-International Classification of Diseases)	Total			White			Nonwhite		
	Under 1 year	Under 28 days	28 days - 11 months	Under 1 year	Under 28 days	28 days - 11 months	Under 1 year	Under 28 days	28 days - 11 months
Northeast									
All causes	238.3	182.0	56.3	218.1	168.1	50.1	415.0	304.2	110.8
Infective and parasitic diseases	1.9	0.2	1.7	1.8	0.2	1.6	2.9	0.3*	2.6
Influenza and pneumonia, including pneumonia of newborn	25.5	7.2	18.3	21.6	6.2	15.3	60.0	15.4	44.6
All other diseases of respiratory system	4.5	0.6	3.9	4.2	0.6	3.6	7.7	0.9	6.9
Gastritis, duodenitis, enteritis and colitis, including diarrhea of newborn[2]	3.3	0.7	2.6	2.5	0.5	2.1	9.9	2.7	7.2
All other diseases of digestive system	3.9	2.6	1.3	3.8	2.6	1.2	4.5	2.5	2.0
Congenital malformations	37.0	24.3	12.7	37.6	24.9	12.7	32.0	19.2	12.8
Birth injuries	22.4	22.4	0.0*	21.8	21.8	0.0*	28.0	28.0	0.0*
Intracranial and spinal injury at birth	7.8	7.8	-	7.2	7.2	-	13.1	13.1	-
Other birth injury	14.7	14.6	0.0*	14.6	14.6	0.0*	14.9	14.8	0.0*
Postnatal asphyxia and atelectasis	45.4	44.5	0.9	41.2	40.5	0.7	82.3	79.7	2.6
Hemolytic disease of newborn	5.7	5.7	0.1*	6.1	6.1	0.1*	2.3	2.2	0.1*
Immaturity unqualified	47.4	47.2	0.2	40.9	40.7	0.2	104.0	103.5	0.5*
Neonatal disorders arising from certain diseases of mother, etc.[3]	22.3	21.1	1.2	19.9	19.0	0.9	43.1	39.4	3.7
Accidents	6.4	1.0	5.5	5.9	1.0	4.9	11.6	1.4	10.2
Residual	12.5	4.7	7.8	10.9	4.2	6.7	26.7	9.1	17.6
Metropolitan Counties									
All causes	239.0	183.4	55.6	214.9	166.7	48.2	414.7	305.2	109.5
Infective and parasitic diseases	1.8	0.2	1.6	1.7	0.2	1.5	2.9	0.3*	2.6
Influenza and pneumonia, including pneumonia of newborn	25.7	7.4	18.4	21.1	6.3	14.8	59.2	15.2	44.0
All other diseases of respiratory system	4.4	0.6	3.8	4.0	0.5	3.4	7.7	0.9	6.8
Gastritis, duodenitis, enteritis and colitis, including diarrhea of newborn[2]	3.0	0.6	2.4	2.2	0.4	1.8	9.1	2.4	6.8

All other diseases of digestive system	3.9	2.6	1.3	3.8	2.6	1.2	4.4	2.5	1.9
Congenital malformations	36.6	23.9	12.7	37.2	24.5	12.7	32.3	19.2	13.1
Birth injuries	21.3	21.3	0.0*	20.5	20.4	0.0*	27.6	27.6	0.0*
Intracranial and spinal injury at birth	7.9	7.9	-	7.1	7.1	-	13.3	13.3	-
Other birth injury	13.5	13.4	0.0*	13.3	13.3	0.0*	14.3	14.3	0.0*
Postnatal asphyxia and atelectasis	46.4	45.4	1.0	41.3	40.5	0.8	83.4	80.7	2.7
Hemolytic disease of newborn	5.7	5.6	0.1*	6.2	6.1	0.1*	2.2	2.1	0.1*
Immaturity unqualified	48.9	48.7	0.2	41.3	41.1	0.2	104.9	104.4	0.6*
Neonatal disorders arising from certain diseases of mother, etc.[3]	22.5	21.4	1.1	19.7	18.9	0.8	43.2	39.6	3.7
Accidents	5.8	0.9	4.9	5.1	0.8	4.2	11.0	1.4	9.7
Residual	12.9	4.8	8.1	11.0	4.2	6.8	26.8	9.1	17.7
Nonmetropolitan Counties									
All causes	235.7	176.6	59.2	229.8	173.0	56.9	419.5	289.0	130.5
Infective and parasitic diseases	2.3	0.1*	2.2	2.3	0.1*	2.1	2.8*	-	2.8*
Influenza and pneumonia, including pneumonia of newborn	24.6	6.4	18.2	23.1	6.0	17.1	72.1	18.2	54.0
All other diseases of respiratory system	5.1	0.7	4.4	5.0	0.7	4.3	8.8*	0.6*	8.3*
Gastritis, duodenitis, enteritis and colitis, including diarrhea of newborn[2]	4.3	1.0	3.4	3.8	0.7	3.1	21.5	8.3	13.2
All other diseases of digestive system	3.7	2.3	1.4	3.6	2.3	1.3	6.6*	2.2*	4.4*
Congenital malformations	38.9	26.1	12.8	39.2	26.2	13.0	28.1	20.4	7.7*
Birth injuries	26.8	26.7	0.1*	26.6	26.5	0.1*	33.6	33.6	-
Intracranial and spinal injury at birth	7.4	7.4	-	7.3	7.3	-	10.5*	10.5*	-
Other birth injury	19.4	19.3	0.1*	19.3	19.2	0.1*	23.1	23.1	-
Postnatal asphyxia and atelectasis	41.4	41.0	0.5	40.7	40.2	0.5	65.5	65.0	0.6*
Hemolytic disease of newborn	5.9	5.9	0.0*	5.9	5.9	0.0*	4.4*	4.4*	-
Immaturity unqualified	41.2	41.0	0.2*	39.6	39.4	0.3*	89.7	89.7	-
Neonatal disorders arising from certain diseases of mother, etc.[3]	21.4	19.9	1.5	20.7	19.4	1.4	41.8	36.9	5.0*
Accidents	9.0	1.4	7.6	8.7	1.4	7.3	20.4	1.7*	18.7
Residual	11.1	4.3	6.8	10.7	4.2	6.5	24.2	8.3*	16.0

NOTE: Source and footnotes are the same as for the table on United States.

Table I.10c   Average annual infant mortality rates per 10,000 live births for selected causes of death by age at death and color, in metropolitan and nonmetropolitan counties: United States and each geographic region, 1959-61 — continued.

Cause of Death (7th Revision-International Classification of Diseases)	Total			White			Nonwhite		
	Under 1 year	Under 28 days	28 days - 11 months	Under 1 year	Under 28 days	28 days - 11 months	Under 1 year	Under 28 days	28 days - 11 months
North Central									
All causes	237.0	177.6	59.4	220.8	167.9	52.9	387.9	267.7	120.1
Infective and parasitic diseases	2.3	0.2	2.0	2.1	0.2	1.9	3.6	0.4*	3.2
Influenza and pneumonia, including pneumonia of newborn	27.9	7.5	20.4	22.6	6.3	16.4	77.3	19.6	57.6
All other diseases of respiratory system	5.5	0.7	4.8	5.1	0.7	4.4	9.7	1.1	8.6
Gastritis, duodenitis, enteritis, and colitis, including diarrhea of newborn2	4.0	0.7	3.3	3.1	0.5	2.6	11.8	2.2	9.5
All other diseases of digestive system	3.5	2.2	1.3	3.5	2.3	1.2	3.8	2.0	1.7
Congenital malformations	37.2	24.5	12.7	37.9	25.1	12.8	30.7	18.9	11.9
Birth injuries	24.7	24.7	0.0*	24.5	24.4	0.0*	27.1	27.1	-
Intracranial and spinal injury at birth	6.5	6.5	-	6.0	6.0	-	10.7	10.7	-
Other birth injury	18.2	18.2	0.0*	18.4	18.4	0.0*	16.5	16.5	-
Postnatal asphyxia and atelectasis	47.0	46.5	0.5	42.5	42.1	0.5	88.4	87.2	1.2
Hemolytic disease of newborn	5.8	5.7	0.0*	6.1	6.1	0.0*	2.4	2.3	0.1*
Immaturity unqualified	40.2	40.0	0.2	37.0	36.8	0.2	70.1	69.5	0.6
Neonatal disorders arising from certain diseases of mother, etc.3	21.1	19.8	1.4	19.8	18.8	1.1	33.1	29.0	4.1
Accidents	7.0	1.0	6.0	6.6	1.0	5.6	10.7	1.4	9.4
Residual	11.0	4.1	6.9	10.1	3.8	6.3	19.3	7.1	12.2
Metropolitan Counties									
All causes	242.2	182.5	59.7	219.5	168.2	51.2	380.9	269.5	111.4
Infective and parasitic diseases	1.9	0.2	1.7	1.8	0.2	1.6	2.7	0.4*	2.3
Influenza and pneumonia, including pneumonia of newborn	30.2	8.3	21.9	22.8	6.4	16.4	74.9	19.6	55.3
All other diseases of respiratory system	6.0	0.7	5.3	5.5	0.7	4.8	9.3	1.0	8.3
Gastritis, duodenitis, enteritis, and colitis, including diarrhea of newborn2	3.6	0.6	3.1	2.7	0.4	2.3	9.6	1.7	7.8

	Col 1	Col 2	Col 3	Col 4	Col 5	Col 6	Col 7	Col 8	Col 9
All other diseases of digestive system	3.3	2.2	1.1	3.3	2.2	1.1	3.7	2.1	1.6
Congenital malformations	36.2	23.8	12.4	37.2	24.7	12.5	30.3	18.3	12.0
Birth injuries	24.2	24.1	0.0*	23.8	23.7	0.0*	26.7	26.7	-
Intracranial and spinal injury at birth	6.8	6.8	-	6.1	6.1	-	11.0	11.0	-
Other birth injury	17.4	17.4	0.0*	17.7	17.6	0.0*	15.7	15.7	1.2
Postnatal asphyxia and atelectasis	53.8	53.3	0.6	47.6	47.2	0.5	91.8	90.6	0.1*
Hemolytic disease of newborn	5.8	5.8	0.0*	6.3	6.3	0.0*	2.4	2.4	0.6
Immaturity unqualified	40.3	40.1	0.2	35.3	35.1	0.2	70.7	70.1	
Neonatal disorders arising from certain diseases of mother, etc.[3]	20.1	18.7	1.4	18.1	17.1	1.0	32.4	28.7	3.7
Accidents	5.7	0.7	5.0	5.1	0.6	4.5	9.4	1.3	8.1
Residual	11.0	4.1	6.9	10.1	3.7	6.4	17.0	6.7	10.4

Nonmetropolitan Counties

	Col 1	Col 2	Col 3	Col 4	Col 5	Col 6	Col 7	Col 8	Col 9
All causes	228.4	169.5	58.9	222.7	167.4	55.3	453.6	251.4	202.2
Infective and parasitic diseases	2.8	0.3	2.5	2.6	0.3	2.3	12.4	0.9*	11.5
Influenza and pneumonia, including pneumonia of newborn	24.3	6.4	17.9	22.4	6.0	16.3	100.0	20.1	79.9
All other diseases of respiratory system	4.6	0.7	4.0	4.4	0.7	3.8	12.9	1.2*	11.8
Gastritis, duodenitis, enteritis and colitis, including diarrhea of newborn[2]	4.6	0.9	3.6	3.8	0.8	3.1	32.8	7.2	25.6
All other diseases of digestive system	3.8	2.3	1.5	3.8	2.3	1.5	4.0*	1.2*	2.9*
Congenital malformations	38.9	25.6	13.2	39.0	25.7	13.3	34.8	23.8	10.9
Birth injuries	25.6	25.6	0.0*	25.5	25.4	0.0*	31.6	31.6	-
Intracranial and spinal injury at birth	6.0	6.0	-	5.9	5.9	-	7.8	7.8	-
Other birth injury	19.6	19.6	0.0*	19.5	19.5	0.0*	23.8	23.8	0.9*
Postnatal asphyxia and atelectasis	35.6	35.2	0.4	35.1	34.7	0.4	55.7	54.9	0.3*
Hemolytic disease of newborn	5.7	5.7	0.0*	5.8	5.8	0.0*	1.7*	1.4*	0.3*
Immaturity unqualified	40.0	39.8	0.1	39.4	39.2	0.1*	64.1	63.8	0.3*
Neonatal disorders arising from certain diseases of mother, etc.[3]	22.8	21.5	1.3	22.4	21.3	1.1	39.6	31.6	8.0
Accidents	9.0	1.5	7.5	8.6	1.5	7.1	23.3	2.0*	21.3
Residual	10.8	4.0	6.8	10.1	3.8	6.3	40.8	11.8	29.0

NOTE: Source and footnotes are the same as for the table on UNITED STATES.

Table I.10d   Average annual infant mortality rates per 10,000 live births for selected causes of death by age at death and color, in metropolitan and nonmetropolitan counties: United States and each geographic region, 1959-61 – continued.

Cause of Death (7th Revision-International Classification of Diseases)	Total			White			Nonwhite		
	Under 1 year	Under 28 days	28 days – 11 months	Under 1 year	Under 28 days	28 days – 11 months	Under 1 year	Under 28 days	28 days – 11 months
South									
All causes	300.3	204.4	95.9	242.0	180.0	62.0	458.4	270.6	-187.8
Infective and parasitic diseases	5.8	1.0	4.8	4.0	0.5	3.5	10.9	2.3	8.5
Influenza and pneumonia, including pneumonia of newborn	39.1	11.1	28.1	22.8	7.3	15.6	83.5	21.4	62.1
All other diseases of respiratory system	6.5	0.8	5.7	4.3	0.6	3.7	12.3	1.4	11.0
Gastritis, duodenitis, enteritis and colitis, including diarrhea of newborn[2]	13.0	1.8	11.2	6.2	0.7	5.6	31.6	5.0	26.6
All other diseases of digestive system	4.1	2.4	1.7	3.7	2.4	1.3	5.2	2.3	3.0
Congenital malformations	35.7	23.2	12.5	38.1	25.5	12.5	29.2	16.7	12.5
Birth injuries	23.1	23.0	0.1	22.1	22.0	0.0*	25.7	25.6	0.1*
Intracranial and spinal injury at birth	8.3	8.3	0.0*	7.4	7.4	-	10.7	10.6	0.0*
Other birth injury	14.8	14.7	0.1	14.7	14.6	0.0*	15.0	14.9	0.1*
Postnatal asphyxia and atelectasis	46.0	45.3	0.7	42.3	41.8	0.5	55.8	54.6	1.1
Hemolytic disease of newborn	3.9	3.9	0.0	4.6	4.6	0.0*	2.1	2.0	0.1*
Immaturity unqualified	52.0	51.5	0.5	42.5	42.3	0.2	77.6	76.3	1.3
Neonatal disorders arising from certain diseases of mother, etc.[3]	32.2	27.1	5.1	26.4	24.0	2.4	47.3	35.3	12.4
Accidents	12.2	2.2	10.0	8.8	1.4	7.4	21.5	4.3	17.3
Residual	26.7	11.3	15.5	16.1	6.8	9.4	55.4	23.5	31.9
Metropolitan Counties									
All causes	278.1	202.3	75.9	230.5	178.0	52.5	418.9	274.0	145.0
Infective and parasitic diseases	3.7	0.5	3.3	2.7	0.3	2.4	7.0	1.0	6.0
Influenza and pneumonia, including pneumonia of newborn	30.3	9.5	20.8	18.4	6.4	12.0	65.6	18.8	46.8
All other diseases of respiratory system	7.0	0.7	6.3	4.6	0.5	4.1	14.0	1.1	12.9
Gastritis, duodenitis, enteritis and colitis, including diarrhea of newborn[2]	7.9	0.9	7.0	4.3	0.5	3.9	18.5	2.2	16.3

All other diseases of digestive system	4.0	2.5	1.5	3.5	2.5	1.0	5.6	2.7	2.8
Congenital malformations	36.7	24.0	12.7	38.4	25.9	12.5	31.6	18.2	13.4
Birth injuries	22.1	22.0	0.0*	21.0	21.0	0.0*	25.1	25.0	0.1*
Intracranial and spinal injury at birth	8.5	8.5	-	7.4	7.4	-	11.7	11.7	-
Other birth injury	13.5	13.5	0.1*	13.6	13.5	0.0*	13.4	13.3	0.1*
Postnatal asphyxia and atelectasis	51.1	50.5	0.6	44.7	44.3	0.5	69.8	68.7	1.1
Hemolytic disease of newborn	4.1	4.0	0.0*	4.7	4.7	0.0*	2.0	2.0	0.0*
Immaturity unqualified	51.3	50.9	0.4	41.9	41.7	0.2	78.9	78.1	0.8
Neonatal disorders arising from certain diseases of mother, etc.3	30.5	27.0	3.5	24.8	23.2	1.7	47.2	38.5	8.7
Accidents	9.3	1.5	8.3	7.5	1.0	6.4	16.8	3.0	13.8
Residual	19.7	8.2	11.5	13.9	6.1	7.9	36.8	14.6	22.2
Nonmetropolitan Counties									
All causes	322.4	206.5	115.9	254.1	182.1	72.0	493.3	267.6	225.7
Infective and parasitic diseases	7.9	1.5	6.4	5.4	0.7	4.6	14.3	3.5	10.8
Influenza and pneumonia, including pneumonia of newborn	48.0	12.6	35.4	27.4	8.2	19.3	99.3	23.7	75.6
All other diseases of respiratory system	6.0	1.0	5.0	4.1	0.8	3.3	10.8	1.6	9.2
Gastritis, duodenitis, enteritis and colitis, including diarrhea of newborn2	18.2	2.8	15.4	8.2	0.9	7.3	43.1	7.5	35.6
All other diseases of digestive system	4.2	2.2	1.9	3.9	2.4	1.5	5.0	1.8	3.1
Congenital malformations	34.7	22.4	12.3	37.7	25.2	12.6	27.1	15.4	11.7
Birth injuries	24.1	24.0	0.1*	23.2	23.2	0.0*	26.2	26.0	0.2*
Intracranial and spinal injury at birth	8.1	8.1	0.0*	7.4	7.4	-	9.7	9.7	0.0*
Other birth injury	16.0	15.9	0.1*	15.8	15.8	0.0*	16.5	16.4	0.2*
Postnatal asphyxia and atelectasis	40.8	40.0	0.8	39.8	39.2	0.6	43.3	42.1	1.2
Hemolytic disease of newborn	3.8	3.8	0.1*	4.5	4.5	0.1*	2.1	2.0	0.1*
Immaturity unqualified	52.6	52.0	0.6	43.2	42.9	0.2	76.4	74.7	1.7
Neonatal disorders arising from certain diseases of mother, etc.3	33.9	27.1	6.8	28.1	24.9	3.2	48.2	32.5	15.8
Accidents	14.6	2.9	11.8	10.2	1.9	8.4	25.7	5.4	20.3
Residual	33.7	14.3	19.4	18.5	7.5	11.0	71.9	31.4	40.6

NOTE: Source and footnotes are the same as for the table on United States.

Table I.10e   Average annual infant mortality rates per 10,000 live births for selected causes of death by age at death and color, in metropolitan and nonmetropolitan counties: United States and each geographic region, 1959-61 – continued.

Cause of Death (7th Revision-International Classification of Diseases)	Total			White			Nonwhite		
	Under 1 year	Under 28 days	28 days - 11 months	Under 1 year	Under 28 days	28 days - 11 months	Under 1 year	Under 28 days	28 days - 11 months
West[1]									
All causes	246.8	178.9	67.9	235.5	174.2	61.3	338.0	216.6	121.4
Infective and parasitic diseases	2.9	0.3	2.6	2.4	0.2	2.2	6.9	0.8*	6.1
Influenza and pneumonia, including pneumonia of newborn	28.4	7.6	20.8	25.4	7.0	18.5	52.3	12.7	39.6
All other diseases of respiratory system	9.3	0.7	8.5	8.7	0.7	8.0	14.1	1.3	12.8
Gastritis, duodenitis, enteritis and colitis, including diarrhea of newborn[2]	5.3	0.9	4.5	3.9	0.6	3.3	17.0	2.8	14.3
All other diseases of digestive system	3.6	2.4	1.2	3.5	2.4	1.1	4.1	2.4	1.7
Congenital malformations	35.4	23.5	11.9	35.6	24.0	11.6	33.4	19.0	14.4
Birth injuries	26.3	26.3	0.0*	25.7	25.7	0.0*	31.2	31.1	0.1*
Intracranial and spinal injury at birth	7.6	7.6	-	7.0	7.0	-	12.3	12.3	-
Other birth injury	18.8	18.7	0.0*	18.7	18.7	0.0*	19.0	18.9	0.1*
Postnatal asphyxia and atelectasis	43.2	42.7	0.5	42.2	42.2	0.5	47.5	46.9	0.6*
Hemolytic disease of newborn	4.9	4.9	0.0*	5.2	5.2	0.0*	2.7	2.7	0.0*
Immaturity unqualified	39.0	38.8	0.2	36.9	36.7	0.2	56.5	56.4	0.1*
Neonatal disorders arising from certain diseases of mother, etc.[3]	26.1	24.7	1.5	25.2	24.1	1.1	34.1	29.4	4.7
Accidents	8.8	1.2	7.6	8.4	1.1	7.3	12.2	2.1	10.1
Residual	13.5	5.0	8.5	12.0	4.5	7.5	26.0	8.9	17.0
Metropolitan Counties									
All causes	235.9	175.9	59.9	227.4	170.5	56.9	299.6	216.9	82.7
Infective and parasitic diseases	2.2	0.2	2.0	2.0	0.2	1.9	3.3	0.4*	2.9
Influenza and pneumonia, including pneumonia of newborn	25.8	7.5	18.3	24.0	6.9	17.1	39.3	12.4	26.9
All other diseases of respiratory system	10.1	0.7	9.5	9.5	0.6	8.9	14.7	1.1*	13.6
Gastritis, duodenitis, enteritis and colitis, including diarrhea of newborn[2]	3.3	0.6	2.7	2.7	0.5	2.3	7.5	1.8	5.8

All other diseases of digestive system	3.5	2.4	1.1	3.5	2.4	1.1	3.3	2.2	1.1*
Congenital malformations	34.4	22.9	11.6	34.8	23.4	11.4	31.8	18.7	13.1
Birth injuries	26.1	26.1	0.0*	25.4	25.4	0.0*	31.2	31.1	0.1*
Intracranial and spinal injury at birth	7.9	7.9	-	7.2	7.2	-	12.8	12.8	-
Other birth injury	18.3	18.2	0.0*	18.2	18.2	0.0*	18.4	18.3	0.1*
Postnatal asphyxia and atelectasis	45.5	45.1	0.4	44.6	44.2	0.4	52.2	51.7	0.5*
Hemolytic disease of newborn	4.8	4.8	0.0*	5.1	5.1	0.0*	2.9	2.9	-
Immaturity unqualified	36.3	36.2	0.1*	33.6	33.4	0.1*	56.6	56.6	-
Neonatal disorders arising from certain diseases of mother, etc.[3]	25.1	24.2	0.9	24.1	23.4	0.7	32.4	30.2	2.2
Accidents	7.2	0.9	6.3	7.1	0.8	6.2	8.0	1.4	6.6
Residual	11.5	4.5	7.1	10.9	4.2	6.7	16.4	6.4	10.0

Nonmetropolitan Counties

All causes	273.7	186.1	87.6	255.0	183.2	71.9	460.7	215.5	245.3
Infective and parasitic diseases	4.6	0.4	4.2	3.2	0.2*	3.0	18.6	2.1*	16.6
Influenza and pneumonia, including pneumonia of newborn	34.8	7.8	26.9	28.9	7.3	21.6	93.8	13.6	80.1
All other diseases of respiratory system	7.1	0.8	6.3	6.6	0.7	5.9	12.1	2.1*	10.1
Gastritis, duodenitis, enteritis and colitis, including diarrhea of newborn[2]	10.3	1.4	8.9	6.6	1.0	5.7	47.5	6.2	41.4
All other diseases of digestive system	3.8	2.5	1.3	3.5	2.4	1.1	6.7	3.2*	3.5*
Congenital malformations	37.8	25.0	12.8	37.7	25.4	12.2	38.8	20.1	18.6
Birth injuries	26.8	26.8	0.0*	26.4	26.4	0.0*	31.1	31.1	-
Intracranial and spinal injury at birth	6.9	6.9	-	6.5	6.5	-	10.4	10.4	-
Other birth injury	20.0	19.9	0.0*	19.9	19.9	0.0*	20.7	20.7	-
Postnatal asphyxia and atelectasis	37.5	36.8	0.7	38.0	37.3	0.7	32.2	31.3	0.9*
Hemolytic disease of newborn	5.1	5.1	0.1*	5.4	5.4	0.1*	2.1*	1.9*	0.2*
Immaturity unqualified	45.8	45.4	0.4	44.8	44.4	0.4	56.1	55.5	0.6*
Neonatal disorders arising from certain diseases of mother, etc.[3]	28.8	25.9	2.8	27.7	25.8	1.9	39.5	26.8	12.7
Accidents	12.9	1.9	11.0	11.6	1.7	10.0	25.5	4.5	21.1
Residual	18.4	6.3	12.1	14.6	5.2	9.4	56.7	17.2	39.5

NOTE: Source and footnotes are the same as for the table on UNITED STATES.

Table I.11a   Average annual infant mortality rates per 1,000 live births by age at death and color for cities over 250,000 population: United States, 1950 and 1960-61.

Area	1960-61 Under 1 year	Under 28 days	Under 1 day	1 - 6 days	7 - 27 days	28 days - 11 mos.	1950 Under 1 year	Under 28 days	28 day 11 mo
United States, Total	25.7	18.6	10.3	6.3	2.0	7.1	29.2	20.5	8.7
Individual Cities by Size[1]									
1,000,000 or more									
New York, N. Y.[2]	26.0	19.4	11.5	6.2	1.7	6.5	24.9	19.2	5.7
Chicago, Ill.[2]	28.4	19.8	11.7	6.2	2.0	8.6	25.4	18.9	6.4
Los Angeles, Calif.[2]	24.1	18.3	10.5	6.1	1.7	5.8	24.8	20.1	4.7
Philadelphia, Pa.[2]	30.7	23.4	14.6	7.1	1.7	7.3	31.1	23.5	7.6
Detroit, Mich.[2]	29.4	22.6	13.7	6.9	2.0	6.7	26.9	20.2	6.7
500,000 - 1,000,000									
Baltimore, Md.[2]	32.6	24.3	13.0	8.4	2.9	8.3	24.8	18.6	6.2
Houston, Tex.[2]	27.2	19.0	9.8	7.1	2.1	8.2	28.7	23.6	5.1
Cleveland, Ohio[2]	29.5	23.4	14.3	7.2	2.0	6.0	25.6	19.5	6.1
Washington, D. C.[2]	36.0	27.3	17.6	7.6	2.1	8.6	30.4	24.5	5.9
St. Louis, Mo.[2]	32.0	23.8	14.7	6.8	2.3	8.3	25.7	19.2	6.6
Milwaukee, Wis.[2]	24.8	19.4	12.6	5.5	1.3	5.4	25.4	20.0	5.4
San Francisco, Calif.[2]	23.8	17.8	11.1	5.1	1.6†	6.0	21.7	17.2	4.5
Boston, Mass.[2]	24.5	18.5	11.6	4.9	2.0	6.0	25.2	20.1	5.0
Dallas, Tex.[2]	27.6	21.1	11.6	7.6	2.0	6.5	26.9	21.3	5.6
New Orleans, La.	32.4	23.7	12.7	8.5	2.5	8.7	30.1	23.3	6.8
Pittsburg, Pa.	29.1	23.4	15.0	6.8	1.6†	5.8	26.4	22.4	4.0
San Antonio, Tex.[2]	30.3	21.0	11.3	7.5	2.1	9.3	38.0	22.4	15.5
San Diego, Calif.[2]	25.7	19.3	11.0	6.3	1.9	6.4	29.3	21.1	8.2
Seattle, Wash.[2]	23.6	17.1	10.7	5.0	1.4†	6.5	25.2	19.8	5.5
Buffalo, N. Y.[2]	25.9	20.1	12.1	6.4	1.6†	5.9	25.6	20.1	5.6
Cincinnati, Ohio[2]	24.2	18.3	9.5	6.9	1.9	5.9	26.4	19.0	7.5
250,000 - 500,000									
Memphis, Tenn.	30.3	22.7	12.9	7.2	2.5	7.5	33.6	24.1	9.5
Denver, Col.	27.2	21.7	14.2	5.7	1.8†	5.5	28.7	22.8	6.0
Atlanta, Ga.	34.0	24.3	13.0	9.0	2.3	9.7	31.1	23.7	7.5
Minneapolis, Minn.	24.6	18.9	11.7	5.6	1.6†	5.7	24.4	20.1	4.3
Indianapolis, Ind.	27.8	20.4	12.4	5.9	2.1	7.4	27.5	18.9	8.6
Kansas City, Mo.[3]	26.2	18.8	3	3	3	7.4	30.7	24.2	6.4
Columbus, Ohio	24.3	18.4	10.3	6.2	1.9†	5.9	25.4	18.6	6.8
Phoenix, Ariz.	27.0	19.1	10.4	6.3	2.4†	7.9	41.6	31.2	10.4
Newark, N. J.	37.4	25.9	11.9	10.9	3.0	11.6	31.1	24.5	6.0
Louisville, Ky.	27.9	21.8	12.0	7.4	2.3†	6.1	30.3	23.4	6.9
Portland, Ore.	24.9	18.3	12.0	4.7	1.7†	6.6	20.0	16.7	3.3
Oakland, Calif.	26.9	20.3	11.8	6.7	1.8†	6.6	24.5	19.2	5.3
Fort Worth, Tex.	27.5	18.8	11.0	6.2	1.7†	8.6	31.5	25.0	6.5
Long Beach, Calif.	25.6	19.0	10.7	6.6	1.8†	6.6	23.3	18.5	4.7
Birmingham, Ala.	29.6	21.4	11.3	8.1	2.1†	8.2	31.2	23.5	7.8
Oklahoma City, Okla.	26.2	20.0	10.8	7.5	1.7†	6.2	25.4	19.4	6.0
Rochester, N. Y.	22.9	18.0	10.9	5.8	1.3†	4.9	25.3	21.5	3.7
Toledo, Ohio	23.6	17.9	10.3	6.1	1.6†	5.7	26.3	19.6	6.7
St. Paul, Minn.	24.1	18.0	11.1	5.3	1.6†	6.1	24.0	18.1	5.8
Norfolk, Va.	31.2	23.3	11.8	8.9	2.6†	7.9	34.1	26.2	7.9
Omaha, Neb.	25.3	20.3	11.8	7.0	1.5†	5.0	26.0 5	21.5 5	4.5
Honolulu, Hawaii[5]	21.9	17.8	10.9	5.7	1.2†	4.0			
Miami, Fla.	28.3	21.7	13.7	6.2	1.9†	6.6	26.3	22.4	3.
Akron, Ohio	24.9	19.5	11.1	7.0	1.4†	5.4	25.6	20.6	5.
El Paso, Tex.	25.0	18.9	9.4	7.6	2.0†	6.1	37.5	23.5	14.
Jersey City, N. J.	28.9	21.4	14.7	5.4	1.2*	7.5	26.7	21.6	5.
Tampa, Fla.	32.9	25.6	15.5	7.9	2.2†	7.3	30.3	25.6	4.
Dayton, Ohio	29.5	22.9	13.3	7.8	1.8†	6.7	29.0	23.1	5.
Tulsa, Okla.	25.9	19.5	11.4	6.6	1.5*	6.4	29.5	22.1	7.
Wichita, Kan.	25.7	19.1	11.5	5.5	2.1†	6.5	28.0	21.0	7.0

Source: Annual volumes Vital Statistics of the United States, National Center for Health Statistics, Public Health Service, Washington, and special tabulations. 1960 Census of Population, Bureau of the Census, U. S. Department of Commerce.

*Rate based on less than 20 deaths.
†Rate based on between 20 and 49 deaths.

[1] Individual cities classified by size according to 1960 census.
[2] Number of nonwhite inhabitants increased by at least one-third between 1950-1960. (Only those cities with population of 500,000 or more are so identified.)
[3] Based on 1960 data only. Data not available by detailed age.
[4] Data not available by color.
[5] For 1950, data not available for Honolulu by place of residence.

Table I.11b   Average annual infant mortality rates per 1,000 live births by age at death and color for cities over 250,000 population: United States, 1950 and 1960-61 - continued.

Area	1960-61						1950		
	Under 1 year	Under 28 days	Under 1 day	1 - 6 days	7 - 27 days	28 days - 11 mos.	Under 1 year	Under 28 days	28 days - 11 mos.
United States, White	22.7	17.1	9.6	5.9	1.6	5.6	26.8	19.4	7.4
Individual cities by size[1]									
1,000,000 or more									
New York, N. Y.[2]	21.5	16.2	9.2	5.4	1.5	5.3	22.4	17.2	5.2
Chicago, Ill.[2]	23.1	16.9	9.9	5.3	1.6	6.3	23.0	17.4	5.6
Los Angeles, Calif.[2]	22.1	16.9	9.5	5.9	1.5	5.2	23.1	18.9	4.2
Philadelphia, Pa.[2]	24.8	19.5	11.6	6.4	1.5	5.3	25.7	20.1	5.6
Detroit, Mich.[2]	24.7	19.3	11.4	6.5	1.4	5.5	24.9	18.8	6.1
500,000 - 1,000,000									
Baltimore, Md.[2]	25.3	19.3	10.5	6.9	1.8†	6.0	23.8	18.1	5.7†
Houston, Tex.[2]	22.9	17.8	9.2	6.8	1.8	5.1	25.6	21.2	4.4
Cleveland, Ohio[2]	24.8	19.5	11.7	6.2	1.6†	5.3	23.1	17.9	5.2
Washington, D. C.[2]	28.3	22.4	12.9	7.7	1.8†	5.9	30.5	26.0	4.5
St. Louis, Mo.[2]	24.5	18.6	11.3	5.6	1.8†	5.9	21.2	16.2	5.0
Milwaukee, Wis.[2]	23.2	18.4	11.7	5.5	1.2†	4.8	24.9	19.8	5.1
San Francisco, Calif.[2]	22.8	17.0	10.5	5.1	1.4†	5.8	21.2	17.1	4.1
Boston, Mass.[2]	22.5	17.2	10.5	4.8	1.9†	5.3	24.4	19.7	4.7
Dallas, Tex.[2]	23.9	19.4	11.0	6.8	1.6†	4.4	24.0	18.9	5.0†
New Orleans, La.	23.4	19.0	10.5	6.9	1.6†	4.5	27.0	21.6	5.3†
Pittsburgh, Pa.	26.2	21.7	13.6	6.5	1.6†	4.5	24.1	20.6	3.5
San Antonio, Tex.[2]	29.6	20.3	11.0	7.3	2.0	9.2	38.2	22.1	16.1
San Diego, Calif.[2]	24.3	18.4	10.3	6.4	1.8†	5.9	28.0	20.6	7.4
Seattle, Wash.[2]	23.0	16.8	10.5	4.9	1.3†	6.2	24.0	18.9	5.1
Buffalo, N. Y.[2]	23.3	18.1	10.3	6.5	1.2†	5.2	25.5	20.5	5.0
Cincinnati, Ohio[2]	20.3	15.0	7.3	6.1	1.6†	5.3	23.9	16.8	7.0
250,000 - 500,000									
Memphis, Tenn.	23.7	19.6	9.8	7.7	2.1†	4.1	28.8[4]	22.3[4]	6.5†[4]
Denver, Col.	26.0	20.8	13.7	5.6	1.6†	5.1	[4]	[4]	[4]
Atlanta, Ga.	29.2	22.8	12.3	8.8	1.8†	6.4	23.9[4]	19.5[4]	4.3†[4]
Minneapolis, Minn.	24.2	18.7	11.5	5.6	1.6†	5.5	[4]	[4]	[4]
Indianapolis, Ind.	24.3	17.8	11.2	5.1	1.5†	6.5	25.3	18.0	7.3
Kansas City, Mo.[3]	22.4	16.3	3	3	3	6.1	28.3	23.4	4.9†
Columbus, Ohio	22.1	17.2	9.6	5.5	2.1†	5.0	23.8	18.1	5.8†
Phoenix, Ariz.	26.0	18.7	10.1	6.4	2.1†	7.4	[4]	[4]	[4]
Newark, N. J.	27.9	18.8	8.7	8.3	1.8*	9.1	25.0	19.5	5.5†
Louisville, Ky.	25.2	20.2	11.6	6.9	1.7†	5.0	29.3	23.4	5.8
Portland, Ore.	24.5	18.4	11.9	4.7	1.8†	6.1	19.4	16.1	3.3†
Oakland, Calif.	22.4	17.6	9.1	6.8	1.7*	4.8†	21.9	17.7	4.3†
Fort Worth, Tex.	21.8	16.1	9.2	5.5	1.4*	5.7	28.5[4]	22.9[4]	5.6†[4]
Long Beach, Calif.	25.0	18.8	10.6	6.4	1.8†	6.2	[4]	[4]	[4]
Birmingham, Ala.	23.4	18.6	9.9	7.7	1.0*	4.8†	26.1	21.1	5.0†
Oklahoma City, Okla.	22.9	17.9	9.2	7.3	1.4†	4.9	24.5	18.5	5.9†
Rochester, N. Y.	21.6	17.8	10.5	6.2	1.2*	3.8†	[4]	[4]	[4]
Toledo, Ohio	22.0	16.6	9.3	5.8	1.4*	5.4	24.3[4]	17.9[4]	6.4†[4]
St. Paul, Minn.	[4]	[4]	[4]	[4]		[4]			
Norfolk, Va.	23.7	18.4	9.9	6.8	1.7†	5.3	25.1	20.0	5.1*
Omaha, Neb.	24.5	19.8	11.4	6.9	1.4†	4.7	25.0[5]	21.2[5]	3.9†[5]
Honolulu, Hawaii[5]	21.9	18.5	10.3†	7.1†	1.0*	3.4*	[5]	[5]	[5]
Miami, Fla.	23.9	19.8	11.7	6.4†	1.7*	4.2†	22.1	19.0	3.1*
Akron, Ohio	21.9	17.8	9.6	6.9	1.3*	4.1†	22.8	19.4	3.4†
El Paso, Tex.	[4]	[4]	[4]	[4]	[4]	[4]	[4]	[4]	[4]
Jersey City, N. J.	25.3	19.1	13.2	5.0†	0.9*	6.2	22.3	18.0	4.3†
Tampa, Fla.	26.5	21.7	14.4	5.9	1.4*	4.8†	27.3	24.1	3.2*
Dayton, Ohio	24.6	19.2	10.7	6.9	1.6*	5.5	27.7	22.8	4.8†
Tulsa, Okla.	23.3	18.4	10.8	5.9	1.8*	4.9	25.4[4]	20.2[4]	5.3†[4]
Wichita, Kan.	25.0	19.7	11.8	5.8	2.1†	5.4	[4]	[4]	[4]

Note: Source and footnotes are the same as on the table for TOTAL.

Table I.11c Average annual infant mortality rates per 1,000 live births by age at death and color for cities over 250,000 population: United States, 1950 and 1960-61 - continued.

Area	1960-61						1950		
	Under 1 year	Under 28 days	Under 1 day	1 - 6 days	7 - 27 days	28 days - 11 mos.	Under 1 year	Under 28 days	28 days 11 mos
United States, Nonwhite	42.0	26.5	14.3	8.4	3.9	15.4	44.5	27.5	16.9
Individual cities by size[1]									
1,000,000 or more									
New York, N. Y.[2]	41.3	30.5	19.4	8.8	2.3	10.8	39.1	30.4	8.7
Chicago, Ill.[2]	37.9	25.2	14.9	7.7	2.5	12.7	34.8	25.0	9.8
Los Angeles, Calif.[2]	29.9	22.4	13.4	6.7	2.3	7.5	34.9	27.6	7.3
Philadelphia, Pa.[2]	41.2	30.3	19.9	8.2	2.2	11.0	46.9	33.4	13.5
Detroit, Mich.[2]	37.0	28.1	17.6	7.5	3.0	8.8	34.6	25.8	8.9
500,000 - 1,000,000									
Baltimore, Md.[2]	40.3	29.6	15.6	9.9	4.1	10.8	33.8†	23.1*	10.8*
Houston, Tex.[2]	36.9	21.6	11.3	7.6	2.7†	15.2	38.5	31.1	7.4*
Cleveland, Ohio[2]	38.0	30.6	19.1	8.9	2.6†	7.4	34.9	25.6	9.3†
Washington, D. C.[2]	39.4	29.5	19.7	7.6	2.2	9.9	30.3	22.6	7.7
St. Louis, Mo.[2]	43.9	31.8	20.0	8.7	3.1†	12.0	40.9	29.3	11.6
Milwaukee, Wis.[2]	34.0	25.2	17.7	5.6†	1.9*	8.9	33.2†	22.9†	10.3*
San Francisco, Calif.[2]	26.3	19.6	12.6	4.9†	2.1*	6.7	24.1	17.9	6.2*
Boston, Mass.[2]	35.4	25.5	17.2	5.7†	2.6*	9.9	34.7†	25.6†	7.4*
Dallas, Tex.[2]	36.9	25.3	13.0	9.4	2.9†	11.6	44.8	35.4	9.3*
New Orleans, La.	41.9	28.7	15.0	10.3	3.5	13.2	34.5	25.7	8.8
Pittsburg, Pa.	39.2	29.0	19.5	7.9†	1.6*	10.2	43.6	36.3	7.3*
San Antonio, Tex.[2]	39.5	29.1	15.8†	10.1†	3.2*	10.4†	34.2†	26.9†	7.3*
San Diego, Calif.[2]	35.2	25.5	16.1	6.2†	3.2*	9.7†	44.9*	26.9*	18.0*
Seattle, Wash.[2]	27.9	19.7	11.9†	6.1*	1.7*	8.2†	42.6†	31.4†	11.2*
Buffalo, N. Y.[2]	35.8	27.5	19.0	5.7†	2.8*	8.3†	26.5†	15.1*	11.3*
Cincinnati, Ohio[2]	35.7	28.1	15.9	9.6	2.7*	7.6	38.3	28.7	9.6†
250,000 - 500,000									
Memphis, Tenn.	37.4	26.1	16.4	6.7	3.1†	11.3	39.4 [4]	26.4 [4]	13.1 [4]
Denver, Col.	38.3	29.7	19.2†	6.9*	3.7*	8.6†	4	4	4
Atlanta, Ga.	39.0	25.8	13.8	9.2	2.8†	13.2	42.7	30.2	12.5†
Minneapolis, Minn.	31.2†	23.0†	15.6*	5.8*	1.6*	8.2*	4	4	4
Indianapolis, Ind.	38.5	28.2	16.1 [3]	8.2 [3]	3.9† [3]	10.2	40.0	24.1†	15.9†
Kansas City, Mo.[3]	37.4	26.3				11.1†	44.9	29.0†	15.9†
Columbus, Ohio	33.5	23.7	13.5	9.2†	1.0*	9.8†	34.8†	21.8†	12.9*
Phoenix, Ariz.	36.7	23.7†	13.5†	4.9*	5.4*	12.9†	4	4	4
Newark, N. J.	46.7	32.8	15.1	13.5	4.2†	13.9	48.5	38.7	9.8†
Louisville, Ky.	37.1	27.2	13.5	9.4†	4.3*	9.8†	35.5	22.9†	12.6†
Portland, Ore.	29.0†	18.1†	13.0*	4.3*	0.7*	10.9*	33.7*	28.8*	4.8*
Oakland, Calif.	34.2	24.6	16.1	6.5†	1.9*	9.6	33.9	24.9†	9.0*
Fort Worth, Tex.	48.4	29.0	17.5	8.9†	2.7*	19.4	50.3 [4]	38.2† [4]	12.1* [4]
Long Beach, Calif.	31.1†	21.0†	11.7*	7.8*	1.6*	10.1*	4	4	4
Birmingham, Ala.	36.6	24.5	12.8	8.5	3.2†	12.1	37.2	26.2	11.0†
Oklahoma City, Okla.	41.3	29.4	17.8	8.6†	3.1*	11.9†	32.7†	26.1†	6.5*
Rochester, N. Y.	30.0	18.9†	12.9†	3.7*	2.3*	11.1†	4	4	4
Toledo, Ohio	31.3 [4]	24.4 [4]	14.9†	7.2*	2.3*	6.9*	44.9†	35.0†	10.0*
St. Paul, Minn.	4	4					4	4	4
Norfolk, Va.	49.2	35.0	16.2	14.0	4.7†	14.2	52.0	38.4	13.6†
Omaha, Neb.	30.8	24.1	14.3†	7.6*	2.1*	6.8*	36.4† [5]	25.5* [5]	10.9* [5]
Honolulu, Hawaii[5]	21.9	17.6	11.1	5.3	1.3*	4.2			
Miami, Fla.	34.7	24.6	16.7	5.9†	2.1*	10.0	38.7	32.5†	6.2*
Akron, Ohio	39.9	28.0	18.3†	7.6*	2.1*	11.9†	48.6†	30.2†	18.4*
El Paso, Tex.	4	4	4	4	4	4	4	4	4
Jersey City, N. J.	40.1	28.6	19.7	6.7†	2.2*	11.5†	60.6†	49.6†	11.0*
Tampa, Fla.	53.8	38.3	19.0	14.5†	4.8*	15.5†	43.0†	31.9†	11.1*
Dayton, Ohio	42.0	32.3	20.0	10.0†	2.2*	9.7†	37.6†	24.8†	12.8*
Tulsa, Okla.	40.7	25.9†	14.9†	10.5*	0.6*	14.9†	60.3† [4]	36.6† [4]	23.8* [4]
Wichita, Kan.	30.0	15.6†	9.4*	3.9*	2.2*	14.4†	4	4	4

Note: Source and footnotes are the same as on the table for TOTAL.

Table I.12a   Fetal death ratios by gestation, sex and color and perinatal mortality rates by sex and color: United States, 1942-1964.

Year	Fetal death ratio I[1]	Fetal death ratio II[2]								
		Total			White			Nonwhite		
		Total	Male	Female	Total	Male	Female	Total	Male	Female
1964[3]	12.3	16.4	17.2	15.5	14.1	14.7	13.4	28.2	30.4	26.1
1963[3]	11.8	15.8	16.4	15.1	13.7	14.1	13.2	26.7	28.5	24.8
1962[3]	11.5	15.9	16.8	15.0	13.9	14.6	13.3	26.7	28.9	24.5
1961[3]	11.6	16.1	17.0	15.2	14.1	14.7	13.5	27.0	29.4	24.6
1960[3]	11.6	16.1	16.9	15.2	14.1	14.7	13.5	26.8	29.1	24.4
1959[3]	11.7	16.2	17.0	15.3	14.2	14.8	13.5	27.3	29.6	25.0
1958	11.9	16.5	17.4	15.6	14.5	15.1	13.9	27.5	30.1	24.9
1957	12.0	16.3	17.3	15.4	14.5	15.2	13.8	26.8	29.2	24.4
1956	12.1	16.5	17.4	15.5	14.6	15.3	13.9	27.2	29.4	24.9
1955	12.6	17.1	18.0	16.2	15.2	15.8	14.5	28.4	31.0	25.8
1954	12.9	17.5	18.4	16.4	15.5	16.3	14.7	28.9	31.2	26.5
1953	13.4	17.8	18.7	16.8	15.9	16.6	15.1	29.6	32.2	27.0
1952	13.8	18.3	19.4	17.2	16.1	16.8	15.3	32.2	35.6	28.9
1951	14.3	18.8	20.0	17.6	16.7	17.6	15.8	32.1	35.4	28.7
1950	14.6	19.2	20.5	17.9	17.1	18.0	16.1	32.5	36.0	28.9
1949	15.1	19.8	21.1	18.5	17.5	18.5	16.6	34.6	38.0	31.2
1948	15.5	20.6	21.8	19.4	18.3	19.3	17.2	36.5	39.6	33.3
1947	16.1	21.1	22.5	19.6	18.7	19.8	17.4	39.6	43.1	36.0
1946	17.2	22.8	24.3	21.2	20.4	21.7	19.1	40.9	44.6	37.2
1945	18.5	23.9	25.5	22.3	21.4	22.6	20.1	42.0	46.3	37.6
1944[4]	19.0	24.5	---	---	---	---	---	---	---	---
1943[4]	19.3	24.5	---	---	---	---	---	---	---	---
1942[4]	20.1	25.6	---	---	---	---	---	---	---	---

Source: Annual volumes Vital Statistics of the United States, National Center for Health Statistics, Public Health Service, Washington, and special tabulations.

Note: Fetal deaths with sex not stated distributed proportionately.

[1]Fetal death ratio I is defined as fetal deaths of 28 weeks or more gestation and a proportionate number of fetal deaths of unknown gestation per 1,000 live births.

[2]Fetal death ratio II differs from fetal death ratio I in that it includes fetal deaths of 20 weeks or more gestation plus all not stated gestation age.

[3]Hawaii not available by sex for 1959. Therefore, 1959 does not include Hawaii but includes Alaska. Alaska and Hawaii included beginning 1960. New Jersey excluded from data by color for 1962 and 1963; color not reported.

[4]For 1942-44, data not available by color or sex.

Table I.12b   Fetal death ratios by gestation, sex and color and perinatal
mortality rates by sex and color: United States, 1942-1964 -
continued.

Year	Perinatal mortality rate I[1]	Perinatal mortality rate II[2]								
		Total			White			Nonwhite		
		Total	Male	Female	Total	Male	Female	Total	Male	Female
1964[3]	28.0	33.7	36.8	30.4	29.8	32.7	26.9	53.2	58.2	48.1
1963[3]	27.9	33.5	36.6	30.2	29.9	32.8	27.0	51.4	56.2	46.6
1962[3]	27.7	33.7	37.0	30.2	30.4	33.4	27.2	51.4	56.2	46.4
1961[3]	28.0	34.0	37.0	30.6	30.6	33.5	27.5	51.8	56.9	46.7
1960[3]	28.2	34.3	37.5	30.8	30.9	33.9	27.8	52.2	57.5	46.9
1959[3]	28.4	34.6	38.0	31.1	31.2	34.3	27.9	53.5	58.5	48.4
1958	28.9	35.4	38.6	32.0	31.9	34.8	28.7	55.0	60.3	49.6
1957	28.5	34.8	38.2	31.3	31.6	34.7	28.3	53.2	58.2	47.9
1956	28.6	34.8	38.2	31.2	31.6	34.8	28.3	52.8	58.1	47.3
1955	29.3	35.6	39.0	32.1	32.4	35.5	29.1	54.1	59.4	48.7
1954	29.5	35.9	39.4	32.2	32.8	36.1	29.4	54.3	59.5	48.9
1953	30.3	36.7	40.2	33.0	33.6	37.0	30.1	55.3	60.3	50.2
1952	30.8	37.4	41.1	33.6	34.1	37.4	30.6	58.4	64.8	51.8
1951	31.5	38.1	42.0	34.1	35.0	38.5	31.3	57.6	64.2	50.8
1950	32.2	39.0	42.9	34.8	35.8	39.5	32.0	58.1	64.4	51.7
1949	33.1	40.5	44.6	36.1	37.2	41.0	33.2	61.1	67.5	54.4
1948	34.1	41.9	46.1	37.5	38.7	42.6	34.6	63.3	69.3	57.2
1947	35.1	42.9	47.3	38.4	39.6	43.7	35.3	67.9	74.4	61.2
1946	36.9	45.8	50.3	41.0	42.6	46.9	38.0	69.6	76.2	62.9
1945	37.8	47.2	51.8	42.3	43.7	48.0	39.2	71.0	78.6	63.2
1944[4]	38.6	44.5	---	---	---	---	---	---	---	---
1943[4]	38.8	48.1	---	---	---	---	---	---	---	---
1942[4]	40.5	50.0	---	---	---	---	---	---	---	---

Source: Derived from annual volumes Vital Statistics of the United States, National
Center for Health Statistics, Public Health Service, Washington, and special tabulations.

Note: Fetal deaths with sex not stated distributed proportionately.

[1]Perinatal mortality rate I is defined as infant deaths under 1 week plus fetal deaths
of 28 weeks or more gestation and a proportionate number of fetal deaths of unknown
gestation per 1,000 live births plus specified fetal deaths.

[2]Perinatal mortality rate II differs from perinatal mortality rate I in that it includes
infant deaths under 28 days plus fetal deaths of 20 weeks or more gestation plus all not
stated gestation age.

[3]Hawaii not available by sex for 1959. Therefore, 1959 does not include Hawaii but
includes Alaska. Alaska and Hawaii included beginning 1960. New Jersey excluded from data
by color for 1962 and 1963; color not reported.

[4]For 1942-44, data not available by color or sex.

Table I.13   Average annual fetal death ratios and
perinatal mortality rates by color: United States,
each geographic division and State, 1959-61.

Area	Fetal death ratio			Perinatal mortality rate		
	Total	White	Non-white	Total	White	Non-white
United States[1]	16.1	14.1	27.0	34.3	30.9	52.4
New England	13.6	13.4	20.1	30.3	29.7	46.4
Connecticut	12.7	12.1	20.9	29.4	27.8	53.3
Maine	14.5	14.6	*	32.9	33.0	22.2[†]
Massachusetts	13.4	13.2	19.6	29.7	29.2	42.8
New Hampshire	13.8	13.7	*	30.9	30.8	*
Rhode Island	14.5	14.2	22.3	31.2	30.6	43.7
Vermont	17.0	17.0	-	35.0	35.0	-
Middle Atlantic[2]	19.6	17.4	35.8	37.4	33.6	64.2
New Jersey	15.2	13.9	24.0	33.2	30.1	53.0
New York[3]	23.1	19.9	44.8	40.6	35.7	72.2
Pennsylvania	16.8	15.6	27.3	35.0	32.4	56.8
East North Central	14.4	13.3	23.2	31.9	29.8	48.9
Illinois	14.8	13.2	23.3	32.3	29.4	47.2
Indiana	13.9	13.0	23.9	30.8	29.2	49.3
Michigan	14.8	13.6	24.5	32.6	30.3	50.5
Ohio	14.5	13.6	21.7	32.5	30.4	50.1
Wisconsin	12.9	12.4	24.0	29.6	28.8	48.5
West North Central	13.2	12.5	23.1	29.9	28.6	48.5
Iowa	11.6	11.5	17.5	27.6	27.4	40.5
Kansas	12.9	12.3	22.5	29.6	28.5	44.0
Minnesota	12.6	12.4	19.7	28.3	28.2	36.5
Missouri	15.0	13.4	25.0	32.6	29.3	52.8
Nebraska	12.6	12.4	18.2	29.7	29.2	41.7
North Dakota	12.7	12.5	18.2[†]	30.6	30.2	41.0
South Dakota	13.7	13.1	21.3	31.0	29.7	47.6
South Atlantic	19.0	15.0	28.5	38.9	32.5	54.2
Delaware	14.3	12.2	23.6	32.1	27.3	52.1
District of Columbia	18.9	15.3	20.6	45.5	38.1	48.8
Florida	16.5	12.7	26.8	36.9	30.9	53.1
Georgia	20.5	15.3	29.9	40.5	32.7	54.3
Maryland	16.0	13.8	23.3	35.4	30.6	51.8
North Carolina	19.3	14.2	30.4	39.2	31.2	56.2
South Carolina	20.4	12.8	30.7	39.6	29.4	53.3
Virginia	23.3	20.3	32.6	43.2	37.7	59.6
West Virginia	16.5	16.0	25.2	34.6	34.2	43.7
East South Central	19.8	14.9	31.5	40.1	33.0	56.8
Alabama	21.6	15.0	32.7	41.5	32.3	56.6
Kentucky	15.7	14.8	25.6	34.9	33.1	52.8
Mississippi	26.2	16.0	34.9	49.2	34.7	61.4
Tennessee	16.8	14.3	25.7	36.8	32.8	50.5

Table I.13, continued.

Area	Fetal death ratio			Perinatal mortality rate		
	Total	White	Non-white	Total	White	Non-white
West South Central	15.7	13.2	24.8	34.6	30.4	49.9
Arkansas	17.0	13.2	25.9	33.8	29.1	44.9
Louisiana	16.5	11.3	24.6	37.9	28.2	52.8
Oklahoma	13.3	11.9	21.5	30.5	28.2	44.4
Texas	15.6	14.0	25.2	34.4	31.6	49.9
Mountain	13.4	13.2	16.6	32.2	31.6	39.4
Arizona	13.6	12.9	17.3	33.3	32.0	40.2
Colorado	16.7	16.5	22.3	37.0	36.5	50.5
Idaho	11.4	11.2	*	28.2	28.0	36.6[†]
Montana	11.5	11.2	15.8	28.7	28.0	36.5
Nevada	12.7	12.7	12.5[†]	33.8	33.6	34.9
New Mexico	13.6	13.5	14.4	33.8	33.5	35.7
Utah	10.6	10.6	13.3[†]	25.4	25.2	33.3
Wyoming	12.8	12.8	*	33.2	32.8	43.2[†]
Pacific[1]	13.0	12.4	16.9	29.9	28.9	37.5
Alaska	12.4	11.8	13.5	35.2	31.5	42.9
California	12.8	12.2	17.6	29.8	28.7	38.5
Hawaii	15.0	16.5	14.3	32.5	33.6	32.0
Oregon	15.5	15.3	22.0	31.9	31.6	38.7
Washington	11.6	11.2	18.6	28.3	27.6	40.5

Source: Annual volumes Vital Statistics of the United States, National Center for Health Statistics, Public Health Service, Washington, and special tabulations. Annual vital statistics summary of the New York City Department of Health.

Note: Fetal death ratios are all reported fetal deaths of 20 weeks or more gestation (plus not stated) per 1,000 live births. Perinatal mortality rates are reported fetal deaths (20 weeks or more gestation plus not stated) plus neonatal deaths per 1,000 live births plus fetal deaths.

[1]Include Alaska and Hawaii

[2]By excluding New York City, the following fetal death ratios and perinatal mortality rates result for the Middle Atlantic division:

	Total	White	Nonwhite
Fetal death ratios	15.8	14.8	25.6
Perinatal mortality rates	33.5	31.2	54.9

[3]By excluding New York City, the following fetal death ratios and perinatal mortality rates result for New York State:

	Total	White	Nonwhite
Fetal death ratios	15.0	14.4	24.6
Perinatal mortality rates	31.9	30.6	53.5

*Rates not computed, based on less than 20 deaths.

†Rates based on between 20 and 49 deaths.

Table I.14   Average annual fetal death ratios and perinatal mortality rates by
              color for metropolitan and nonmetropolitan counties and population-
              size groups: United States, 1960-61.

Area	Total		White		Nonwhite	
	Fetal death ratio	Perinatal mortality rate	Fetal death ratio	Perinatal mortality rate	Fetal death ratio	Perinatal mortality rate
United States	16.1	34.1	14.1	30.8	26.9	52.0
Metropolitan counties	16.1	34.0	14.2	30.6	26.0	51.5
Nonmetropolitan counties	16.1	34.3	13.9	31.0	28.5	53.1
Cities by size[1]						
1,000,000 or more	24.1	43.2	20.8	37.0	32.3	58.1
250,000-1,000,000	16.8	37.1	14.5	32.7	22.9	48.7
100,000-250,000	16.0	35.3	13.6	31.1	26.5	52.6

Source: Annual volumes Vital Statistics of the United States, National Center
for Health Statistics, Public Health Service, Washington, and special tabulations.

Note: Fetal death ratios are all reported fetal deaths of 20 weeks or more
gestation (plus not stated) per 1,000 live births. Perinatal mortality rates are
reported fetal deaths (20 weeks or more gestation plus not stated) plus neonatal
deaths per 1,000 live births plus fetal deaths.

[1]Cities are classified by their size according to 1960 census.

Table I.15   Average annual fetal death ratios and perinatal mortality rates by color for cities over 250,000 population: United States, 1960-61.

Area	Total		White		Nonwhite	
	Fetal death ratio	Perinatal mortality rate	Fetal death ratio	Perinatal mortality rate	Fetal death ratio	Perinatal mortality rate
United States	16.1	34.1	14.1	30.8	26.9	52.0
Individual cities by size[1]						
1,000,000 or more						
New York, N. Y.	28.0	46.2	24.6	39.8	39.8	67.6
Chicago, Ill.	17.6	36.8	14.6	31.0	23.3	47.4
Los Angeles, Calif.	14.7	32.5	13.1	29.6	19.2	40.8
Philadelphia, Pa.	19.1	41.7	15.2	34.2	26.1	55.0
Detroit, Mich.	19.8	41.6	15.7	34.4	26.4	53.1
500,000 - 1,000,000						
Baltimore, Md.	18.7	42.2	15.5	34.3	22.1	50.5
Houston, Tex.	16.6	35.0	13.2	30.6	24.2	44.8
Cleveland, Ohio	16.8	39.6	15.4	34.4	19.4	49.0
Washington, D. C.	19.3	45.7	15.7	37.5	20.9	49.4
St. Louis, Mo.	20.4	43.3	14.6	32.8	29.5	59.6
Milwaukee, Wis.	14.0	32.9	11.5	29.6	28.5	52.1
San Francisco, Calif.	13.3	30.7	12.9	29.6	14.2	33.4
Boston, Mass.	15.2	33.2	14.2	30.9	20.6	45.2
Dallas, Tex.	14.6	35.2	12.6	31.6	19.7	44.1
New Orleans, La.	16.5	39.6	10.3	28.9	23.1	50.7
Pittsburg, Pa.	27.5	49.5	26.6	47.1	30.6	57.8
San Antonio, Tex.	17.6	38.0	17.3	37.0	21.2	49.2
San Diego, Calif.	12.3	31.3	11.4	29.5	18.5	43.3
Seattle, Wash.	11.7	28.5	11.0	27.4	16.7†	35.8
Buffalo, N. Y.	17.2	36.6	14.8	32.3	26.1	52.3
Cincinnati, Ohio	14.0	31.9	12.5	27.2	18.4	45.7
250,000 - 500,000						
Memphis, Tenn.	19.8	41.7	13.2	32.4	26.9	51.6
Denver, Col.	22.7	43.5	22.9	42.8	20.8	49.5
Atlanta, Ga.	19.4	42.9	16.9	39.1	22.1	46.8
Minneapolis, Minn.	12.9	31.4	13.2	31.4	9.0*	31.8†
Indianapolis, Ind.	15.5	35.4	14.0	31.4	20.2	47.5
Kansas City, Mo.[2]	12.6	31.1	11.3	27.3	16.5	42.1
Columbus, Ohio	13.5	31.5	12.6	29.4	17.3	40.3
Phoenix, Ariz.	13.6	32.3	12.7	31.0	22.7†	45.4
Newark, N. J.	22.4	47.2	18.9	36.9	25.9	57.2
Louisville, Ky.	15.9	37.1	14.1	33.8	22.2	48.3
Portland, Ore.	20.0	37.6	19.2	36.8	28.3†	45.1
Oakland, Calif.	16.7	36.4	12.2	29.4	24.0	47.4
Fort Worth, Tex.	16.3	34.6	11.8	27.6	32.8	59.9
Long Beach, Calif.	12.1	30.8	12.2	30.6	11.7*	32.3†
Birmingham, Ala.	21.7	42.2	11.6	29.8	33.1	55.8
Oklahoma City, Okla.	12.9	32.4	11.3	28.9	20.2	48.6
Rochester, N. Y.	15.1	32.6	14.7	32.1	17.5†	35.8
Toledo, Ohio	17.4	34.7	16.6	32.6	21.0	44.5
St. Paul, Minn.	11.9	29.6	3	3	3	3
Norfolk, Va.	36.0	57.2	31.1	48.0	48.0	79.2
Omaha, Neb.	12.1	32.0	11.1	30.5	19.0†	42.2
Honolulu, Hawaii	15.1	32.5	19.5	37.2	13.7	30.9
Miami, Fla.	20.0	40.9	16.9	36.0	24.5	47.9
Akron, Ohio	13.5	32.6	12.1	29.5	20.4†	47.4
El Paso, Tex.	15.6	34.0	3	3	3	3
Jersey City, N. J.	18.4	39.1	16.6	35.1	23.9	51.3
Tampa, Fla.	19.5	44.3	14.8	36.0	34.8	70.6
Dayton, Ohio	21.0	43.0	20.2	38.6	23.1	54.1
Tulsa, Okla.	12.3	31.5	10.1	28.2	25.3†	49.9
Wichita, Kan.	13.1	31.8	11.6	30.9	23.9†	38.5

Sources: Annual volumes Vital Statistics of the United States, National Center for Health Statistics, Public Health Service, Washington, and special tabulations. 1960 Census of Population, Bureau of the Census, U. S. Dept. of Commerce.

Note: Fetal death ratios are all reported fetal deaths of 20 weeks or more gestation (plus not stated) per 1,000 live births. Perinatal mortality rates are reported fetal deaths (20 weeks or more gestation plus not stated) plus neonatal deaths per 1,000 live births plus fetal deaths.

*Rate based on less than 20 deaths.
†Rate based on between 20 and 49 deaths.
[1]Individual cities classified by size according to the 1960 census.
[2]Based on 1960 data only.
[3]Data not available by color.

Table I.16   Percent distribution of live births by birth weight and
                    selected characteristics: United States, 1950, 1960 and 1964.

Birth Weight[1]	Total	Plurality		Sex		Color	
		Single	Plural	Male	Female	White	Nonwhite
1964							
Total	100.0	100.0	100.0	100.0	100.0	100.0	100.0
1,000 grams or less	0.6	0.5	5.1	0.6	0.5	0.5	1.1
1,001 - 1,500 grams	0.7	0.6	6.1	0.7	0.6	0.6	1.2
1,501 - 2,000 grams	1.5	1.3	14.6	1.5	1.6	1.3	2.7
2,001 - 2,500 grams	5.4	4.9	29.9	4.8	6.1	4.8	8.9
2,501 - 3,000 grams	19.3	19.1	28.5	16.6	22.2	18.0	26.1
3,001 - 3,500 grams	38.2	38.8	13.0	36.7	39.9	38.5	37.1
3,501 - 4,000 grams	25.8	26.3	2.4	28.6	22.9	27.4	17.9
4,001 - 4,500 grams	7.0	7.1	0.3	8.7	5.2	7.6	4.0
4,501 grams or more	1.4	1.5	0.0	1.9	0.9	1.5	1.0
2,500 grams or less	8.2	7.2	55.7	7.5	8.9	7.1	13.9
2,501 grams or more	91.8	92.8	44.3	92.5	91.1	92.9	86.1
Median birth weight[2]	3290	3310	2410	3350	3240	3320	3140
1960							
Total	100.0	100.0	100.0	100.0	100.0	100.0	100.0
1,000 grams or less	0.5	0.5	4.7	0.6	0.5	0.5	1.0
1,001 - 1,500 grams	0.6	0.5	5.4	0.6	0.6	0.5	1.1
1,501 - 2,000 grams	1.4	1.2	14.0	1.4	1.5	1.3	2.5
2,001 - 2,500 grams	5.1	4.6	29.5	4.5	5.7	4.5	8.3
2,501 - 3,000 grams	18.5	18.3	29.6	15.8	21.3	17.3	25.3
3,001 - 3,500 grams	38.0	38.5	13.9	36.3	39.8	38.1	37.1
3,501 - 4,000 grams	26.8	27.3	2.6	29.5	23.9	28.2	18.9
4,001 - 4,500 grams	7.5	7.6	0.3	9.2	5.6	8.0	4.6
4,501 grams or more	1.6	1.6	0.0	2.1	1.0	1.6	1.3
2,500 grams or less	7.7	6.8	53.7	7.1	8.4	6.8	12.8
2,501 grams or more	92.3	93.2	46.3	92.9	91.6	93.2	87.2
Median birth weight[2]	3310	3320	2440	3370	3250	3340	3150
1950[3]							
Total	100.0	100.0	100.0	100.0	100.0	100.0	100.0
1,000 grams or less	0.5	0.4	4.0	0.5	0.5	0.4	0.6
1,001 - 1,500 grams	0.6	0.5	5.9	0.6	0.6	0.6	0.9
1,501 - 2,000 grams	1.4	1.2	14.1	1.4	1.5	1.3	2.0
2,001 - 2,500 grams	5.1	4.6	30.0	4.5	5.7	4.8	6.8
2,501 - 3,000 grams	18.3	18.1	29.0	15.6	21.2	17.8	21.4
3,001 - 3,500 grams	37.9	38.4	13.8	36.2	39.6	38.3	35.3
3,501 - 4,000 grams	26.8	27.3	2.7	29.6	23.9	27.5	22.7
4,001 - 4,500 grams	7.5	7.6	0.3	9.3	5.6	7.6	6.9
4,501 grams or more	1.9	2.0	0.1	2.5	1.3	1.7	3.3
2,500 grams or less	7.6	6.6	54.1	7.0	8.3	7.2	10.4
2,501 grams or more	92.4	93.4	45.9	93.0	91.7	92.8	89.6
Median birth weight[2]	3310	3330	2440	3380	3250	3320	3250

Source: Annual volumes Vital Statistics of the United States, National Center for
Health Statistics, Public Health Service, Washington.

[1]Figures for birth weight not stated are distributed.

[2]Computed to nearest 10 grams.

[3]In 1950, excludes births to residents of Connecticut and Massachusetts since birth
weight data were not available for births in these States.

Table I.17   Neonatal mortality per 1,000 live births by birth weight and
selected characteristics: United States, January-March 1950.
(Excludes data for Massachusetts)

Birth weight	Total	Plurality		Sex		Color	
		Single	Plural	Male	Female	White	Nonwhi
Total	20.0	18.3	98.6	22.7	17.1	18.9	26
1,000 grams or less	871.7	871.7	871.5	894.2	848.0	883.3	821
1,001-1,500 grams	551.3	562.3	503.7	621.8	478.2	562.1	507
1,501-2,000 grams	211.0	228.9	145.4	265.0	160.5	214.6	195
2,001-2,500 grams	50.4	52.8	32.9	67.4	36.6	50.6	49
2,501-3,000 grams	12.6	12.6	11.3	16.6	9.5	12.0	15
3,001-3,500 grams	6.7	6.7	10.4	8.1	5.3	6.2	9
3,501-4,000 grams	5.6	5.6	18.7*	6.4	4.6	4.9	10
4,001-4,500 grams	7.5	7.4	38.1*	7.7	7.2	6.7	12
4,501 grams or more	14.2	14.2	-	13.7	15.1	12.0	20
2,500 grams or less	173.7	173.4	175.6	213.9	138.9	175.8	164
2,501 grams or more	7.8	7.7	11.8	9.1	6.4	7.1	11

Source: Shapiro, S. Influence of birth weight, sex, and plurality on neonatal loss in
the United States. Am. J. Pub. Health 44:1142-1153, Sept. 1954.

Note: Figures for birth weight not stated are distributed.

*Rates based on less than 20 deaths.

Table I.18   Percent of live births at birth weights of 2,500 grams or less, by age of mother, color, and total-birth order: United States, January-March 1950.

Age of mother and color	Total	Birth order				
		First	Second	Third	Fourth	Fifth and over
Total						
All ages	7.4	7.7	6.9	7.2	7.5	7.7
15-19	9.0	8.5	9.6	12.0	13.9	18.3
20-24	7.3	6.9	6.9	8.0	9.1	10.5
25-29	6.7	7.1	5.9	6.5	7.2	8.0
30-34	7.2	9.1	6.6	6.5	6.8	7.6
35-39	7.7	11.0	8.1	7.2	6.9	7.1
40-44	7.7	13.7	8.2	7.0	7.8	6.8
White						
All ages	7.0	7.2	6.5	6.9	7.4	7.4
15-19	8.0	7.6	8.6	12.5	16.7	*
20-24	6.9	6.5	6.5	7.8	9.2	10.7
25-29	6.5	6.9	5.7	6.4	7.1	8.0
30-34	7.0	8.9	6.4	6.3	6.8	7.3
35-39	7.5	10.9	8.1	7.1	6.8	6.7
40-44	7.5	13.1	7.9	6.5	7.6	6.7
Nonwhite						
All ages	9.7	11.8	10.1	8.9	8.3	8.5
15-19	12.0	12.2	11.5	11.5	12.4	16.3
20-24	9.6	11.1	9.6	8.6	8.7	10.2
25-29	8.4	11.0	8.9	8.0	7.4	7.9
30-34	8.8	11.6	9.8	9.1	7.5	8.3
35-39	9.0	13.2	8.3	9.8	8.4	8.7
40-44	8.9	*	13.0	16.2	10.0	7.5

Source: National Office of Vital Statistics: Weight at birth and survival of newborn, by age of mother and total-birth order, by J. Loeb. Vital Statistics--Special Reports, Vol. 47, No. 2. Public Health Service, Washington, 1958.

Notes: Total-birth order refers to number of children ever born to mother, including fetal deaths. Excludes data for Massachusetts. Figures for birth weight, birth order, and age of mother not stated are distributed. Figures for age of mother under 15 years of age and 45 years and over are not shown separately but are included in totals for groups.

*Rates not computed, less than 10 deaths.

Table I.19   Neonatal mortality rates per 1,000 live births by total-birth order, color, and age of mother: United States, January-March 1950.

Birth order and color	All ages	Age of mother, years					
		15-19	20-24	25-29	30-34	35-39	40-44
Total							
Total	20.0	23.8	19.0	17.6	20.0	23.6	27.2
First	19.1	21.2	16.6	17.3	24.1	28.7	30.9
Second	17.8	28.1	18.2	14.3	16.1	20.3	25.3
Third	19.7	35.3	22.0	17.7	16.9	19.8	26.4
Fourth	21.1	45.2	24.9	19.6	18.8	21.5	23.6
Fifth and over	26.9	68.8	35.8	25.5	25.5	26.1	28.0
White							
Total	18.9	22.3	18.0	16.7	18.9	22.6	26.1
First	17.8	19.8	15.5	16.4	22.3	28.1	29.8
Second	16.9	27.2	17.5	14.0	15.2	20.2	26.3
Third	19.3	41.4	22.5	17.1	16.8	19.9	25.5
Fourth	20.3	49.0	25.9	18.8	18.5	20.1	22.1
Fifth and over	26.0	*	37.5	25.9	24.4	24.9	26.5
Nonwhite							
Total	26.7	28.3	24.8	24.6	28.7	29.9	35.0
First	28.9	26.6	27.7	31.8	49.2	37.2	*
Second	25.4	29.9	23.5	20.3	32.6	22.5	*
Third	22.3	28.6	20.5	23.9	18.7	19.0	*
Fourth	25.0	43.2	22.9	23.6	21.7	38.3	*
Fifth and over	29.1	*	34.3	24.9	28.7	30.3	34.5

Source: National Office of Vital Statistics: Weight at birth and survival of newborn by age of mother and total-birth order, by J. Loeb. Vital Statistics--Special Reports, Vol. 47, No. 2. Public Health Service, Washington, 1958.

Notes: Based on deaths under 28 days among children born January 1 to March 31, 1950. Total-birth order refers to number of children ever born to mother, including fetal deaths. Excludes data for Massachusetts. Figures for birth order and age of mother not stated are distributed. Figures for age of mother under 15 years of age and 45 years and over are not shown separately but are included in totals for groups.

*Rates not computed, less than 10 deaths.

Table I.20   Average fetal death rates per 1,000 live births and fetal deaths by age of mother, color, and total-birth order: United States, 1960-61.

Color and birth order	All ages[1]	Age of mother, years					
		15-19	20-24	25-29	30-34	35-39	40-44
Total							
Total	15.8	13.7	11.9	14.2	19.0	26.8	38.5
First	15.5	13.8	13.0	17.8	30.0	46.6	60.2
Second	11.2	12.2	9.4	10.7	14.6	21.0	32.2
Third	13.2	16.3	11.3	11.5	14.5	21.4	32.2
Fourth	16.0	23.1	14.4	13.9	15.8	21.9	31.0
Fifth	19.1	47.3	17.3	16.2	18.7	23.8	33.0
Sixth and over	28.8	72.7	23.3	22.4	25.2	31.6	43.4
White							
Total	13.9	11.7	10.6	12.6	16.6	23.4	34.3
First	13.8	12.1	11.8	16.3	26.9	41.8	56.2
Second	10.1	10.0	8.5	9.9	13.3	19.2	29.7
Third	12.1	12.7	10.2	10.6	13.4	19.7	30.3
Fourth	14.7	17.4	12.6	12.7	14.6	20.3	29.4
Fifth	17.5	30.4	15.1	14.6	16.7	22.0	30.7
Sixth and over	24.0	41.2	20.3	19.0	21.0	26.3	37.5
Nonwhite							
Total	26.2	20.9	19.7	24.1	33.1	45.5	61.7
First	26.5	21.2	25.1	32.4	57.6	88.4	96.7
Second	19.0	18.3	16.4	19.5	27.9	39.3	63.3
Third	20.5	22.1	16.3	20.6	27.5	41.6	54.6
Fourth	23.3	28.7	19.5	21.7	27.9	39.0	50.0
Fifth	26.1	60.1	21.0	22.0	31.5	38.4	57.4
Sixth and over	36.5	101.0	26.2	27.7	34.4	46.4	62.4

Source: Annual volumes Vital Statistics of the United States, National Center for Health Statistics, Public Health Service, Washington.

Notes: Includes only fetal deaths for which the period of gestation was given as 20 weeks (or 5 months) or more or was not stated. Total-birth order refers to number of children ever born to mother, including fetal deaths. Data for Massachusetts are included only in the totals by age of mother because this State did not require the reporting of birth order. Figures for birth order not stated (for States other than Massachusetts) and for age of mother not stated are distributed.

[1]Includes data for age groups under 15 years and 45 years and over.

Table I.21a   Infant mortality rates per 1,000 live births, cohort and adjusted, by month: United States, 1940-61.

Year of birth	Month of birth[1]												
	Total	Jan.	Feb.	Mar.	Apr.	May	June	July	Aug.	Sept.	Oct.	Nov.	Dec
1961	25.2	25.0	23.0	23.6	24.8	25.7	26.2	26.2	26.3	25.6	25.6	25.4	25.
1960	25.9	25.5	24.4	24.1	25.4	27.3	27.6	26.6	25.9	25.6	26.9	26.2	25.
1959	26.3	26.2	24.6	24.5	25.6	27.3	27.3	27.2	27.4	26.3	26.3	26.3	26
1958	27.0	26.2	24.5	25.4	26.2	27.1	27.9	28.3	28.4	27.2	27.8	27.9	27
1957	26.5	25.5	24.8	25.0	25.9	27.2	27.7	27.6	27.5	26.6	26.8	26.6	26.
1956	26.2	24.9	24.1	24.3	26.4	27.7	27.6	27.4	27.2	25.5	26.6	26.5	26.
1955	26.4	25.5	24.6	25.0	26.4	27.3	27.9	27.4	27.1	26.7	26.2	26.4	25.
1954	26.5	25.6	24.9	25.4	26.8	27.3	28.1	27.3	27.6	26.6	26.9	25.9	25.
1953	27.5	27.3	25.6	26.1	27.7	29.1	29.2	28.3	28.0	27.4	27.7	26.9	26.
1952	28.4	28.3	26.9	26.6	28.5	29.6	30.5	29.6	28.7	28.3	28.4	27.7	27
1951	28.5	28.7	27.3	27.4	28.3	28.5	29.2	29.4	28.9	28.3	28.9	29.0	28.
1950	29.3	28.4	27.6	28.5	30.3	30.6	29.7	29.5	29.6	29.4	29.0	29.5	29.
1949	30.8	31.6	29.5	29.2	31.6	32.4	32.2	31.6	31.6	30.2	30.0	29.8	29
1948	31.9	32.6	30.2	29.4	31.2	33.1	34.5	32.3	32.2	31.1	32.0	32.2	32
1947	32.0	31.9	30.2	30.4	31.5	31.6	31.2	31.5	33.5	32.4	32.8	33.7	33.
1946	34.6	36.2	34.5	34.0	35.5	37.1	36.9	34.8	34.8	33.5	33.8	33.4	33.
1945	37.0	38.7	36.7	35.8	36.9	37.8	37.8	36.1	37.4	36.7	37.0	36.5	37
1944	39.0	39.7	37.3	39.1	39.3	40.0	40.0	38.4	38.7	39.1	39.3	38.7	39.
1943	39.7	40.1	38.3	38.4	38.5	39.7	39.9	39.8	40.3	39.4	39.9	41.3	41.
1942	41.3	44.6	40.9	39.6	41.6	41.7	41.3	41.4	42.0	41.2	39.6	40.9	41.
1941	44.5	49.4	45.7	44.4	44.6	45.5	44.6	42.0	42.1	42.3	44.2	45.3	45
1940	47.7	49.7	47.7	46.2	46.4	46.4	46.7	45.8	46.3	46.9	48.6	50.4	51.

Source: Guralnick, L. and Winter, E.: A note on cohort infant mortality rates. Public Health Reports, Vol. 80, No. 8, August, 1965.

[1] Rates are based on birth cohorts classified by month of birth.

[2] Rates are adjusted for changing number of births.

Table I.21b   Infant mortality rates per 1,000 live births, cohort and adjusted, by month: United States, 1940-61- continued.

Year of death	Month of Death[2]												
	Total	Jan.	Feb.	Mar.	Apr.	May	June	July	Aug.	Sept.	Oct.	Nov.	Dec.
1961	25.3	28.5	25.9	24.9	24.9	25.0	24.6	23.9	23.5	23.7	25.0	25.7	27.1
1960	26.0	27.9	26.8	26.2	25.9	26.6	26.2	24.6	23.1	23.3	26.0	26.6	28.7
1959	26.4	29.4	27.1	26.1	25.7	26.9	25.9	24.8	24.7	24.9	25.2	27.0	27.4
1958	27.0	29.1	28.0	27.1	26.8	26.8	26.4	26.3	25.1	24.4	26.3	27.4	29.6
1957	26.4	29.0	26.5	26.3	25.8	26.0	26.0	25.1	24.3	24.4	26.4	27.1	27.7
1956	26.1	27.7	25.3	25.3	26.7	27.9	26.5	25.3	24.9	22.7	25.6	26.5	28.3
1955	26.4	28.8	27.3	25.6	25.8	25.8	26.1	25.7	24.9	24.8	25.5	27.2	28.7
1954	26.7	28.4	26.6	26.2	27.3	27.0	27.4	25.8	24.8	24.5	26.0	26.6	28.3
1953	27.8	30.9	28.7	27.4	27.7	28.0	27.7	26.0	26.1	26.5	27.7	27.8	28.5
1952	28.5	29.8	28.8	28.9	28.8	27.9	30.7	27.9	26.0	26.3	28.3	28.6	29.5
1951	28.6	31.5	31.0	29.3	28.4	27.7	28.1	27.1	26.5	25.9	28.1	29.2	29.7
1950	29.2	30.1	29.6	31.1	30.9	29.8	29.1	27.0	26.8	27.1	27.7	29.6	31.2
1949	31.4	34.8	33.7	32.1	30.6	30.7	30.1	30.9	30.9	29.3	29.8	30.7	31.7
1948	31.8	36.2	34.8	32.2	31.7	32.7	32.2	29.7	30.2	28.7	31.0	31.1	32.7
1947	32.8	36.7	35.1	34.7	32.8	31.3	29.9	29.1	29.9	29.3	29.6	31.4	34.3
1946	34.6	39.7	39.5	36.7	37.0	38.1	36.5	33.5	32.4	31.2	32.1	32.7	35.4
1945	38.1	41.3	43.1	39.8	36.9	36.2	36.5	34.4	37.1	37.2	35.9	36.4	41.1
1944	39.4	43.7	40.3	41.8	40.9	39.1	39.3	37.3	37.1	38.1	39.7	37.8	39.4
1943	40.7	44.5	43.8	44.0	39.4	38.1	38.7	38.1	37.8	36.2	37.3	39.8	44.3
1942	41.2	47.4	47.4	45.3	42.1	40.6	39.9	40.4	37.8	38.3	38.1	38.4	42.2
1941	45.9	57.4	52.4	50.3	45.2	43.6	43.3	43.8	42.1	41.7	44.3	44.0	43.2
1940	47.4	56.1	52.1	49.5	46.8	45.5	44.0	44.4	41.7	41.7	44.4	49.1	53.1

Table I.22a Specified complications of pregnancy and delivery per 1,000 single births by age of mother, birth order and color: Upstate New York, 1960-62.

Complication, birth order, and color	Total[1]	Age of mother, years					
		Under 20	20-24	25-29	30-34	35-39	40 and over
White							
Complications A-E							
Total	86	100	83	75	83	103	133
1	127	113	118	140	172	231	310
2 and 3	69	63	61	64	76	100	138
4 and 5	74	63	63	65	72	90	115
6 or more	91	*	63	70	87	101	122
Complication A							
Total	12	20	11	8	11	18	32
1	21	24	19	17	28	44	49
2 and 3	8	8	6	6	9	17	34
4 and 5	10	*	7	6	10	15	28
6 or more	15	-	*	7	12	18	33
Complication C							
Total	19	14	15	18	22	27	34
1	14	14	13	16	16	24	33
2 and 3	10	14	15	15	18	22	30
4 and 5	23	*	21	21	23	27	31
6 or more	32	*	30	29	31	33	40
Complication E							
Total	51	66	55	46	46	54	65
1	92	75	86	107	131	173	234
2 and 3	41	37	36	38	45	58	71
4 and 5	36	*	30	33	35	41	51
6 or more	39	-	23	30	39	44	47

Source: Special tabulations, New York State Department of Health.

Note: Included are live births and all reported fetal deaths of 20 weeks or more gestation. Complications are as follows: A--pre-eclampsia, eclampsia and hypertension; C--placenta previa and premature separation; E--dystocias. Complications B (diabetes) and D (prolapse of cord) included in "Complications A-E" but not shown separately. Birth order refers to number of children ever born to mother including fetal deaths.

[1]Not stated ages are included in totals but not distributed.

*Rates not computed, less than 10 cases.

Table I.22b Specified complications of pregnancy and delivery per 1,000 single births by age of mother, birth order and color: Upstate New York, 1960-62 - continued.

Complication, birth order, and color	Total[1]	Age of mother, years					
		Under 20	20-24	25-29	30-34	35-39	40 and over
Nonwhite							
Complications A-E							
Total	100	98	85	94	114	146	214
1	135	115	128	182	207	299	400
2 and 3	79	73	68	82	101	137	200
4 and 5	87	70	69	80	104	130	189
6 or more	115	*	93	91	116	142	214
Complication A							
Total	28	33	20	21	34	58	98
1	41	46	37	30	35	116	*
2 and 3	18	14	14	17	31	54	*
4 and 5	23	*	15	20	31	41	98
6 or more	40	*	24	25	38	63	102
Complication C							
Total	21	17	18	22	27	26	37
1	19	15	18	26	32	*	*
2 and 3	17	21	16	17	16	*	*
4 and 5	24	*	22	23	27	21	*
6 or more	30	-	31	27	32	31	*
Complication E							
Total	46	46	44	44	49	59	75
1	77	55	76	129	152	152	*
2 and 3	39	33	36	40	52	55	*
4 and 5	35	*	27	32	39	62	*
6 or more	39	-	34	30	39	47	80

Note: The source and footnotes are the same as on the table for WHITE.

Table I.23   Selected complications of pregnancy and delivery per 1,000 single births by birth weight and color: Upstate New York, 1960-62.

Birth weight and color	A-E[1]	A	B	C	D	E
White						
Total[2]	86	12	2	19	2	51
1,000 grams or less	460	22	6	315	27	99
1,001-1,500	429	52	9	264	20	107
1,501-2,000	310	47	7	175	10	83
2,001-2,500	162	24	3	74	5	60
2,501-3,500	73	10	1	13	2	47
3,501-4,500	74	12	2	6	1	53
4,501 or more	129	28	14	4	4	92
2,500 or less	242	30	4	133	9	73
2,501 or more	74	11	2	10	2	51
Nonwhite						
Total[2]	100	28	3	21	4	46
1,000 grams or less	397	41	*	226	41	102
1,001-1,500	392	69	*	205	23	119
1,501-2,000	258	72	*	119	*	72
2,001-2,500	126	43	4	40	5	43
2,501-3,500	75	22	2	10	2	39
3,501-4,500	95	29	5	6	3	55
4,501 or more	250	98	49	-	*	132
2,500 or less	214	50	4	96	12	64
2,501 or more	81	25	3	9	2	44

Source: Special tabulations, New York State Department of Health.

Note: Included are live births and all reported fetal deaths of 20 weeks or more gestation or gestation not stated. Complications are as follows: A--pre-eclampsia, eclampsia and hypertension; B--diabetes; C--placenta previa and premature separation: D--prolapse of cord; E--dystocias.

[1]Sum of figures for individual complications per 1,000 births of specified weight is greater than the total because more than 1 complication was reported for some pregnancies.

[2]Not stated birth weights included in totals but not distributed.

*Rates not computed, less than 10 cases

Table I.24   Neonatal, fetal and perinatal mortality rates per 1,000 single white births by selected complications of labor and delivery; total and Caesarian section deliveries: Upstate New York, 1951-52 and 1960-62.

Decennium and Complication	Neonatal[1]		Fetal[2]		Perinatal[3]	
	Total	With CS[4]	Total	With CS[4]	Total	With CS[4]
1960-62						
Total	12	40	13	22	25	61
A-E	57	54	68	36	122	88
A	22	51	65	47	86	96
B	87	115	149	53	223	163
C	162	137	179	91	312	216
D	100	45	269	74	342	117
E	31	15	20	7	50	22
None of above	8	27	8	8	16	35
1951-52						
Total	15	42	15	31	30	72
A-E	50	49	66	42	113	89
A	36	81	81	42	114	119
B	124	133	180	*	281	169
C	172	133	216	132	351	247
D	119	*	466	182	530	218
E	29	16	18	8	46	24
None of above	11	29	9	14	19	46

Source: Special tabulations, New York State Department of Health.

Note: Included are live births and all reported fetal deaths of 20 weeks or more gestation or gestation not stated. Complications are as follows: A--pre-eclampsia, eclampsia and hypertension; B--diabetes; C--placenta previa and premature separation; D--prolapse of cord; E--dystocias.

[1]Number of deaths under 4 weeks per 1,000 live births.

[2]Number of fetal deaths of 20 weeks or more gestation per 1,000 live births plus fetal deaths.

[3]Number of neonatal deaths plus fetal deaths per 1,000 live births plus fetal deaths.

[4]"CS" refers to Caesarian section.

*Rates not computed, less than 10 deaths.

Table I.25   Neonatal, fetal and perinatal mortality per 1,000 single white Caesarian section births by whether previous section was performed, birth order and obstetrical complications and neonatal deaths as a percent of perinatal deaths: Upstate New York, 1962.

Caesarian Section	Total	Birth order			Complications A-E	None of specified complications
		1	2 and 3	4 or more		
With previous Caesarian section						
Neonatal mortality[1]	24	-	22	26	40	20
Fetal mortality[2]	7	-	4	11	18	4
Perinatal mortality[3]	30	-	26	37	58	23
No previous Caesarian section						
Neonatal mortality[1]	50	21	66	85	52	44
Fetal mortality[2]	37	20	45	57	45	*
Perinatal mortality[3]	85	41	108	137	95	52
Neonatal deaths as a percent of perinatal deaths						
With previous Caesarian section	78	-	84	71	68	85
No previous Caesarian section	57	50	59	59	53	83

Source: Special tabulations, New York State Department of Health.

Note: Included are live births and all reported fetal deaths of 20 weeks or more gestation or gestation not stated.   Complications are as follows: A--pre-eclampsia, eclampsia and hypertension; B--diabetes; C--placenta previa and premature separation; D--prolapse of cord; E--dystocias.   Birth order refers to number of children ever born to mother including fetal deaths.

[1]Number of deaths under 4 weeks per 1,000 live births.
[2]Number of fetal deaths of 20 weeks or more gestation per 1,000 live births plus fetal deaths.
[3]Number of neonatal deaths plus fetal deaths per 1,000 live births plus fetal deaths.
*Rate not computed, less than 10 deaths.

Table II.1   Maternal mortality rates per 10,000 live births, by color: Birth-registration States or United States, 1915-1964.

Year	Total	White	Nonwhite	Year	Total	White	Nonwhite
1964	3.3	2.2	9.0	1939	40.4	35.3	76.2
1963	3.6	2.4	9.7	1938	43.5	37.7	84.9
1962	3.5	2.4	9.6	1937	48.9	43.6	85.8
1961	3.7	2.5	10.1	1936	56.8	51.2	97.2
1960	3.7	2.6	9.8	1935	58.2	53.1	94.6
1959	3.7	2.6	10.2	1934[1]	59.3	54.4	89.7
1958	3.8	2.6	10.2	1933[1]	61.9	56.4	96.7
1957	4.1	2.8	11.8	1932[1]	63.3	58.1	97.6
1956	4.1	2.9	11.1	1931	66.1	60.1	111.4
1955	4.7	3.3	13.0	1930	67.3	60.9	117.4
1954	5.2	3.7	14.4	1929	69.5	63.1	119.9
1953	6.1	4.4	16.6	1928	69.2	62.7	121.0
1952	6.8	4.9	18.8	1927	64.7	59.4	113.3
1951	7.5	5.5	20.1	1926	65.6	61.9	107.1
1950	8.3	6.1	22.2	1925	64.7	60.3	116.2
1949	9.0	6.8	23.5	1924	65.6	60.7	117.9
1948	11.7	8.9	30.1	1923	66.5	62.6	109.5
1947	13.5	10.9	33.5	1922	66.4	62.8	106.8
1946	15.7	13.1	35.9	1921	68.2	64.4	107.7
1945	20.7	17.2	45.5	1920	79.9	76.0	128.1
1944	22.8	18.9	50.6	1919	73.7	69.6	124.4
1943	24.5	21.1	51.0	1918	91.6	88.9	139.3
1942	25.9	22.2	54.4	1917	66.2	63.2	117.7
1941	31.7	26.6	67.8	1916	62.2	60.8	117.9
1940	37.6	32.0	77.3	1915	60.8	60.1	105.6

Source: Annual volumes Vital Statistics of the United States, National Center for Health Statistics, Public Health Service, Washington.

Note: Refers only to deaths occurring within the specified area. Prior to 1933, data are for birth-registration States only. Deaths are classified according to the International Classification of Diseases used at the time. Alaska included in data beginning 1959 and Hawaii, 1960. New Jersey excluded from data by color for 1962 and 1963; color not reported.

[1]For 1932-1934, Mexicans included with nonwhite.

Table II.2 Average annual maternal mortality rates per 100,000 live births for selected causes of death by age of mother: United States, selected decennium periods.

Cause of death and decennium	All ages¹	Under 20	20-24	25-29	30-34	35-39	40-44	45 and over
1959-61								
Deliveries and complications of pregnancy, childbirth and the puerperium (640-689)	37.1	23.4	20.1	29.7	52.3	90.1	143.3	280.3
Sepsis of pregnancy, childbirth, and puerperium (640, 641, 681, 682, 684)	4.0	3.3	2.3	3.0	5.0	10.2	13.8	31.8*
Toxemias of pregnancy and puerperium except abortion with toxemia (642, 685, 686)	7.1	7.6	4.2	4.7	7.2	17.2	31.2	63.7*
Hemorrhage of pregnancy and childbirth (643, 644, 670-672)	6.3	2.2	2.5	4.4	10.1	18.2	36.3	70.1*
Ectopic pregnancy (645)	2.6	0.9*	1.4	2.5	4.7	5.8	5.8*	6.4*
Abortion without mention of sepsis or toxemia (650)	2.1	1.2	1.2	2.1	3.5	3.7	6.2*	12.7*
Abortion with sepsis (651)	4.6	3.2	2.9	5.1	5.7	7.3	7.6	31.8*
Abortion with toxemia, without mention of sepsis (652)	0.3	0.2*	0.2*	0.3*	0.2*	0.3*	1.5*	6.4*
Other complications of pregnancy, childbirth, and puerperium and delivery without mention of complication (646-649, 660, 673-680, 683, 687-689)	10.1	4.9	5.4	7.6	14.9	27.3	41.0	57.3*
1949-51								
Deliveries and complications of pregnancy, childbirth and the puerperium	82.7	71.8	47.6	64.8	106.1	180.6	323.7	627.2
Sepsis of pregnancy, childbirth and puerperium	11.7	10.7	7.1	8.4	15.4	23.9	50.5	73.4*
Toxemias of pregnancy and puerperium, except abortion with toxemia	26.8	33.5	15.6	19.2	29.5	55.6	113.7	253.5
Hemorrhage of pregnancy and childbirth	14.6	6.2	7.3	11.8	20.4	37.9	66.8	126.8*
Ectopic pregnancy	5.3	2.1	2.3	5.6	9.0	11.7	11.0	20.0*
Abortion without mention of sepsis or toxemia	2.5	1.8	1.7	2.1	3.1	5.9	7.4*	20.0*

Abortion with sepsis	5.9	6.0	4.5	5.3	6.2	9.5	17.1	13.3*
Abortion with toxemia, without mention of sepsis (652)	0.9	0.5*	0.6	0.8	1.0*	2.0*	1.8*	13.3*
Other complications of pregnancy, childbirth and puerperium and delivery without mention of complication 1939-41	15.0	11.0	8.4	11.6	21.5	34.0	55.3	106.8*
Deliveries and complications of pregnancy, childbirth and the puerperium	363.9	355.2	238.9	288.9	442.3	708.3	988.7	1481.0
Sepsis of pregnancy, childbirth, and puerperium	91.1	87.0	62.5	74.5	111.1	171.9	219.3	342.2
Toxemias of pregnancy and puerperium, except abortion with toxemia	87.4	131.3	59.3	60.8	92.2	156.7	209.4	348.1
Hemorrhage of pregnancy and childbirth	46.3	25.0	24.3	36.2	62.3	116.5	178.6	212.4
Ectopic pregnancy	15.7	4.0	7.6	16.8	24.4	36.6	33.6	59.0*
Abortion without mention of sepsis or toxemia [2]	11.7	9.3	6.7	9.8	12.8	24.0	31.3	36.9*
Abortion with sepsis	52.4	50.9	40.7	44.0	65.4	77.9	115.2	141.6
Abortion with toxemia, without mention of sepsis [2]	3.8	1.0*	2.0	3.5	5.2	8.8	14.0*	9.2*
Other complications of pregnancy, childbirth and puerperium and delivery without mention of complication	55.5	44.8	35.4	43.8	67.6	114.8	179.7	330.4

Source: Annual volumes Vital Statistics of the U. S., National Center for Health Statistics, Public Health Service, Washington, and special tabulations.

Note: Alaska and Hawaii included in 1959-61 deaths. Numbers after causes of death are category numbers of the Seventh Revision of the International Classification of Diseases, 1955. Deaths are classified according to the Sixth Revision, 1948 for 1949-51 and Fifth Revision, 1938 for 1939-41. The effect that the changes in the rules of the I.C.D. had upon the comparability of the rates for the decenniums is discussed in the "NOTE" following Table 7.2.

[1]Deaths for age not stated distributed among age groups.
[2]Data not available by age for these causes for 1939. Rates for "all ages" based on 3-year figures; rates for individual age groups based on 1940 and 1941 data.
*Rates based on less than 20 deaths.

Table II.3   Average annual maternal mortality rates per 100,000 live births by race: United States, each geographic division and State, 1959-61.

Area	Total	White	Nonwhite Total	Nonwhite Negro	Area	Total	White	Nonwhite Total	Nonwhite Negro
United States[1, 3]	37.1	25.5	100.0	104.6	South Atlantic-continued				
					West Virginia	37.3	34.0	*	*
New England	22.9	20.5	84.5	84.4	North Carolina	50.2	23.3	108.3	109.5
Maine	31.5	30.4	*	-	South Carolina	64.4	21.2	123.4	123.9
New Hampshire	29.1†	29.3†	-	-	Georgia	60.3	24.4	125.1	125.5
Vermont	*	*	-	-	Florida	49.9	22.2	124.7	125.8
Massachusetts	22.3	19.8	85.8†	86.6†					
Rhode Island	*	*	-	-	East South Central	62.1	35.0	127.1	127.7
Connecticut	22.3	16.9	100.8†	103.8†	Kentucky	47.8	42.3	105.9	107.8
					Tennessee	44.1	30.1	92.8	93.2
Middle Atlantic	38.1	27.8	111.3	113.4	Alabama	75.9	34.7	144.7	145.0
New York	44.4	32.4	124.0	127.8	Mississippi	85.8	29.1	134.2	134.8
New Jersey	35.1	22.0	119.7	120.7					
Pennsylvania	30.3	24.2	82.1	82.4	West South Central	45.6	31.3	98.4	100.5
					Arkansas	58.1	31.5	120.2	120.8
East North Central	29.9	23.8	78.3	79.5	Louisiana	48.9	20.7	92.8	93.3
Ohio	28.7	23.6	72.1	73.2	Oklahoma	39.1	31.1	88.8†	112.1†
Indiana	28.7	24.8	71.5	72.6	Texas	43.6	34.1	98.4	99.2
Illinois	26.2	20.6	55.2	56.6					
Michigan	36.5	24.9	129.7	131.4	Mountain[3]	32.2	28.7	76.0	86.9
Wisconsin	29.7	27.7	*	*	Montana	19.1†	*	*	*
					Idaho	21.5†	19.9†	-	-
West North Central	23.7	21.1	63.9	69.4	Wyoming	*	*	-	-
Minnesota	14.1	13.6	*	*	Colorado	32.4	31.3	*	*
Iowa	21.3	21.1	*	*	New Mexico	52.8	50.6	*	*
Missouri	35.4	29.2	74.4	75.4	Arizona	34.2	24.1	87.9†	*
North Dakota	27.9†	24.9†	*	*	Utah	26.8	23.5†	*	-
South Dakota	25.5†	22.3†	*	-	Nevada	*	*	*	-
Nebraska	20.4	19.3†	*	*					
Kansas	22.2	19.6	*	*	Pacific[1, 3]	26.7	22.1	59.5	74.2
					Washington	19.9	18.9	*	*
South Atlantic	51.2	24.8	114.2	114.9	Oregon	24.9	23.0	*	*
Delaware	48.3†	*	*	*	California[3]	27.9	22.5	71.1	76.5
Maryland	36.2	22.3	83.9	85.5	Alaska	*	*	*	*
District of Columbia	71.3	*	84.5	83.3	Hawaii[2]	23.1†	*	*	-
Virginia	50.5	26.3	122.9	122.8					

Source: Annual volumes Vital Statistics of the United States, National Center for Health Statistics, Public Health Service, Washington, and special tabulations.

[1]Includes Alaska and Hawaii.

[2]Live births in Hawaii in 1959 not tabulated by race: births for Negro and other races for that year estimated on the basis of the 1960-61 distribution.

[3]There were less than 20 deaths from maternal causes tabulated for other races in all the geographic divisions except Mountain and Pacific and in all the States except California. Rates for other races in these areas were 70.7 (Mountain), 42.9 (Pacific) and 57.9 (California). The United States rate for other races was 48.6.

*Rates not computed, based on less than 10 deaths.

†Rates based on between 10 and 19 deaths.

Table II.4a   Average annual maternal mortality rates per 100,000 live births for selected causes of death by color in metropolitan and nonmetropolitan counties: United States and each geographic region, 1959-61.

Cause of Death and Area (7th Revision-International Classification of Diseases)	Total			White			Nonwhite		
	All counties	Metropolitan counties	Nonmetropolitan counties	All counties	Metropolitan counties	Nonmetropolitan counties	All counties	Metropolitan counties	Nonmetropolitan counties
United States[1]									
Deliveries and complications of pregnancy, childbirth, and the puerperium (640-689)	37.1	33.0	44.3	25.5	22.7	30.5	100.0	87.6	123.4
Sepsis of pregnancy, childbirth, and puerperium (640, 641, 681, 682, 684)	4.0	3.4	5.0	3.1	2.7	3.7	8.9	7.2	12.2
Toxemias of pregnancy and puerperium, except abortion with toxemia (642, 685, 686)	7.1	4.8	11.1	4.4	3.4	6.1	21.5	12.0	39.4
Hemorrhage of pregnancy and childbirth (643, 644, 670-672)	6.3	4.4	9.6	4.5	3.3	6.7	15.8	10.5	25.9
Ectopic pregnancy (645)	2.6	2.8	2.3	1.2	1.3	1.2	10.3	11.2	8.6
Abortion (650, 651, 652)	7.0	8.2	4.9	4.1	4.7	3.1	22.7	26.6	15.3
Other complications of pregnancy, childbirth, and puerperium and delivery without mention of complication (646-649, 660, 673-680, 683, 687-689)	10.1	9.3	11.5	8.1	7.3	9.7	20.9	20.2	22.1

Source: Special tabulations of the Division of Vital Statistics, National Center for Health Statistics, Public Health Service, Washington.

[1] Includes Alaska and Hawaii.

*Rates based on less than 20 deaths.

Table II.4b   Average annual maternal mortality rates per 100,000 live births for selected causes of death by color in metropolitan and nonmetropolitan counties: United States and each geographic region, 1959-61 - continued.

Cause of Death and Area (7th Revision-International Classification of Diseases)	Total			White			Nonwhite		
	All counties	Metro-politan counties	Nonmet-ropolitan counties	All counties	Metro-politan counties	Nonmet-ropolitan counties	All counties	Metro-politan counties	Nonmet-ropolitan counties
Northeast									
Deliveries and complications of pregnancy, childbirth, and the puerperium	34.4	36.4	26.4	25.9	26.3	24.5	108.9	110.2	88.1*
Sepsis of pregnancy, childbirth, and puerperium	3.3	3.3	3.2*	2.8	2.7	3.0*	7.7	7.5	11.0*
Toxemias of pregnancy and puerperium, except abortion with toxemia	4.2	4.0	5.1	3.8	3.4	5.1	8.4	8.5	5.5*
Hemorrhage of pregnancy and childbirth	4.9	5.1	4.1	4.2	4.1	4.2	11.0	11.7	-
Ectopic pregnancy	2.9	3.1	2.2*	1.8	1.8	1.8*	13.0	12.8	16.5*
Abortion	8.9	10.4	2.7*	4.7	5.4	2.1*	46.1	47.6	22.0*
Other complications of pregnancy, childbirth, and puerperium and delivery without mention of complication	10.2	10.4	9.0	8.7	8.9	8.3	22.7	22.0	33.0*
North Central									
Deliveries and complications of pregnancy, childbirth, and the puerperium	28.1	27.6	28.9	23.0	20.0	27.3	75.6	73.8	91.9
Sepsis of pregnancy, childbirth, and puerperium	3.8	3.9	3.6	3.3	3.3	3.3	8.0	7.3	14.4*
Toxemias of pregnancy and puerperium, except abortion with toxemia	4.1	3.9	4.5	3.3	2.8	4.0	11.9	10.4	25.9*
Hemorrhage of pregnancy and childbirth	4.7	3.3	7.0	4.5	2.9	6.8	6.6	5.5*	17.2*
Ectopic pregnancy	2.0	2.5	1.1*	1.1	1.2	0.9*	10.5	10.7	8.6*
Abortion	4.1	5.4	1.9	2.5	3.1	1.7	18.4	19.5	8.6*
Other complications of pregnancy, childbirth, and puerperium and delivery without mention of complication	9.4	8.5	10.8	8.2	6.5	10.6	20.1	20.4	17.2*

NOTE: Source and footnotes are the same as for the table on UNITED STATES

Table II.4c — Average annual maternal mortality rates per 100,000 live births for selected causes of death by color in metropolitan and nonmetropolitan counties: United States and each geographic region, 1959-61 - continued.

Cause of Death and Area (7th Revision-International Classification of Diseases)	Total			White			Nonwhite		
	All counties	Metropolitan counties	Nonmetropolitan counties	All counties	Metropolitan counties	Nonmetropolitan counties	All counties	Metropolitan counties	Nonmetropolitan counties
South									
Deliveries and complications of pregnancy, childbirth, and the puerperium	51.8	39.7	63.9	29.2	22.0	34.6	113.3	92.2	132.1
Sepsis of pregnancy, childbirth, and puerperium	5.3	3.6	7.0	3.5	2.4	4.6	10.1	7.0	12.9
Toxemias of pregnancy and puerperium, except abortion with toxemia	13.1	7.5	18.6	6.4	4.3	8.6	31.1	16.0	43.7
Hemorrhage of pregnancy and childbirth	9.8	5.6	14.0	5.7	3.1	8.5	20.9	13.2	27.7
Ectopic pregnancy	3.7	3.9	3.4	1.2	1.2*	1.2*	10.4	12.0	8.9
Abortion	8.3	8.9	7.6	4.2	4.1	4.3	19.3	23.0	16.1
Other complications of pregnancy, childbirth, and puerperium and delivery without mention of complication	11.7	10.2	13.2	8.1	6.8	9.4	21.5	20.2	22.7
West[1]									
Deliveries and complications of pregnancy, childbirth, and the puerperium	28.2	26.9	31.4	24.0	22.1	28.4	62.6	60.9	61.5
Sepsis of pregnancy, childbirth, and puerperium	2.8	2.7	3.0*	2.4	2.2	3.0*	6.2*	7.0*	3.7*
Toxemias of pregnancy and puerperium, except abortion with toxemia	4.4	3.6	6.4	4.0	3.3	5.8	7.5*	5.8*	13.0*
Hemorrhage of pregnancy and childbirth	4.2	3.6	5.9	3.2	2.7	4.5	12.4	9.9*	20.5*
Ectopic pregnancy	1.3	1.3*	1.2*	0.7*	0.5*	1.1*	5.8*	7.0*	1.9*
Abortion	7.2	8.1	4.9	6.4	7.0	4.6	14.2	16.3	7.4*
Other complications of pregnancy, childbirth, and puerperium and delivery without mention of complication	8.2	7.5	10.0	7.2	6.3	9.5	16.4	16.9	14.9*

NOTE: Source and footnotes are the same as for the table on UNITED STATES

Table III.1a

Childhood mortality*, ages 1-4 years, by color and sex:
United States, 1900-64.

Area and year	Total			White			Nonwhite		
	Both sexes	Male	Female	Both sexes	Male	Female	Both sexes	Male	Female
United States[1]									
1964	1.0	1.0	0.9	0.8	0.9	0.8	1.6	1.7	1.5
1963[2]	1.0	1.1	0.9	0.9	0.9	0.8	1.8	1.9	1.6
1962[2]	1.0	1.0	0.9	0.9	0.9	0.8	1.7	1.8	1.5
1961	1.0	1.1	0.9	0.9	1.0	0.8	1.7	1.8	1.6
1960	1.1	1.2	1.0	1.0	1.0	0.9	1.9	2.1	1.7
1959	1.1	1.2	1.0	0.9	1.0	0.8	1.9	2.1	1.7
1958	1.1	1.2	1.0	1.0	1.1	0.9	1.9	2.0	1.9
1957	1.1	1.2	1.0	1.0	1.1	0.9	1.9	2.1	1.8
1956	1.1	1.2	1.0	1.0	1.1	0.9	1.9	2.0	1.8
1955	1.1	1.2	1.0	1.0	1.1	0.9	2.0	2.1	1.9
1954	1.2	1.3	1.1	1.1	1.1	1.0	2.0	2.2	1.9
1953	1.3	1.4	1.2	1.2	1.3	1.1	2.2	2.4	2.0
1952	1.4	1.5	1.3	1.3	1.4	1.2	2.5	2.7	2.3
1951	1.4	1.5	1.3	1.2	1.3	1.1	2.5	2.7	2.3
1950	1.4	1.5	1.3	1.2	1.4	1.1	2.5	2.7	2.3
1949	1.5	1.6	1.4	1.4	1.5	1.2	2.5	2.7	2.3
1948	1.6	1.7	1.5	1.5	1.6	1.3	2.6	2.7	2.4
1947	1.6	1.8	1.5	1.5	1.6	1.3	2.6	2.7	2.4
1946	1.8	2.0	1.7	1.7	1.8	1.5	2.9	3.1	2.6
1945	2.0	2.2	1.9	1.9	2.0	1.7	3.3	3.5	3.1
1944	2.3	2.5	2.2	2.1	2.3	1.9	3.9	4.1	3.7
1943	2.6	2.8	2.4	2.3	2.5	2.1	4.2	4.5	3.9
1942	2.4	2.6	2.3	2.2	2.4	2.0	4.1	4.4	3.9
1941	2.8	3.0	2.6	2.5	2.7	2.3	5.0	5.2	4.8
1940	2.9	3.1	2.7	2.6	2.8	2.4	4.8	5.3	4.4
1939	3.2	3.4	2.9	2.9	3.1	2.6	5.3	5.7	4.9
1938	3.8	4.1	3.6	3.5	3.7	3.3	6.3	6.7	5.8
1937	4.2	4.5	3.9	3.8	4.1	3.6	6.6	7.1	6.1
1936	4.4	4.7	4.1	4.1	4.4	3.8	6.6	7.1	6.1
1935	4.4	4.7	4.1	4.1	4.4	3.8	6.7	7.1	6.3
1934	5.1	5.4	4.7	4.7	5.0	4.4	8.1	8.8	7.4
1933	4.7	5.0	4.4	4.4	4.7	4.1	7.0	7.4	6.6

Source: Annual volumes Vital Statistics of the United States, National Center for Health Statistics, Public Heatlh Service, Washington.

[1]Alaska included beginning 1959, and Hawaii, 1960.

[2]Figures by color exclude data for residents of New Jersey.

*Rates per 1,000 population residing in area for specified group, enumerated as of April 1 for 1940, 1950 and 1960 and estimated as of July 1 for all other years.

Table III.1b Childhood mortality rates*, ages 1-4 years, by color and sex
United States, 1900-64 - continued.

Area and year	Total			White			Nonwhite		
	Both sexes	Male	Female	Both sexes	Male	Female	Both sexes	Male	Female
Death Registration States[1]									
1932	4.6	4.9	4.4	4.3	4.6	4.1	6.9	7.2	6.5
1931	5.3	5.6	4.9	4.8	5.2	4.5	8.6	9.1	8.0
1930	5.6	6.0	5.2	5.2	5.5	4.8	9.3	10.0	8.7
1929	6.3	6.6	5.9	5.8	6.1	5.5	9.7	10.3	9.2
1928	6.5	6.8	6.1	6.0	6.3	5.6	10.5	11.1	9.9
1927	5.9	6.2	5.6	5.4	5.7	5.1	10.4	11.0	9.7
1926	7.2	7.6	6.8	6.7	7.0	6.3	12.5	13.1	11.9
1925	6.4	6.7	6.1	5.9	6.2	5.6	11.0	11.4	10.6
1924	6.8	7.2	6.4	6.2	6.6	5.8	12.6	13.2	12.0
1923	8.1	8.5	7.7	7.5	7.9	7.1	13.4	13.9	12.8
1922	7.4	7.9	6.9	7.1	7.5	6.6	10.7	11.4	9.9
1921	8.0	8.4	7.6	7.7	8.1	7.2	11.8	12.2	11.5
1920	9.9	10.3	9.5	9.4	9.8	9.0	14.6	15.0	14.2
1919	9.3	9.7	8.8	8.7	9.2	8.3	15.0	15.6	14.3
1918	15.7	16.0	15.5	14.7	15.0	14.5	28.4	28.8	27.9
1917	10.7	11.2	10.1	10.0	10.5	9.4	19.7	20.5	18.9
1916	11.1	11.7	10.5	10.6	11.2	10.1	17.8	18.8	16.8
1915	9.2	9.7	8.8	8.9	9.4	8.4	17.8	18.1	17.4
1914	10.2	10.7	9.7	9.9	10.4	9.4	19.1	19.5	18.8
1913	11.9	12.5	11.4	11.6	12.1	11.1	20.2	20.9	19.4
1912	10.9	11.5	10.4	10.7	11.2	10.1	21.6	22.2	20.9
1911	11.8	12.2	11.3	11.4	11.8	10.9	25.4	26.7	24.2
1910	14.0	14.6	13.4	13.7	14.2	13.0	28.3	30.1	26.6
1909	13.5	14.1	12.9	13.1	13.7	12.5	28.9	29.6	28.2
1908	14.0	14.6	13.4	13.6	14.2	13.0	30.3	31.7	29.1
1907	14.7	15.3	14.1	14.2	14.8	13.6	33.7	35.2	32.2
1906	15.8	16.4	15.2	15.3	15.8	14.7	36.4	38.3	34.5
1905	15.0	15.8	14.2	14.6	15.4	13.8	38.7	41.1	36.4
1904	15.9	16.6	15.2	15.5	16.2	14.8	39.8	42.4	37.3
1903	15.4	15.9	14.9	15.0	15.5	14.5	39.4	41.6	37.4
1902	16.6	17.1	16.0	16.2	16.8	15.6	37.4	38.4	36.4
1901	16.9	17.7	16.2	16.6	17.4	15.9	34.8	36.0	33.8
1900	19.8	20.5	19.1	19.4	20.2	18.7	43.5	43.4	43.5

Source: Annual volumes Vital Statistics of the United States, National Center for Health Statistics, Public Health Service, Washington.

[1]Increased in number from 10 States and the District of Columbia in 1900 to the entire conterminous United States in 1933.

*Rates per 1,000 population residing in area for specified group, enumerated as of April 1 for 1940, 1950 and 1960 and estimated as of July 1 for all other years.

Table III.2a

Childhood mortality rates*, ages 5-14 years, by color and sex:
United States, 1900-64.

Area and year	Total			White			Nonwhite		
	Both sexes	Male	Female	Both sexes	Male	Female	Both sexes	Male	Female
United States[1]									
1964	0.4	0.5	0.3	0.4	0.5	0.3	0.6	0.7	0.5
1963[2]	0.4	0.5	0.4	0.4	0.5	0.3	0.6	0.7	0.5
1962[2]	0.4	0.5	0.4	0.4	0.5	0.3	0.6	0.7	0.5
1961	0.4	0.5	0.4	0.4	0.5	0.3	0.6	0.7	0.5
1960	0.5	0.6	0.4	0.4	0.5	0.3	0.6	0.8	0.5
1959	0.5	0.6	0.4	0.4	0.6	0.3	0.7	0.8	0.5
1958	0.5	0.6	0.4	0.4	0.5	0.4	0.6	0.7	0.5
1957	0.5	0.6	0.4	0.5	0.6	0.4	0.7	0.8	0.6
1956	0.5	0.6	0.4	0.4	0.5	0.4	0.6	0.8	0.5
1955	0.5	0.6	0.4	0.5	0.6	0.4	0.7	0.8	0.5
1954	0.5	0.6	0.4	0.5	0.6	0.4	0.7	0.8	0.6
1953	0.6	0.7	0.4	0.5	0.6	0.4	0.7	0.9	0.6
1952	0.6	0.7	0.5	0.6	0.7	0.5	0.8	0.9	0.7
1951	0.6	0.7	0.5	0.6	0.7	0.4	0.9	1.0	0.7
1950	0.6	0.7	0.5	0.6	0.7	0.5	0.9	1.0	0.8
1949	0.7	0.8	0.5	0.6	0.7	0.5	0.9	1.0	0.8
1948	0.7	0.8	0.5	0.6	0.7	0.5	0.9	1.0	0.9
1947	0.7	0.8	0.5	0.6	0.8	0.5	1.0	1.1	0.9
1946	0.8	0.9	0.6	0.7	0.9	0.6	1.1	1.2	1.0
1945	0.8	1.0	0.7	0.8	1.0	0.6	1.2	1.2	1.1
1944	0.9	1.0	0.7	0.8	1.0	0.6	1.3	1.4	1.2
1943	0.9	1.1	0.8	0.9	1.0	0.7	1.3	1.4	1.2
1942	0.9	1.0	0.7	0.8	1.0	0.6	1.4	1.5	1.2
1941	1.0	1.1	0.8	0.9	1.0	0.7	1.5	1.6	1.4
1940	1.0	1.2	0.9	1.0	1.1	0.8	1.5	1.6	1.4
1939	1.1	1.3	0.9	1.0	1.2	0.8	1.6	1.8	1.5
1938	1.2	1.4	1.1	1.1	1.3	1.0	1.8	1.9	1.7
1937	1.4	1.5	1.2	1.3	1.5	1.1	1.9	2.0	1.8
1936	1.5	1.7	1.3	1.4	1.6	1.2	2.1	2.2	1.9
1935	1.5	1.7	1.4	1.5	1.6	1.3	2.1	2.2	2.0
1934	1.5	1.7	1.4	1.5	1.6	1.3	2.2	2.2	2.1
1933	1.5	1.7	1.3	1.4	1.6	1.2	2.2	2.2	2.1

Source: Annual volumes Vital Statistics of the United States, National Center for Health Statistics, Public Health Service, Washington.

[1]Alaska included beginning 1959, and Hawaii, 1960.

[2]Figures by color exclude data for residents of New Jersey.

*Rates per 1,000 population residing in area for specified group, enumerated as of April 1 for 1940, 1950 and 1960 and estimated as of July 1 for all other years.

Table III.2b   Childhood mortality rates*, ages 5-14 years, by color and sex:
United States, 1900-64 - continued.

Area and year	Total			White			Nonwhite		
	Both sexes	Male	Female	Both sexes	Male	Female	Both sexes	Male	Female
Death Registration States[1]									
1932	1.5	1.7	1.4	1.5	1.6	1.3	2.2	2.3	2.1
1931	1.7	1.8	1.5	1.6	1.8	1.4	2.4	2.5	2.4
1930	1.7	1.9	1.5	1.6	1.8	1.4	2.6	2.7	2.6
1929	1.9	2.1	1.7	1.8	2.0	1.6	2.7	2.8	2.5
1928	1.9	2.1	1.7	1.8	2.0	1.6	2.8	2.9	2.8
1927	1.9	2.1	1.7	1.8	2.0	1.6	2.8	2.9	2.7
1926	1.9	2.1	1.7	1.8	2.0	1.6	2.9	3.0	2.9
1925	2.0	2.2	1.8	1.9	2.1	1.6	3.0	3.1	2.9
1924	2.0	2.2	1.8	1.9	2.1	1.7	2.9	2.9	2.9
1923	2.1	2.3	2.0	2.1	2.3	1.9	2.9	2.8	2.9
1922	2.1	2.3	2.0	2.1	2.3	1.9	2.7	2.7	2.7
1921	2.5	2.7	2.3	2.4	2.6	2.2	3.1	3.1	3.1
1920	2.6	2.8	2.5	2.5	2.7	2.3	3.8	3.7	3.9
1919	2.7	2.8	2.5	2.5	2.7	2.3	4.4	4.1	4.6
1918	4.1	4.2	4.1	3.9	3.9	3.8	7.0	6.5	7.4
1917	2.6	2.7	2.4	2.4	2.6	2.2	4.3	4.1	4.5
1916	2.5	2.6	2.3	2.3	2.5	2.1	3.8	3.6	4.0
1915	2.3	2.4	2.2	2.2	2.4	2.1	4.4	4.3	4.5
1914	2.5	2.6	2.4	2.4	2.6	2.3	4.6	4.4	4.8
1913	2.7	2.8	2.5	2.6	2.7	2.4	4.7	4.4	5.0
1912	2.5	2.6	2.3	2.4	2.5	2.3	5.0	4.7	5.2
1911	2.7	2.8	2.6	2.6	2.7	2.5	5.7	5.5	5.9
1910	2.9	3.0	2.9	2.9	3.0	2.8	5.7	5.4	5.9
1909	2.8	2.9	2.7	2.7	2.9	2.6	6.3	5.7	6.8
1908	3.0	3.1	2.9	2.9	3.0	2.8	6.9	6.8	6.9
1907	3.2	3.3	3.0	3.1	3.2	2.9	6.8	6.5	7.1
1906	3.3	3.4	3.2	3.1	3.3	3.0	7.8	7.3	8.3
1905	3.4	3.4	3.3	3.3	3.4	3.2	8.1	6.9	9.3
1904	3.7	3.7	3.6	3.6	3.6	3.6	8.1	7.4	8.7
1903	3.4	3.5	3.4	3.4	3.5	3.3	7.2	6.3	8.0
1902	3.3	3.4	3.2	3.2	3.4	3.1	7.1	7.1	7.2
1901	3.5	3.7	3.4	3.5	3.6	3.3	7.4	7.2	7.5
1900	3.9	3.8	3.9	3.8	3.8	3.8	9.0	7.8	10.1

Source: Annual volumes Vital Statistics of the United States, National Center for Health
Statistics, Public Health Service, Washington.

[1]Increased in number from 10 States and the District of Columbia in 1900 to the entire
conterminous United States in 1933.

*Rates per 1,000 population residing in area for specified group, enumerated as of April 1 for
1940, 1950 and 1960 and estimated as of July 1 for all other years.

Table III.3   Childhood mortality rates by age, color and sex per 1,000 population:*
United States, selected years.

Age, color and sex	1964	1963	1962	1961	1960	1959	1958	1957	1956	1955	1950
1-4											
Total	0.96	1.00	0.98	1.02	1.09	1.07	1.12	1.12	1.10	1.14	1.39
Male	1.05	1.08	1.05	1.11	1.20	1.16	1.19	1.20	1.19	1.23	1.52
Female	0.87	0.91	0.91	0.93	0.98	0.98	1.04	1.04	1.02	1.04	1.27
White	0.84	0.86	0.86	0.90	0.95	0.94	0.98	0.99	0.98	1.01	1.24
Male	0.92	0.94	0.93	0.99	1.05	1.02	1.06	1.06	1.06	1.10	1.36
Female	0.75	0.78	0.80	0.81	0.85	0.86	0.90	0.91	0.89	0.91	1.12
Nonwhite	1.62	1.76	1.67	1.69	1.91	1.86	1.93	1.94	1.92	1.97	2.51
Male	1.75	1.88	1.79	1.80	2.07	2.04	2.00	2.07	2.04	2.09	2.71
Female	1.49	1.64	1.55	1.59	1.74	1.68	1.86	1.82	1.80	1.85	2.30
5-14											
Total	0.43	0.44	0.44	0.44	0.47	0.47	0.46	0.48	0.47	0.48	0.60
Male	0.52	0.52	0.52	0.53	0.56	0.57	0.55	0.58	0.56	0.58	0.71
Female	0.34	0.35	0.35	0.35	0.37	0.37	0.37	0.38	0.37	0.38	0.49
White	0.41	0.41	0.42	0.42	0.44	0.44	0.44	0.45	0.44	0.46	0.56
Male	0.49	0.49	0.50	0.50	0.53	0.54	0.52	0.55	0.53	0.56	0.67
Female	0.32	0.32	0.33	0.33	0.35	0.34	0.35	0.36	0.35	0.36	0.45
Nonwhite	0.59	0.61	0.60	0.57	0.64	0.63	0.60	0.67	0.64	0.65	0.86
Male	0.71	0.69	0.70	0.68	0.75	0.73	0.69	0.79	0.75	0.75	0.97
Female	0.48	0.52	0.50	0.46	0.53	0.53	0.50	0.56	0.53	0.54	0.75

Source: Annual volumes Vital Statistics of the United States, National Center for Health Statistics, Public Health Service, Washington.

Note: Alaska included beginning 1959 and Hawaii 1960. New Jersey excluded from data by color for 1962 and 1963.

*Enumerated as of April 1 for 1950 and 1960 and estimated as of July 1 for other years.

Table III.4a   Average annual childhood mortality rates per 100,000 population for selected causes of death by age, color and sex: United States, selected decennium periods.

Cause of Death (7th Revision - International Classification of Diseases)	1 - 14 years			1 - 4 years			5 - 14 years		
	1959– 1961	1949– 1951	1939– 1941	1959– 1961	1949– 1951	1939– 1941	1959– 1961	1949– 1951	1939– 1941
Total									
All childhood causes	65.0	90.3	157.2	105.9	143.3	296.8	46.3	61.9	104.1
Infective and parasitic diseases (001-138)	3.7	12.8	29.8	7.5	21.7	63.0	2.0	7.9	17.2
Tuberculosis, all forms (001-019)	0.3	3.3	7.7	0.7	6.1	12.9	0.1	1.7	5.7
Malignant neoplasms, including neoplasms of lymphatic and hematopoietic tissues (140-205)	8.2	8.3	6.1	10.6	11.6	9.5	7.0	6.5	4.8
Malignant neoplasms of brain and other parts of nervous system (193)	1.7	1.6	1.0	2.2	2.0	1.3	1.6	1.4	0.8
Leukemia and aleukemia (204)	3.9	3.9	2.7	5.3	5.8	4.6	3.3	2.8	1.9
Allergic, endocrine system, metabolic and nutritional diseases (240-289)	1.2	1.7	2.7	1.8	3.0	4.5	0.9	1.0	2.1
Diabetes mellitus (260)	0.3	0.5	1.2	0.2	0.4	0.8	0.4	0.5	1.4
Avitaminoses and nutritional deficiency states (280-286)	0.2	0.3	0.5	0.6	0.7	1.2	0.1	0.1	0.2
All other allergic, endocrine system, metabolic, nutritional diseases (240-254, 270-277, 287-289)	0.6	1.0	1.0	1.0	2.0	2.4	0.4	0.4	0.5
Diseases of blood and blood-forming organs (290-299)	1.0	0.9	1.1	1.6	1.4	2.0	0.7	0.7	0.7
Anemias (290-293)	0.7	0.6	0.4	1.2	0.9	0.9	0.5	0.4	0.3
Diseases of nervous system and sense organs (330-398)	4.6	5.8	8.2	7.8	9.4	14.2	3.2	3.8	6.0
Vascular lesions affecting central nervous systems (330-334)	0.7	0.7	1.0	0.9	0.9	1.4	0.7	0.5	0.8
Meningitis, except meningococcal and tuberculous (340)	1.1	1.5	1.8	2.6	3.0	3.8	0.4	0.6	1.1
Cerebral spastic infantile paralysis (351)	0.7	1.0	——	0.9	1.5	——	0.6	0.7	——
Diseases of circulatory system (400-468)	1.4	3.4	9.0٭	1.5	2.0	5.1	1.4	4.1	10.5
Rheumatic fever and chronic rheumatic heart disease (400-416)	0.5	2.2	5.6	0.2	0.6	1.8	0.7	3.1	7.1
Diseases of respiratory system (470-527)	8.4	12.1	27.8	19.6	25.7	71.6	3.3	4.8	11.1
Influenza and pneumonia, except pneumonia of newborn (480-493)	6.3	8.9	24.3	14.9	19.4	63.5	2.4	3.2	9.5
Bronchitis (500-502)	0.7	1.1	1.2	1.9	2.5	3.5	0.2	0.3	0.3
Other diseases of respiratory system except acute upper respiratory infections[1] (510-527)	1.0	1.4	1.1	1.9	2.2	2.3	0.5	1.0	0.7
Diseases of digestive system (530-587)	3.1	5.0	23.2	6.0	9.8	49.5	1.8	2.5	13.2
Appendicitis (550-553)	0.4	1.2	7.4	0.3	1.3	6.9	0.4	1.1	7.7
Gastritis, duodenitis, enteritis and colitis, except diarrhea of newborn (543-571, 572)	1.2	2.3	9.1	3.3	5.8	30.6	0.3	0.5	0.9
Fibrocystic disease of pancreas[2] (587B)	0.7 }	1.5	6.7	1.0 }	2.7	12.0	0.6 }	0.9	4.6
All other diseases of digestive system (530-542, 544-570, 573-587A)	0.8 }			1.4 }			0.5 }		
Diseases of genito-urinary system (590-637)	1.0	2.3	3.5	0.9	2.7	4.4	1.0	2.0	3.1
Nephritis and nephrosis (590-594)	0.8	2.0	2.8	0.7	2.4	3.3	0.8	1.8	2.7
Congenital malformations (750-759)	6.4	5.6	4.4	12.3	11.6	10.4	3.7	2.4	2.1
Congenital hydrocephalus and other congenital malformations, etc.[3] (752, 753)	1.4	1.5	1.8	3.0	3.3	4.7	0.6	0.5	0.7
Congenital malformations of circulatory system (754)	3.9	2.6	2.1	6.9	5.0	4.5	2.5	1.2	1.2
Other congenital malformations (750, 751, 755-759)	1.1	1.5	0.5	2.4	3.2	1.3	0.5	0.6	0.2
Accidents[4] (E800-E936)	22.5	28.0	34.6	30.7	37.2	49.6	18.8	23.2	28.9
Motor vehicle accidents (E810-E835)	8.4	10.0	11.9	9.7	11.6	13.0	7.8	9.1	11.5
Accidental poisoning (E870-E895)	1.0	1.2	1.4	2.6	3.1	4.3	0.2	0.3	0.3
Accidental falls (E900-E904)	1.0	1.1	1.8	1.8	1.7	2.6	0.6	0.8	1.5
Accident caused by fire and explosion of combustible material (E916)	3.5	4.4	6.3	6.5	7.7	14.6	2.2	2.6	3.1
Accident caused by firearm (E919)	1.0	1.3	1.7	0.5	0.6	0.9	1.2	1.6	1.9
Accidental drowning (E929)	3.8	4.8	5.6	4.2	5.1	6.4	3.6	4.6	5.4
All other accidents[4] (E800-E802, E840-E866, E910-E915, E917, E918, E920-E928, E930-E936)	3.8	5.3	5.8	5.4	7.3	7.7	3.1	4.2	5.1
Residual (210-239, 300-326, 640-749, 760-795, E940-E999)	3.5	4.4	6.9	5.5	7.1	13.0	2.6	3.0	4.6

Source: Annual volumes <u>Vital Statistics of the United States,</u> National Center for Health Statistics, Public Health Service, Washington, and special tabulations.

Note: Alaska and Hawaii included in 1959-61 deaths. Numbers after causes of death are category numbers of the Seventh Revision of the International Classification of Diseases, 1955. Deaths are classified according to the Sixth Revision, 1948, for 1949-1951 and Fifth Revision, 1938, for 1939-1941. The more important sources of incomparability are footnoted to the affected categories.

[1]Fifth Revision includes "asthma" and "hemorrhagic infarction and thrombosis." In Sixth and Seventh Revision, these diseases were included, respectively, with "all other allergic, etc." and "diseases of circulatory system."
[2]Fibrocystic disease of pancreas (587B) not tabulated **separately prior to Seventh Revision.**
[3]Includes other congenital malformations of nervous system and sense organs.
[4]Sixth Revision includes "late effects of motor vehicle accidents, accidental poisoning and other accidental injury" (960-962). In Seventh Revision, those deaths included with "Residual." In Fifth Revision, there was no comparable category.
٭Rate based on less than 20 deaths.

Table III.4b

Average annual childhood mortality rates per 100,000 population for selected causes of death by age, color and sex: United States, selected decennium periods - continued.

Cause of Death (7th Revision - International Classification of Diseases)	1 - 14 years			1 - 4 years			5 - 14 years		
	1959-1961	1949-1951	1939-1941	1959-1961	1949-1951	1939-1941	1959-1961	1949-1951	1939-1941
White									
All childhood causes	59.0	82.7	143.4	92.9	128.3	266.4	43.8	58.2	96.8
Infective and parasitic diseases	3.2	11.1	24.4	6.2	18.4	52.6	1.8	7.2	13.7
Tuberculosis, all forms	0.2	2.3	4.9	0.4	4.4	9.3	0.1	1.1	3.2
Malignant neoplasms, including neoplasms of lymphatic and hematopoietic tissues	8.6	8.7	6.4	11.3	12.2	10.1	7.4	6.8	5.0
Malignant neoplasms of brain and other parts of nervous system	1.8	1.6	1.0	2.2	2.0	1.4	1.6	1.4	0.9
Leukemia and aleukemia	4.2	4.2	2.9	5.7	6.3	5.0	3.5	3.0	2.1
Allergic, endocrine system, metabolic and nutritional diseases	1.0	1.6	2.6	1.4	2.7	4.3	0.8	1.0	2.0
Diabetes mellitus	0.3	0.5	1.2	0.2	0.4	0.9	0.4	0.5	1.3
Avitaminoses and nutritional deficiency states	0.1	0.2	0.4	0.3	0.5	1.0	0.1	0.1	0.1
All other allergic, endocrine system, metabolic, nutritional diseases	0.5	0.9	1.0	0.9	1.8	2.4	0.4	0.4	0.5
Diseases of blood and blood-forming organs	0.8	0.8	1.1	1.1	1.2	2.0	0.6	0.6	0.7
Anemias	0.5	0.4	0.4	0.7	0.7	0.8	0.4	0.3	0.3
Diseases of nervous system and sense organs	4.3	5.4	8.0	7.0	8.7	13.8	3.0	3.7	5.8
Vascular lesions affecting central nervous systems	0.7	0.6	0.9	0.8	0.8	1.4	0.6	0.5	0.7
Meningitis, except meningococcal and tuberculous	1.0	1.3	1.7	2.2	2.6	3.6	0.4	0.6	0.9
Cerebral spastic infantile paralysis	0.7	1.0	---	0.9	1.4	---	0.6	0.7	---
Diseases of circulatory system	1.1	2.9	8.5	1.1	1.7	4.8	1.1	3.5	9.9
Rheumatic fever and chronic rheumatic heart disease	0.4	1.8	5.3	0.1	0.5	1.6	0.5	2.6	6.7
Diseases of respiratory system	6.9	10.3	24.3	15.6	21.5	62.3	3.0	4.3	9.9
Influenza and pneumonia, except pneumonia of newborn	5.0	7.2	20.9	11.2	15.4	54.1	2.1	2.8	8.3
Bronchitis	0.7	1.0	1.2	1.8	2.4	3.5	0.2	0.3	0.4
Other diseases of respiratory system except acute upper respiratory infections[1]	0.9	1.4	1.1	1.7	2.2	2.4	0.5	0.9	0.7
Diseases of digestive system	2.8	4.5	21.7	5.2	8.5	45.1	1.8	2.3	12.9
Appendicitis	0.3	1.1	7.6	0.3	1.3	7.4	0.3	1.0	7.7
Gastritis, duodenitis, enteritis and colitis, except diarrhea of newborn	1.0	2.0	7.7	2.6	4.8	26.1	0.2	0.4	0.8
Fibrocystic disease of pancreas[2]	0.8	} 1.4	6.4	1.1	} 2.5	11.6	0.7	} 0.9	4.4
All other diseases of digestive system	0.7			1.2			0.5		
Diseases of genito-urinary system	0.9	2.1	3.2	0.8	2.5	4.0	1.0	1.9	2.9
Nephritis and nephrosis	0.7	1.9	2.6	0.5	2.2	2.9	0.7	1.7	2.5
Congenital malformations	6.3	5.7	4.6	12.0	11.7	11.0	3.7	2.4	2.1
Congenital hydrocephalus and other congenital malformations, etc.[3]	1.3	1.5	1.9	2.9	3.3	4.9	0.6	0.5	0.7
Congenital malformations of circulatory system	3.8	2.6	2.2	6.6	5.1	4.7	2.5	1.2	1.2
Other congenital malformations	1.1	1.6	0.5	2.4	3.3	1.3	0.6	0.7	0.2
Accidents[4]	20.3	26.2	33.6	26.9	34.0	48.1	17.3	22.0	28.1
Motor vehicle accidents	8.3	10.0	12.2	9.6	11.7	13.5	7.7	9.1	11.7
Accidental poisoning	0.7	1.0	1.2	1.9	2.5	3.7	0.2	0.2	0.2
Accidental falls	0.8	1.1	1.9	1.4	1.6	2.6	0.6	0.8	1.6
Accident caused by fire and explosion of combustible material	2.3	3.2	5.4	4.0	5.3	12.6	1.5	2.0	2.7
Accident caused by firearm	0.9	1.2	1.5	0.4	0.5	0.8	1.2	1.5	1.8
Accidental drowning	3.5	4.7	5.7	4.5	5.5	7.0	3.1	4.3	5.2
All other accidents[4]	3.7	5.0	5.8	5.1	6.8	7.9	3.1	4.1	5.0
Residual	2.9	3.5	5.0	4.2	5.5	8.5	2.3	2.5	3.7

Note: Source and footnotes are the same as for the table on TOTAL.

Table III.4c   Average annual childhood mortality rates per 100,000 population for selected causes of death by age, color and sex: United States, selected decennium periods - continued.

Cause of Death (7th Revision - International Classification of Diseases)	1 - 14 years			1 - 4 years			5 - 14 years		
	1959-1961	1949-1951	1939-1941	1959-1961	1949-1951	1939-1941	1959-1961	1949-1951	1939-1941
Nonwhite									
All childhood causes	102.3	144.1	255.0	182.6	251.8	508.2	62.5	88.1	156.4
Infective and parasitic diseases	7.1	24.3	68.1	15.0	46.3	135.4	3.1	12.8	42.0
Tuberculosis, all forms	1.0	10.4	27.4	2.0	18.5	38.3	0.4	6.2	23.2
Malignant neoplasms, including neoplasms of lymphatic and hematopoietic tissues	5.6	5.5	3.3	7.0	7.4	4.8	4.9	4.5	2.8
Malignant neoplasms of brain and other parts of nervous system	1.4	1.3	0.4	1.6	1.6	0.7	1.3	1.1	0.3
Leukemia and aleukemia	2.0	1.7	1.2	2.5	2.2	1.7	1.7	1.5	1.0
Allergic, endocrine system, metabolic and nutritional diseases	2.2	2.9	3.5	4.1	5.7	5.9	1.3	1.5	2.6
Diabetes mellitus	0.3	0.6	1.1	0.3*	0.4*	0.4*	0.4	0.6	1.4
Avitaminoses and nutritional deficiency states	0.8	0.8	1.3	2.1	2.2	3.2	0.2	0.1*	0.6
All other allergic, endocrine system, metabolic, nutritional diseases	1.0	1.5	1.1	1.7	3.1	2.3	0.7	0.7	0.6
Diseases of blood and blood-forming organs	2.3	1.9	1.1	4.3	3.2	2.2	1.3	1.2	0.7
Anemias	2.1	1.6	0.7	4.0	2.8	1.4	1.1	1.0	0.4
Diseases of nervous system and sense organs	6.9	8.1	10.0	12.0	14.5	17.2	4.4	4.8	7.1
Vascular lesions affecting central nervous systems	1.1	0.8	1.2	1.5	1.1	1.7	0.9	0.7	1.1
Meningitis, except meningococcal and tuberculous	2.1	2.8	2.8	4.9	6.3	5.4	0.7	1.0	1.8
Cerebral spastic infantile paralysis	0.8	1.0	----	1.1	1.7	----	0.6	0.7	----
Diseases of circulatory system	3.2	7.1	12.8	3.6	4.2	7.5	3.0	8.6	14.8
Rheumatic fever and chronic rheumatic heart disease	1.5	5.1	7.7	0.7	1.9	3.1	1.9	6.7	9.4
Diseases of respiratory system	17.7	24.9	52.5	43.4	56.5	136.5	5.0	8.5	19.8
Influenza and pneumonia, except pneumonia of newborn	14.7	20.7	49.2	36.2	48.3	128.7	4.0	6.4	18.2
Bronchitis	0.9	1.3	1.0	2.5	3.3	3.0	0.2	0.2	0.2*
Other diseases of respiratory system except acute upper respiratory infections[1]	1.5	1.9	1.1	3.3	2.7	2.0	0.6	1.5	0.7
Diseases of digestive system	4.9	9.0	33.4	10.4	19.1	80.2	2.1	3.8	15.2
Appendicitis	0.6	1.6	6.0	0.5	1.1	3.1	0.7	1.8	7.2
Gastritis, duodenitis, enteritis and colitis, except diarrhea of newborn	2.7	4.9	18.4	7.4	13.3	61.6	0.4	0.6	1.5
Fibrocystic disease of pancreas[2]	0.1 }	} 2.5	} 9.0	0.3 }	} 4.8	} 15.4	0.0* }	} 1.4	} 6.4
All other diseases of digestive system	1.4 }			2.2 }			1.0 }		
Diseases of genito-urinary system	1.7	3.2	5.3	2.0	4.5	7.3	1.6	2.6	4.5
Nephritis and nephrosis	1.4	2.9	4.5	1.6	4.0	6.3	1.4	2.3	3.9
Congenital malformations	7.0	5.2	3.0	14.2	10.7	6.7	3.5	2.3	1.6
Congenital hydrocephalus and other congenital malformations, etc.[3]	1.5	1.6	1.2	3.1	3.5	3.1	0.7	0.6	0.5
Congenital malformations of circulatory system	4.5	2.4	1.3	8.7	4.5	2.8	2.4	1.3	0.8
Other congenital malformations	1.1	1.2	0.5	2.5	2.6	0.9	0.4	0.4	0.3
Accidents[4]	36.4	41.0	41.7	53.6	60.5	60.3	28.0	30.9	34.5
Motor vehicle accidents	9.3	9.7	10.0	10.6	11.0	9.2	8.7	9.1	10.3
Accidental poisoning	2.6	2.8	2.7	7.1	7.4	8.2	0.4	0.4	0.5
Accidental falls	1.7	1.5	1.8	3.8	2.6	2.8	0.7	0.9	1.3
Accident caused by fire and explosion of combustible material	11.4	12.7	12.7	21.3	24.9	28.6	6.5	6.4	6.5
Accident caused by firearm	1.6	1.9	2.8	1.0	1.3	2.1	1.8	2.3	3.1
Accidental drowning	5.4	5.2	5.6	2.2	2.2	2.5	7.0	6.8	6.8
All other accidents[4]	4.4	7.1	6.2	7.6	11.0	6.9	2.9	5.0	5.9
Residual	7.2	10.9	20.2	13.0	19.3	44.2	4.4	6.6	10.9

Note: Source and footnotes are the same as for the table on TOTAL.

Table III.4d

Average annual childhood mortality rates per 100,000 population for selected causes of death by age, color and sex: United States, selected decennium periods - continued.

Cause of Death (7th Revision - International Classification of Diseases)	1 - 14 years			1 - 4 years			5 - 14 years		
	1959-1961	1949-1951	1939-1941	1959-1961	1949-1951	1939-1941	1959-1961	1949-1951	1939-1941
Male									
All childhood causes	74.3	102.2	174.0	115.4	155.4	318.2	55.6	73.7	119.1
Infective and parasitic diseases	3.9	13.3	30.1	7.8	22.2	63.6	2.1	8.5	17.3
Tuberculosis, all forms	0.3	3.1	7.2	0.7	6.1	13.1	0.1	1.5	4.9
Malignant neoplasms, including neoplasms of lymphatic and hematopoietic tissues	9.1	9.2	6.8	11.7	12.7	10.4	7.9	7.3	5.4
Malignant neoplasms of brain and other parts of nervous system	1.9	1.8	1.1	2.4	2.2	1.4	1.7	1.5	1.0
Leukemia and aleukemia	4.4	4.3	3.0	5.8	6.4	5.0	3.8	3.1	2.3
Allergic, endocrine system, metabolic and nutritional diseases	1.2	1.7	2.7	2.0	3.2	4.8	0.8	1.0	1.8
Diabetes mellitus	0.2	0.4	1.1	0.2	0.3	0.8	0.3	0.4	1.2
Avitaminoses and nutritional deficiency states	0.3	0.3	0.5	0.6	0.8	1.2	0.1	0.1	0.2
All other allergic, endocrine system, metabolic, nutritional diseases	0.7	1.1	1.1	1.1	2.1	2.8	0.5	0.5	0.5
Diseases of blood and blood-forming organs	1.0	1.0	1.1	1.6	1.6	2.2	0.7	0.7	0.7
Anemias	0.6	0.6	0.5	1.1	1.0	1.0	0.4	0.4	0.3
Diseases of nervous system and sense organs	5.2	6.4	8.9	8.7	10.3	15.0	3.5	4.2	6.6
Vascular lesions affecting central nervous systems	0.8	0.7	1.0	1.0	1.0	1.4	0.7	0.6	0.8
Meningitis, except meningococcal and tuberculous	1.3	1.7	2.0	3.1	3.5	4.3	0.5	0.7	1.2
Cerebral spastic infantile paralysis	0.8	1.1	----	1.1	1.6	----	0.7	0.8	----
Diseases of circulatory system	1.4	3.2	8.8	1.6	2.0	5.1	1.4	3.9	10.2
Rheumatic fever and chronic rheumatic heart disease	0.5	2.1	5.3	0.2	0.6	1.7	0.6	2.9	6.7
Diseases of respiratory system	8.9	12.8	29.5	21.1	27.2	76.6	3.3	5.1	11.6
Influenza and pneumonia, except pneumonia of newborn	6.6	9.3	25.6	15.7	20.1	67.0	2.5	3.5	9.8
Bronchitis	0.8	1.2	1.4	2.2	2.9	4.2	0.2	0.3	0.4
Other diseases of respiratory system except acute upper respiratory infections[1]	1.0	1.6	1.2	2.2	2.6	2.5	0.5	1.0	0.7
Diseases of digestive system	3.4	5.5	25.3	6.6	10.5	54.3	1.9	2.8	14.2
Appendicitis	0.4	1.4	8.3	0.4	1.5	7.9	0.4	1.3	8.5
Gastritis, duodenitis, enteritis and colitis, except diarrheas of newborn	1.4	2.4	9.7	3.8	5.9	32.6	0.3	0.5	0.9
Fibrocystic disease of pancreas[2]	0.7	} 1.7	} 7.3	0.8	} 3.1	} 13.8	0.6	} 1.0	} 4.8
All other diseases of digestive system	0.9			1.6			0.6		
Diseases of genito-urinary system	1.0	2.4	3.6	1.0	3.0	4.9	1.0	2.1	3.0
Nephritis and nephrosis	0.8	2.2	3.0	0.8	2.7	3.8	0.8	1.9	2.7
Congenital malformations	6.5	5.8	4.5	12.3	11.8	10.8	3.9	2.6	2.1
Congenital hydrocephalus and other congenital malformations, etc.[3]	1.4	1.6	1.8	3.0	3.4	4.8	0.7	0.6	0.7
Congenital malformations of circulatory system	3.9	2.7	2.1	6.7	5.2	4.5	2.7	1.4	1.2
Other congenital malformations	1.2	1.6	0.6	2.6	3.2	1.4	0.6	0.7	0.3
Accidents[4]	28.9	36.0	45.4	35.1	43.0	56.8	26.2	32.3	41.1
Motor vehicle accidents	10.6	12.6	15.7	11.1	13.6	15.0	10.4	12.1	16.0
Accidental poisoning	1.1	1.4	1.5	2.9	3.5	4.7	0.3	0.3	0.3
Accidental falls	1.2	1.5	2.6	2.1	2.1	3.2	0.8	1.2	2.3
Accident caused by fire and explosion of combustible material	3.2	3.9	5.7	6.2	7.2	14.2	1.8	2.1	2.4
Accident caused by firearm	1.6	2.0	2.6	0.6	0.7	1.2	2.1	2.7	3.2
Accidental drowning	5.8	7.4	9.0	5.6	7.2	8.9	5.9	7.5	9.0
All other accidents[4]	5.4	7.1	8.3	6.6	8.6	9.6	4.9	6.4	7.9
Residual	3.9	4.8	7.4	5.8	7.7	13.6	3.0	3.3	5.0

Note: Source and footnotes are the same as for the table on TOTAL.

Table III.4e   Average annual childhood mortality rates per 100,000 population for selected causes of death by age, color and sex: United States, selected decennium periods - continued.

Cause of Death (7th Revision - International Classification of Diseases)	1 - 14 years 1959-1961	1949-1951	1939-1941	1 - 4 years 1959-1961	1949-1951	1939-1941	5 - 14 years 1959-1961	1949-1951	1939-1941
Female									
All childhood causes	55.3	77.9	139.8	96.0	130.7	274.7	36.7	49.7	88.7
Infective and parasitic diseases	3.5	12.2	29.6	7.1	21.3	62.4	1.9	7.3	17.1
Tuberculosis, all forms	0.3	3.4	8.2	0.7	6.2	12.8	0.1	1.9	6.5
Malignant neoplasms, including neoplasms of lymphatic and hematopoietic tissues	7.2	7.4	5.3	9.5	10.5	8.5	6.1	5.7	4.1
Malignant neoplasms of brain and other parts of nervous system	1.6	1.4	0.8	1.9	1.7	1.2	1.4	1.2	0.7
Leukemia and aleukemia	3.3	3.5	2.3	4.7	5.2	4.2	2.7	2.5	1.6
Allergic, endocrine system, metabolic and nutritional diseases	1.1	1.7	2.8	1.6	2.8	4.1	0.9	1.1	2.3
Diabetes mellitus	0.4	0.6	1.3	0.3	0.4	0.8	0.5	0.7	1.5
Avitaminoses and nutritional deficiency states	0.2	0.3	0.5	0.5	0.7	1.2	0.1	0.1	0.2
All other allergic, endocrine system, metabolic, nutritional diseases	0.5	0.8	1.0	0.8	1.8	2.1	0.4	0.3	0.6
Diseases of blood and blood-forming organs	1.0	0.8	1.0	1.6	1.2	1.7	0.7	0.6	0.7
Anemias	0.8	0.6	0.4	1.3	0.8	0.8	0.6	0.4	0.3
Diseases of nervous system and sense organs	4.1	5.1	7.5	6.8	8.3	13.4	2.8	3.4	5.3
Vascular lesions affecting central nervous systems	0.7	0.6	0.9	0.8	0.7	1.4	0.6	0.5	0.7
Meningitis, except meningococcal and tuberculous	0.9	1.2	1.6	2.1	2.5	3.3	0.4	0.5	0.9
Cerebral spastic infantile paralysis	0.6	0.9	---	0.8	1.3	---	0.6	0.7	---
Diseases of circulatory system	1.4	3.5	9.3	1.3	2.0	5.1	1.4	4.4	10.9
Rheumatic fever and chronic rheumatic heart disease	0.5	2.4	5.9	0.2	0.6	1.9	0.7	3.4	7.4
Diseases of respiratory system	7.9	11.3	25.9	18.1	24.1	66.5	3.2	4.5	10.6
Influenza and pneumonia, except pneumonia of newborn	6.0	8.4	23.1	14.0	18.7	59.8	2.3	3.0	9.1
Bronchitis	0.6	0.9	1.0	1.6	2.2	2.8	0.2	0.2	0.3
Other diseases of respiratory system except acute upper respiratory infections[1]	0.9	1.3	1.0	1.7	1.8	2.1	0.5	1.0	0.6
Diseases of digestive system	2.9	4.6	21.0	5.4	9.1	44.5	1.8	2.2	12.0
Appendicitis	0.3	1.0	6.5	0.2	1.1	5.8	0.4	1.0	6.7
Gastritis, duodenitis, enteritis and colitis, except diarrhea of newborn	1.1	2.2	8.4	2.8	5.7	28.4	0.2	0.4	0.8
Fibrocystic disease of pancreas[2]	0.8 }	1.4	6.0	1.2 }	2.3	10.3	0.7 }	0.8	4.5
All other diseases of digestive system	0.7			1.1			0.5		
Diseases of genito-urinary system	1.0	2.1	3.4	0.8	2.3	3.9	1.1	2.0	3.2
Nephritis and nephrosis	0.8	1.9	2.7	0.6	2.1	2.8	0.9	1.7	2.7
Congenital malformations	6.2	5.4	4.2	12.4	11.4	10.1	3.4	2.2	2.0
Congenital hydrocephalus and other congenital malformations, etc.[3]	1.3	1.4	1.7	3.0	3.3	4.6	0.6	0.4	0.7
Congenital malformations of circulatory system	3.8	2.4	2.0	7.1	4.9	4.4	2.4	1.1	1.1
Other congenital malformations	1.0	1.5	0.4	2.3	3.2	1.1	0.5	0.6	0.2
Accidents[4]	15.9	19.7	23.5	26.3	31.2	42.2	11.1	13.6	16.3
Motor vehicle accidents	6.2	7.2	8.0	8.3	9.6	10.9	5.2	5.9	6.9
Accidental poisoning	0.9	1.1	1.2	2.4	2.6	3.8	0.2	0.2	0.2
Accidental falls	0.7	0.8	1.1	1.5	1.3	2.1	0.3	0.5	0.7
Accident caused by fire and explosion of combustible material	3.9	4.8	7.0	6.7	8.2	15.1	2.6	3.0	3.9
Accident caused by firearm	0.4	0.5	0.6	0.4	0.5	0.7	0.4	0.5	0.6
Accidental drowning	1.7	2.0	2.2	2.7	2.9	3.8	1.2	1.6	1.6
All other accidents[4]	2.2	3.4	3.3	4.2	6.0	5.8	1.2	2.0	2.3
Residual	3.2	4.0	6.4	5.2	6.6	12.3	2.2	2.7	4.2

Note: Source and footnotes are the same as for the table on TOTAL.

Table III.5   Average annual childhood mortality rates per 100,000 population by age
and color in metropolitan and nonmetropolitan counties: United States
and each geographic division, 1959-61, and all counties, 1950.

| Area and Color | 1959-61 | | | | | | 1950 | |
| | 1-4 years | | | 5-14 years | | | 1- 4 years | 5-14 years |
	All coun-ties	Metro-politan counties	Nonmet-ropolitan counties	All coun-ties	Metro-politan counties	Nonmet-ropolitan counties	All coun-ties	All coun-ties
United States[1]	105.9	96.5	122.2	46.3	42.7	52.0	139.4	60.1
New England	84.3	79.9	98.3	41.7	39.6	48.3	107.9	45.9
Middle Atlantic	92.5	92.4	93.3	42.1	40.5	48.8	110.1	51.5
East North Central	92.4	90.2	97.0	43.7	42.4	46.2	124.0	59.3
West North Central	94.9	87.8	101.1	45.6	42.9	47.6	135.3	58.0
South Atlantic	127.4	112.6	142.5	51.6	47.6	55.3	153.0	64.6
East South Central	132.0	108.2	146.1	53.0	48.3	55.6	179.8	69.5
West South Central	127.8	115.3	143.8	51.3	47.1	56.1	184.0	66.2
Mountain	131.1	113.4	147.8	53.0	47.6	57.9	191.4	77.0
Pacific[1]	97.7	92.2	118.7	41.8	38.7	52.6	119.9	56.7
White[1]	92.9	86.1	104.5	43.8	40.6	48.9	124.1	56.4
New England	82.4	77.2	98.7	41.0	38.7	48.2	107.8	45.7
Middle Atlantic	84.6	83.0	90.9	40.2	38.1	48.4	102.7	49.3
East North Central	85.8	80.8	95.2	42.8	41.1	45.7	116.0	58.4
West North Central	89.9	81.4	96.7	44.9	42.5	46.6	124.2	56.4
South Atlantic	97.0	88.6	106.1	45.9	42.5	49.2	121.1	57.6
East South Central	104.7	86.2	115.7	47.1	44.8	48.3	154.2	61.6
West South Central	109.1	101.4	119.6	49.0	44.8	53.9	169.7	61.6
Mountain	116.9	107.2	126.3	51.8	47.3	55.9	158.0	69.9
Pacific[1]	94.2	90.0	109.5	40.5	37.9	49.7	115.8	55.5
Nonwhite[1]	182.6	157.1	227.5	62.5	56.5	71.7	250.8	86.0
New England	135.6	142.3	74.5*	64.2	65.2	54.1*	112.3*	57.6*
Middle Atlantic	159.4	158.8	169.2	60.7	60.5	63.8	210.3	82.0
East North Central	148.5	146.2	184.0	53.2	51.8	73.0	244.0	74.0
West North Central	181.9	153.3	267.5	60.7	48.0	94.2	435.1	101.8
South Atlantic	203.4	180.1	223.4	67.0	63.1	69.8	238.1	82.2
East South Central	200.6	163.6	222.6	69.5	57.4	76.2	252.0	92.0
West South Central	199.5	175.5	224.6	60.9	57.8	63.8	245.0	85.5
Mountain	333.0	230.1	394.2	74.1	54.4	84.6	782.5	197.1
Pacific[1]	126.1	108.7	222.6	53.1	45.9	89.2	187.9	79.1

Source: Special tabulations of the Division of Vital Statistics, National Center for Health
Statistics, Public Health Service, Washington.

[1]Includes Alaska and Hawaii in 1959-61.

*Rates based on less than 20 deaths.

Table III.6   Average annual mortality rates per 100,000 population among children 1 to 14 years of age in metropolitan and nonmetropolitan counties by color for the United States and each geographic division and by sex for the United States, 1959-61.

Area	Total			White			Nonwhite		
	All Counties	Metropolitan Counties	Nonmetropolitan Counties	All Counties	Metropolitan Counties	Nonmetropolitan Counties	All Counties	Metropolitan Counties	Nonmetropolitan Counties
UNITED STATES[1]	65.0	60.0	73.2	59.0	55.1	65.6	102.3	91.2	120.1
Male	74.3	68.7	83.4	68.1	63.2	75.9	114.7	104.5	130.7
Female	55.3	50.9	62.5	49.7	46.6	54.8	90.0	77.9	109.3
New England	55.2	52.4	64.1	54.1	50.9	64.1	90.5	93.4	62.1*
Middle Atlantic	57.9	56.8	62.7	54.0	52.0	61.6	94.8	94.5	99.7
East North Central	59.4	58.1	61.8	56.5	54.0	60.9	86.9	85.3	109.8
West North Central	61.2	57.8	63.7	59.0	55.3	61.7	103.6	86.1	152.1
South Atlantic	74.9	68.4	81.0	61.4	57.1	65.7	110.4	102.6	116.4
East South Central	76.8	67.3	82.1	64.1	57.8	67.6	111.1	92.2	121.7
West South Central	75.1	69.2	82.0	67.5	62.9	73.1	106.0	98.0	113.5
Mountain	77.8	68.9	86.0	72.3	66.6	77.7	164.2	118.2	189.7
Pacific[1]	59.3	55.7	72.5	57.2	54.2	67.6	77.8	67.4	132.0

Source: Special tabulations of the Division of Vital Statistics, National Center for Health Statistics, Public Health Service, Washington.

[1]Includes Alaska and Hawaii.

*Rates based on less than 20 deaths.

Table III.7a Average annual childhood mortality rates per 100,000 population for selected causes of death by age and color in metropolitan and nonmetropolitan counties: United States and each geographic region, 1959-61.

Cause of Death (7th Revision-International Classification of Diseases)	1 - 14 years			1 - 4 years			5 - 14 years		
	Total	White	Non-white	Total	White	Non-white	Total	White	Non-white
United States[1]									
All causes	65.0	59.0	102.3	105.9	92.9	182.6	46.3	43.8	62.5
Infective and parasitic diseases (001-138)	3.7	3.2	7.1	7.5	6.2	15.0	2.0	1.8	3.1
Malignant neoplasms including neoplasms of lymphatic and haematopoietic tissues (140-205)	8.2	8.6	5.6	10.6	11.3	7.0	7.0	7.4	4.9
Malignant neoplasm of brain and other parts of nervous system (193)	1.7	1.8	1.4	2.2	2.2	1.6	1.6	1.6	1.3
Leukemia and aleukemia (204)	3.9	4.2	2.0	5.3	5.7	2.5	3.3	3.5	1.7
Diseases of nervous system and sense organs (330-398)	4.6	4.3	6.9	7.8	7.0	12.0	3.2	3.0	4.4
Rheumatic fever and chronic rheumatic heart disease (400-416)	0.5	0.4	1.5	0.2	0.1	0.7	0.7	0.5	1.9
Influenza and pneumonia[2] (480-493)	6.3	5.0	14.7	14.9	11.2	36.2	2.4	2.1	4.0
All other diseases of respiratory system (470-475, 500-527)	2.1	2.0	3.0	4.8	4.4	7.1	0.9	0.9	1.0
Gastritis, duodenitis, enteritis and colitis[3] (543, 571, 572)	1.2	1.0	2.7	3.3	2.6	7.4	0.3	0.2	0.4
All other diseases of digestive system (530-542, 544-570, 573-587)	1.9	1.9	2.1	2.7	2.6	3.0	1.5	1.5	1.7
Congenital malformations (750-759)	6.4	6.3	7.0	12.3	12.0	14.2	3.7	3.7	3.5
Accidents (E800-E936)	22.5	20.3	36.4	30.7	26.9	53.6	18.8	17.3	28.0
Motor vehicle accidents (E810-E835)	8.4	8.3	9.3	9.7	9.6	10.6	7.8	7.7	8.7
Accident caused by fire and explosion of combustible material (E916)	3.5	2.3	11.4	6.5	4.0	21.3	2.2	1.5	6.5
Accidental drowning (E929)	3.8	3.5	5.4	4.2	4.5	2.2	3.6	3.1	7.0
All other accidents (E800-E802, E840-E915, E917-E928, E930-E936)	6.8	6.2	10.3	10.4	8.8	19.5	5.1	5.0	5.8
Residual (210-326, 420-468, 590-749, 760-795, E940-E999)	7.6	6.4	15.2	11.1	8.5	26.3	5.9	5.4	9.7
Metropolitan Counties									
All causes	60.0	55.1	91.2	96.5	86.1	157.1	42.7	40.6	56.5
Infective and parasitic diseases (001-138)	3.2	2.8	5.7	6.1	5.1	11.8	1.8	1.7	2.4
Malignant neoplasms including neoplasms of lymphatic and haematopoietic tissues (140-205)	8.6	8.9	6.2	11.0	11.6	7.7	7.4	7.7	5.5
Malignant neoplasm of brain and other parts of nervous system (193)	1.9	1.9	1.6	2.3	2.3	1.7	1.7	1.7	1.5
Leukemia and aleukemia (204)	4.1	4.4	2.2	5.5	5.9	2.8	3.5	3.7	1.9
Diseases of nervous system and sense organs (330-398)	4.6	4.3	6.7	7.7	7.1	11.6	3.1	3.0	4.2
Rheumatic fever and chronic rheumatic heart disease (400-416)	0.4	0.3	1.2	0.2	0.1	0.5	0.5	0.4	1.5
Influenza and pneumonia[2] (480-493)	5.9	4.8	12.7	13.5	10.6	30.4	2.3	2.1	3.5
All other diseases of respiratory system									

Gastritis, duodenitis, enteritis and colitis³ (543, 571, 572)	0.9	0.8	1.7	2.4	2.1	4.4	0.2	0.2	0.3
All other diseases of digestive system (530-542, 544-570, 573-587)	1.8	1.7	2.0	2.5	2.5	2.9	1.4	1.4	1.5
Congenital malformations (750-759)	6.6	6.4	7.6	12.5	12.1	14.6	3.8	3.8	3.9
Accidents (E800-E936)	18.8	16.9	31.2	25.9	22.5	46.0	15.4	11.2	23.4
Motor vehicle accidents (E810-E835)	7.0	6.9	8.3	8.0	7.8	9.3	6.6	6.4	7.8
Accident caused by fire and explosion of combustible material (E916)	2.8	1.8	9.0	5.1	3.2	16.2	1.7	1.2	5.2
Accidental drowning (E929)	3.3	3.0	4.6	3.7	4.0	1.5	3.1	2.6	6.2
All other accidents (E800-E802, E840-E915, E917-E928, E930-E936)	5.7	5.1	9.3	9.2	7.6	19.0	4.0	4.0	4.2
Residual (210-326, 420-468, 590-749, 760-795, E940-E999)	7.1	6.2	13.1	9.9	8.1	20.5	5.8	5.3	9.2
Nonmetropolitan Counties									
All causes	73.2	65.6	120.1	122.2	104.5	227.5	52.0	48.9	71.7
Infective and parasitic diseases (001-138)	4.6	3.9	9.3	9.9	8.0	20.8	2.4	2.1	4.1
Malignant neoplasms including neoplasms of lymphatic and haematopoietic tissues (140-205)	7.5	8.0	4.5	9.9	10.7	5.6	6.5	6.9	4.0
Malignant neoplasm of brain and other parts of nervous system (193)	1.6	1.6	1.1	2.0	2.1	1.5	1.4	1.5	1.0
Leukemia and aleukemia (204)	3.5	3.8	1.6	4.9	5.4	1.9	2.9	3.2	1.4
Diseases of nervous system and sense organs (330-398)	4.6	4.2	7.1	7.8	7.0	12.8	3.2	3.0	4.6
Rheumatic fever and chronic rheumatic heart disease (400-416)	0.7	0.4	2.1	0.2	0.1	0.9	0.8	0.6	2.6
Influenza and pneumonia² (480-493)	7.0	5.2	17.8	17.2	12.3	46.6	2.6	2.2	4.9
All other diseases of respiratory system (470-475, 500-527)	2.1	1.9	3.0	4.9	4.4	7.9	0.9	0.9	0.8
Gastritis, duodenitis, enteritis and colitis³ (543, 571, 572)	1.7	1.3	4.3	4.9	3.6	12.5	0.3	0.3	0.7
All other diseases of digestive system (530-542, 544-570, 573-587)	2.1	2.1	2.4	2.9	2.9	3.3	1.7	1.7	2.0
Congenital malformations (750-759)	6.0	6.0	6.2	12.0	11.7	13.6	3.4	3.5	2.8
Accidents (E800-E936)	28.5	25.9	44.8	39.0	34.4	66.9	24.0	22.3	34.9
Motor vehicle accidents (E810-E835)	10.7	10.6	10.9	12.8	12.8	12.9	9.8	9.7	10.0
Accident caused by fire and explosion of combustible material (E916)	4.7	3.0	15.3	8.9	5.3	30.3	2.9	2.0	8.5
Accidental drowning (E929)	4.6	4.3	6.7	5.1	5.4	3.3	4.4	3.8	8.2
All other accidents (E800-E802, E840-E915, E917-E928, E930-E936)	8.5	8.0	11.9	12.3	10.9	20.4	6.9	6.7	8.1
Residual (210-326, 420-468, 590-749, 760-795, E940-E999)	8.3	6.7	18.5	13.3	9.4	36.6	6.2	5.5	10.4

Source: Special tabulations of the Division of Vital Statistics, National Center for Health Statistics, Public Health Service, Washington.

¹Includes Alaska and Hawaii.
²Except pneumonia of newborn.
³Except diarrhea of newborn.
*Rate based on less than 20 deaths.

Table III.7b   Average annual childhood mortality rates per 100,000 population for selected causes of death by age and color in metropolitan and nonmetropolitan counties: United States and each geographic region, 1959-61 - continued.

Cause of Death (7th Revision-International Classification of Diseases)	1 - 14 years			1 - 4 years			5 - 14 years		
	Total	White	Non-white	Total	White	Non-white	Total	White	Non-white
Northeast									
All causes	57.3	54.1	94.4	90.5	84.1	157.2	42.0	40.4	61.0
Infective and parasitic diseases	2.8	2.6	5.3	5.0	4.5	10.3	1.8	1.7	2.6
Malignant neoplasms including neoplasms of lymphatic and haematopoietic tissues	8.8	9.0	6.6	11.4	11.8	7.8	7.5	7.7	6.0
Malignant neoplasm of brain and other parts of nervous system	1.9	1.9	1.5	2.5	2.5	1.9*	1.6	1.6	1.3
Leukemia and aleukemia	4.4	4.5	2.5	5.7	6.0	2.7	3.7	3.8	2.3
Diseases of nervous system and sense organs	4.4	4.2	7.0	7.1	6.6	12.6	3.2	3.2	4.0
Rheumatic fever and chronic rheumatic heart disease	0.5	0.4	1.4	0.2*	0.1*	0.3*	0.6	0.5	2.0
Influenza and pneumonia2	6.1	5.6	12.3	13.5	12.1	27.1	2.8	2.6	4.4
All other diseases of respiratory system	2.1	2.0	2.7	4.7	4.6	6.0	0.9	0.9	1.0*
Gastritis, duodenitis, enteritis and colitis3	0.9	0.9	1.5	2.4	2.3	3.8	0.2	0.4	0.3*
All other diseases of digestive system	1.8	1.8	2.5	2.6	2.4	3.2	1.5	1.4	2.0
Congenital malformations	6.2	6.1	7.5	11.6	11.4	13.6	3.7	3.6	4.3
Accidents	17.0	15.5	34.1	22.9	20.1	51.3	14.3	13.5	25.0
Motor vehicle accidents	5.9	5.8	6.8	6.3	6.2	7.1	5.7	5.6	6.6
Accident caused by fire and explosion of combustible material	2.9	2.2	10.6	4.9	3.6	18.2	2.0	1.6	6.5
Accidental drowning	2.9	2.8	4.7	2.9	3.1	1.5*	2.9	2.6	6.5
All other accidents	5.3	4.8	12.0	8.8	7.2	24.5	3.8	3.6	5.3
Residual	6.6	6.0	13.5	9.1	8.0	21.1	5.5	5.1	9.4
Metropolitan Counties									
All causes	55.8	51.8	94.4	89.5	81.5	157.3	40.3	38.2	60.9
Infective and parasitic diseases	2.7	2.4	5.3	4.8	4.1	10.5	1.7	1.6	2.6
Malignant neoplasms including neoplasms of lymphatic and haematopoietic tissues	8.8	9.0	6.7	11.5	12.0	7.9	7.5	7.6	6.0
Malignant neoplasm of brain and other parts of									

Leukemia and aleukemia	4.4	4.6	2.4	5.8	6.1	2.7	3.7	3.9	2.3
Diseases of nervous system and sense organs	4.4	4.1	7.0	7.1	6.5	12.3	3.1	3.0	4.2
Rheumatic fever and chronic rheumatic heart disease	0.5	0.4	1.4	0.1*	0.1*	0.2*	0.6	0.5	2.1
Influenza and pneumonia2	6.2	5.6	12.4	13.8	12.2	27.7	2.7	2.6	4.3
All other diseases of respiratory system	2.1	2.0	2.7	4.8	4.6	6.0	0.9	0.9	0.9*
Gastritis, duodenitis, enteritis and colitis3	0.9	0.8	1.5	2.2	2.1	3.7	0.2	0.2	0.3*
All other diseases of digestive system	1.8	1.7	2.5	2.5	2.4	3.4	1.4	1.4	2.0
Congenital malformations	6.3	6.2	7.6	11.9	11.7	13.6	3.7	3.7	4.4
Accidents	15.5	13.6	33.9	21.3	17.9	50.9	12.9	11.7	24.8
Motor vehicle accidents	5.3	5.1	6.9	5.8	5.6	7.3	5.1	4.9	6.7
Accident caused by fire and explosion of combustible material	2.6	1.7	10.3	4.4	2.9	17.4	1.7	1.2	6.5
Accidental drowning	2.6	2.4	4.6	2.5	2.7	1.3*	2.7	2.3	6.4
All other accidents	5.0	4.3	12.0	8.6	6.7	24.9	3.4	3.2	5.2
Residual	6.7	6.0	13.5	9.3	7.9	21.2	5.5	5.1	9.4

Nonmetropolitan Counties

All causes	63.1	62.3	94.4	94.8	93.1	154.3	48.7	48.4	62.5
Infective and parasitic diseases	3.2	3.2	4.7*	5.9	5.9	8.4*	2.0	2.0	2.7*
Malignant neoplasms including neoplasms of lymphatic and haematopoietic tissues	8.7	8.8	5.8*	11.1	11.2	6.7*	7.6	7.7	5.4*
Malignant neoplasms of brain and other parts of nervous system	1.8	1.9	0.6*	2.5	2.5	-	1.6	1.6	0.9*
Leukemia and aleukemia	4.2	4.3	2.9*	5.6	5.6	3.4*	3.6	3.7	2.7*
Diseases of nervous system and sense organs	4.6	4.6	7.0*	7.1	6.8	16.8*	3.5	3.5	1.8*
Rheumatic fever and chronic rheumatic heart disease	0.5	0.5	1.2*	0.2*	0.1*	1.7*	0.6	0.6	0.9*
Influenza and pneumonia2	5.8	5.7	9.9*	12.2	12.1	18.4*	2.8	2.8	5.4*
All other diseases of respiratory system	2.1	2.1	3.5*	4.5	4.5	5.0*	1.1	1.0	2.7*
Gastritis, duodenitis, enteritis and colitis3	1.2	1.2	2.3*	3.2	3.1	6.7*	0.3*	0.3*	-
All other diseases of digestive system	2.0	2.0	2.3*	2.5	2.6	-	1.8	1.8	3.6*
Congenital malformations	5.6	5.6	7.0*	10.5	10.5	13.4*	3.4	3.4	3.6*
Accidents	22.9	22.5	37.9	29.0	28.2	58.7	20.1	19.9	26.8
Motor Vehicle accidents	8.1	8.2	4.7*	8.4	8.5	3.4*	8.0	8.0	5.4*
Accident caused by fire and explosion of combustible material	4.2	3.9	15.2	6.7	6.0	31.9*	3.0	3.0	6.3*
Accidental drowning	4.1	4.1	6.4*	4.6	4.6	5.0*	3.9	3.8	7.1*
All other accidents	6.5	6.4	11.7	9.4	9.2	18.4*	5.2	5.1	8.0*
Residual	6.3	6.2	12.8	8.5	8.2	18.4*	5.4	5.3	9.8*

Note: Sources and footnotes are the same as for the table on United States.

Table III.7c   Average annual childhood mortality rates per 100,000 population for selected causes of death by age and color in metropolitan and nonmetropolitan counties: United States and each geographic region, 1959-61 - continued.

Cause of Death (7th Revision-International Classification of Diseases)	1 - 14 years			1 - 4 years			5 - 14 years		
	Total	White	Non-white	Total	White	Non-white	Total	White	Non-white
North Central									
All causes	59.9	57.2	89.9	93.1	87.1	154.4	44.3	43.4	54.5
Infective and parasitic diseases	3.0	2.8	5.5	6.0	5.5	11.4	1.7	1.6	2.3
Malignant neoplasms including neoplasms of lymphatic and haematopoietic tissues	8.6	8.8	5.8	11.3	11.7	7.4	7.3	7.5	5.0
Malignant neoplasm of brain and other parts of nervous system	1.9	1.9	1.4	2.2	2.3	1.5	1.7	1.7	1.4
Leukemia and aleukemia	4.0	4.2	2.1	5.5	5.8	2.9	3.3	3.4	1.7
Diseases of nervous system and sense organs	4.4	4.2	6.5	7.0	6.6	10.8	3.2	3.1	4.1
Rheumatic fever and chronic rheumatic heart disease	0.4	0.4	1.1	0.2	0.1*	0.8*	0.5	0.5	1.2
Influenza and pneumonia[2]	5.4	4.6	15.3	12.7	10.4	35.6	2.0	1.8	4.1
All other diseases of respiratory system	1.9	1.8	2.6	4.0	3.9	4.9	0.9	0.8	1.3
Gastritis, duodenitis, enteritis and colitis[3]	1.0	0.9	1.3	2.5	2.4	3.1	0.2	0.2	0.3*
All other diseases of digestive system	1.7	1.8	1.5	2.4	2.4	2.0	1.4	1.4	1.3
Congenital malformations	6.5	6.4	7.6	12.2	12.1	14.0	3.8	3.7	4.1
Accidents	20.7	19.7	31.3	26.6	24.6	46.9	17.9	17.5	22.7
Motor vehicle accidents	8.1	8.1	8.6	9.0	8.9	10.1	7.7	7.7	7.8
Accident caused by fire and explosion of combustible material	2.7	2.2	8.9	4.8	3.7	15.4	1.7	1.4	5.2
Accidental drowning	3.3	3.3	3.9	3.2	3.4	1.5	3.4	3.2	5.2
All other accidents	6.5	6.2	9.9	9.6	8.6	19.8	5.1	5.1	4.5
Residual	6.3	5.9	11.3	8.2	7.3	17.5	5.4	5.2	8.0
Metropolitan Counties									
All causes	58.1	54.3	85.4	89.7	80.9	147.2	42.5	41.4	51.3
Infective and parasitic diseases	2.9	2.6	5.2	5.5	4.7	10.7	1.6	1.6	2.2
Malignant neoplasms including neoplasms of lymphatic and haematopoietic tissues	8.9	9.3	5.7	11.3	11.9	7.4	7.7	8.1	4.8
Malignant neoplasm of brain and other parts of nervous system	1.9	2.0	1.4	2.2	2.3	1.5*	1.8	1.8	1.?

Leukemia and aleukemia	4.2	4.5	2.1	5.6	6.0	2.9	3.5	3.8	1.6
Diseases of nervous system and sense organs	4.6	4.3	6.6	7.1	6.5	10.7	3.3	3.2	4.3
Rheumatic fever and chronic rheumatic heart disease	0.4	0.4	0.9	0.2*	0.1*	0.7*	0.6	0.5	1.1
Influenza and pneumonia2	5.8	4.5	14.7	13.3	10.2	33.9	2.1	1.8	4.1
All other diseases of respiratory system	1.9	1.8	2.5	4.0	3.9	4.6	0.8	0.8	1.3
Gastritis, duodenitis, enteritis and colitis3	0.9	0.8	1.1	2.1	2.1	2.6	0.2	0.2	0.3*
All other diseases of digestive system	1.5	1.5	1.5	2.1	2.1	2.0	1.3	1.3	1.3
Congenital malformations	6.7	6.6	7.7	12.4	12.2	13.8	3.9	3.9	4.3
Accidents	17.8	16.3	28.6	22.9	19.7	44.1	15.3	14.6	20.1
Motor vehicle accidents	6.8	6.7	7.6	7.2	6.9	8.8	6.7	6.6	7.0
Accident caused by fire and explosion of combustible material	2.6	1.8	8.0	4.6	3.1	14.0	1.6	1.2	4.7
Accidental drowning	2.9	2.8	3.5	2.6	2.8	1.4*	3.0	2.7	4.7
All other accidents	5.5	4.9	9.5	8.6	6.9	20.0	4.0	4.0	3.7
Residual	6.7	6.1	10.8	8.7	7.6	16.6	5.7	5.4	7.6

Nonmetropolitan Counties

All causes	62.6	61.2	129.7	98.7	95.8	223.3	46.8	46.1	82.9
Infective and parasitic diseases	3.3	3.2	8.4	6.9	6.6	18.0	1.7	1.7	3.7*
Malignant neoplasms including neoplasms of lymphatic and haematopoietic tissues	8.1	8.1	7.1	11.2	11.3	7.4*	6.8	6.7	6.9*
Malignant neoplasm of brain and other parts of nervous system	1.8	1.8	2.2*	2.3	2.3	1.6*	1.6	1.6	2.5*
Leukemia and aleukemia	3.7	3.7	2.5*	5.4	5.5	2.5*	2.9	2.9	2.5*
Diseases of nervous system and sense organs	4.1	4.1	5.4	6.8	6.7	11.5*	3.0	3.0	2.5*
Rheumatic fever and chronic rheumatic heart disease	0.4	0.3	2.5*	0.2*	0.1*	2.5*	0.5	0.4	4.5*
Influenza and pneumonia2	4.9	4.6	20.2	11.7	10.8	51.5	1.9	1.9	1.6*
All other diseases of respiratory system	1.8	1.8	3.8*	4.0	3.9	8.2*	0.9	0.9	0.4*
Gastritis, duodenitis, enteritis and colitis3	1.1	1.0	2.7*	3.0	2.9	7.4*	0.2	0.2	1.2*
All other diseases of digestive system	2.0	2.0	1.6*	2.9	2.9	2.5*	1.7	1.7	2.5*
Congenital malformations	6.1	6.0	6.8	11.9	11.8	15.5*	3.5	3.5	2.5*
Accidents	25.0	24.4	55.0	32.7	31.7	73.6	21.7	21.2	45.7
Motor vehicle accidents	10.1	9.9	17.4	12.0	11.8	22.9	9.3	9.1	14.7
Accident caused by fire and explosion of combustible material	2.9	2.6	16.6	5.2	4.7	29.4	1.8	1.7	10.2
Accidental drowning	4.1	4.0	7.6	4.3	4.3	3.3*	4.0	3.8	9.8
All other accidents	8.0	7.9	13.3	11.2	11.0	18.0	6.6	6.5	11.0
Residual	5.8	5.5	16.1	7.4	7.0	25.4	5.1	4.9	11.4

Note: Sources and footnotes are the same as for the table on United States.

Table III.7d   Average annual childhood mortality rates per 100,000 population for selected causes of death by age and color in metropolitan and nonmetropolitan counties: United States and each geographic region, 1959-61 - continued.

Cause of Death (7th Revision-International Classification of Diseases)	1 - 14 years			1 - 4 years			5 - 14 years		
	Total	White	Non-white	Total	White	Non-white	Total	White	Non-white
South									
All causes	75.4	64.0	109.5	128.5	102.7	201.7	51.8	47.2	66.1
Infective and parasitic diseases	5.2	4.3	7.9	11.0	8.8	17.4	2.6	2.4	3.5
Malignant neoplasms including neoplasms of lymphatic and haematopoietic tissues	7.2	8.0	4.8	9.5	10.7	6.0	6.2	6.9	4.3
Malignant neoplasm of brain and other parts of nervous system	1.5	1.6	1.3	1.9	2.0	1.5	1.4	1.5	1.2
Leukemia and aleukemia	3.3	3.9	1.5	4.5	5.5	1.9	2.8	3.3	1.4
Diseases of nervous system and sense organs	5.2	4.5	7.0	9.0	7.8	12.2	3.5	3.1	4.5
Rheumatic fever and chronic rheumatic heart disease	0.7	0.4	1.7	0.2	0.1*	0.7	0.9	0.5	2.2
Influenza and pneumonia[2]	7.7	5.1	15.7	19.1	11.7	40.2	2.7	2.2	4.2
All other diseases of respiratory system	2.1	1.8	3.2	5.1	4.0	8.1	0.8	0.8	0.9
Gastritis, duodenitis, enteritis and colitis[3]	1.9	1.3	3.5	5.3	3.8	9.8	0.3	0.3	0.5
All other diseases of digestive system	2.1	2.0	2.3	3.1	3.0	3.5	1.6	1.5	1.8
Congenital malformations	6.3	6.1	6.8	12.9	12.2	14.8	3.4	3.5	3.1
Accidents	27.3	23.3	39.2	37.3	30.3	57.1	22.9	20.3	30.8
Motor vehicle accidents	10.1	10.1	9.9	11.5	11.7	11.2	9.4	9.5	9.3
Accident caused by fire and explosion of combustible material	5.2	2.5	13.3	10.0	4.4	25.8	3.1	1.7	7.4
Accidental drowning	4.4	3.8	5.9	4.1	4.9	1.9	4.5	3.4	7.9
All other accidents	7.7	6.9	10.1	11.7	9.4	18.3	5.9	5.8	6.2
Residual	9.7	7.1	17.4	16.0	10.4	32.0	6.9	5.7	10.5
Metropolitan Counties									
All causes	68.5	59.4	99.2	112.9	93.1	175.5	47.5	43.8	60.5
Infective and parasitic diseases	4.3	3.6	6.6	8.8	7.1	14.4	2.2	2.1	2.7
Malignant neoplasms including neoplasms of lymphatic and haematopoietic tissues	7.9	8.5	5.7	10.1	11.1	7.0	6.8	7.3	5.1
Malignant neoplasm of brain and other parts of	1.8	1.8	.6	2.3	2.4	1.5	1.6	1.6	1.6

Leukemia and aleukemia	3.6	4.1	1.7	4.8	5.7	2.0	3.0	3.4	1.8
Diseases of nervous system and sense organs	5.3	4.8	7.1	9.5	8.4	12.9	3.4	3.2	4.2
Rheumatic fever and chronic rheumatic heart disease	0.5	0.3	1.2	0.2*	0.1*	0.5*	0.6	0.4	1.6
Influenza and pneumonia[2]	6.3	4.4	13.0	15.1	9.6	32.5	2.2	1.9	3.2
All other diseases of respiratory system	2.1	1.7	3.7	4.9	3.7	8.6	0.8	0.8	1.2
Gastritis, duodenitis, enteritis and colitis[3]	1.3	1.0	2.4	3.6	2.7	6.7	0.2	0.2	0.2
All other diseases of digestive system	2.0	1.9	2.2	3.1	3.0	3.5	1.4	1.4	1.6
Congenital malformations	6.7	6.3	7.9	13.0	11.9	16.3	3.7	3.7	3.6
Accidents	23.4	20.3	34.1	31.7	26.5	48.3	19.5	17.4	26.9
Motor vehicle accidents	8.6	8.5	9.2	9.4	9.2	10.2	8.2	8.1	8.7
Accident caused by fire and explosion of combustible material	4.0	2.1	10.6	7.4	3.6	19.7	2.4	1.4	5.9
Accidental drowning	4.3	3.9	5.5	4.5	5.5	1.3	4.2	3.2	7.7
All other accidents	6.5	5.8	8.8	10.4	8.2	17.1	4.6	4.6	4.5
Residual	8.6	6.7	15.2	12.9	9.0	25.0	6.6	5.5	10.3

Nonmetropolitan Counties

All Causes	81.6	68.4	117.2	143.8	112.6	223.4	55.6	50.3	70.2
Infective and parasitic diseases	6.0	5.0	8.9	13.2	10.6	20.0	3.0	2.7	4.0
Malignant neoplasms including neoplasms of lymphatic and haematopoietic tissues	6.7	7.6	4.2	8.8	10.2	5.3	5.8	6.5	3.7
Malignant neoplasm of brain and other parts of nervous system	1.3	1.4	1.1	1.6	1.6	1.5	1.2	1.3	0.8
Leukemia and aleukemia	3.1	3.7	1.4	4.3	5.3	1.8	2.6	3.1	1.2
Diseases of nervous system and sense organs	5.0	4.3	6.9	8.5	7.3	11.7	3.5	3.1	4.8
Rheumatic fever and chronic rheumatic heart disease	0.9	0.5	2.1	0.3	0.1*	0.9*	1.2	0.6	2.6
Influenza and pneumonia[2]	8.9	5.7	17.6	23.0	13.8	46.5	3.1	0.8	4.9
All other diseases of respiratory system	2.1	1.9	2.8	5.3	4.4	7.7	0.8	0.8	0.7
Gastritis, duodenitis, enteritis and colitis[3]	2.3	1.7	4.2	6.9	4.9	12.2	0.4	0.3	0.7
All other diseases of digestive system	2.2	2.1	2.4	3.1	3.0	3.4	1.8	1.7	2.0
Congenital malformations	5.9	5.9	6.0	12.8	12.5	13.5	3.1	3.2	2.6
Accidents	30.8	26.2	43.1	42.7	34.2	64.5	25.8	23.0	33.6
Motor vehicle accidents	11.4	11.7	10.4	13.6	14.2	12.1	10.4	10.7	9.7
Accident caused by fire and explosion of combustible material	6.3	2.9	15.3	12.4	5.2	30.7	3.7	2.0	8.5
Accidental drowning	4.4	3.7	6.2	3.7	4.2	2.3	4.7	3.5	8.0
All other accidents	8.7	7.9	11.0	13.1	10.6	19.3	6.9	6.8	7.4
Residual	10.7	7.6	19.0	19.1	11.8	37.8	7.1	5.9	10.6

Note: Sources and footnotes are the same as for the table on United States

356 / APPENDIX TABLES

Table III.7e Average annual childhood mortality rates per 100,000 population for selected causes of death by age and color in metropolitan and nonmetropolitan counties: United States and each geographic region, 1959-61 - continued.

Cause of Death (7th Revision-International Classification of Diseases)	1 - 14 years			1 - 4 years			5 - 14 years		
	Total	White	Non-white	Total	White	Non-white	Total	White	Non-white
West[1]									
All causes	64.2	61.4	93.0	106.7	100.5	163.4	44.8	43.6	56.7
Infective and parasitic diseases	3.2	2.8	7.1	6.6	5.7	14.9	1.7	1.5	3.0
Malignant neoplasms including neoplasms of lymphatic and haematopoietic tissues	8.4	8.5	7.9	10.6	10.7	9.9	7.4	7.5	6.9
Malignant neoplasm of brain and other parts of nervous system	1.8	1.8	1.8	2.1	2.1	2.0*	1.6	1.6	1.7
Leukemia and aleukemia	4.2	4.2	3.7	5.5	5.6	4.8	3.6	3.6	3.1
Diseases of nervous system and sense organs	4.2	3.9	6.9	7.8	7.3	12.4	2.6	2.4	4.0
Rheumatic fever and chronic rheumatic heart disease	0.3	0.3	1.2	0.2*	0.1*	0.8*	0.4	0.3	1.5
Influenza and pneumonia	5.3	4.6	11.6	12.5	10.7	28.7	2.0	1.9	2.8
All other diseases of respiratory system	2.5	2.4	3.0	5.8	5.6	7.3	0.9	1.0	0.7*
Gastritis, duodenitis, enteritis and colitis[3]	0.9	0.7	2.6	2.2	1.7	6.7	0.3	0.3	0.5*
All other diseases of digestive system	2.0	2.0	1.7	2.6	2.6	2.2*	1.7	1.7	1.4*
Congenital malformations	6.6	6.6	6.8	12.3	12.2	12.7	4.0	4.0	3.7
Accidents	24.0	23.2	32.5	36.7	35.3	49.3	18.2	17.7	23.7
Motor vehicle accidents	9.3	9.2	10.2	12.4	12.4	12.8	7.9	7.8	8.9
Accident caused by fire and explosion of combustible material	2.6	2.2	6.3	5.0	4.2	12.2	1.4	1.3	3.2
Accidental drowning	4.6	4.5	5.5	7.9	8.1	5.9	3.1	2.8	5.3
All other accidents	7.5	7.3	10.4	11.4	10.6	18.5	5.8	5.7	6.3
Residual	6.9	6.4	11.7	9.6	8.7	18.3	5.6	5.4	8.3
Metropolitan Counties									
All causes	58.1	56.6	71.6	96.1	93.4	119.4	40.3	39.7	46.6
Infective and parasitic diseases	2.8	2.6	4.0	5.4	5.1	7.9	1.5	1.5	2.0
Malignant neoplasms including neoplasms of lymphatic and haematopoietic tissues	8.6	8.6	8.3	11.0	11.0	10.7	7.5	7.6	7.1
Malignant neoplasm of brain and other parts of									

Leukemia and aleukemia	4.3	4.3	4.0	5.8	5.9	5.5	3.6	3.6	3.1
Diseases of nervous system and sense organs	4.1	3.9	5.4	7.4	7.3	8.4	2.6	2.4	3.8
Rheumatic fever and chronic rheumatic heart disease	0.3	0.2	1.1*	0.2*	0.1*	0.9*	0.3	0.2	1.2*
Influenza and pneumonia[2]	4.8	4.4	8.4	11.1	9.9	20.6	1.9	1.8	2.1
All other diseases of respiratory system	2.4	2.4	2.5	5.6	5.5	6.2	1.0	1.0	0.6*
Gastritis, duodenitis, enteritis and colitis[3]	0.7	0.6	1.1*	1.5	1.5	2.1*	0.3	0.3	0.5*
All other diseases of digestive system	1.9	1.9	1.5	2.4	2.5	2.1*	1.7	1.7	1.2*
Congenital malformations	6.7	6.8	6.5	12.7	12.8	12.4	3.9	4.0	3.4
Accidents	19.4	19.1	22.6	30.4	29.8	35.2	14.3	14.2	16.0
Motor vehicle accidents	8.1	8.0	8.8	10.8	10.9	10.7	6.8	6.7	7.8
Accident caused by fire and explosion of combustible material	1.9	1.7	3.9	3.7	3.2	8.2	1.0	1.0	1.6*
Accidental drowning	3.5	3.5	3.5	6.0	6.4	3.1*	2.3	2.1	3.7
All other accidents	6.0	6.0	6.4	9.8	9.4	13.2	4.2	4.4	2.9
Residual	6.4	6.0	10.2	8.5	7.9	13.1	5.4	5.1	8.7
Nonmetropolitan Counties									
All causes	78.8	72.3	158.5	132.6	117.5	304.0	55.1	52.6	87.1
Infective and parasitic diseases	4.2	3.2	16.5	9.4	6.9	37.4	2.0	1.6	6.2
Malignant neoplasms including neoplasms of lymphatic and haematopoietic tissues	7.9	8.0	6.7	9.7	9.9	7.7*	7.1	7.2	6.2
Malignant neoplasm of brain and other parts of nervous system	1.6	1.7	1.4*	2.0	2.0	1.6*	1.5	1.5	1.3*
Leukemia and aleukemia	3.9	4.0	2.9*	4.7	4.8	2.7*	3.6	3.6	3.0*
Diseases of nervous system and sense organs	4.5	3.9	11.6	8.8	7.4	25.3	2.6	2.4	4.9*
Rheumatic fever and chronic rheumatic heart disease	0.6	0.5	1.8*	0.3*	0.2*	0.5*	0.7	0.5	2.4*
Influenza and pneumonia[2]	6.4	5.2	21.4	15.9	12.5	54.4	2.3	2.0	5.1*
All other diseases of respiratory system	2.5	2.4	4.3	6.2	5.8	11.0	0.9	0.9	1.1*
Gastritis, duodenitis, enteritis and colitis[3]	1.3	0.9	7.4	3.7	2.2	21.4	0.3*	0.3*	0.5*
All other diseases of digestive system	2.1	2.1	2.4*	2.9	3.0	2.7*	1.8	1.7	2.2*
Congenital malformations	6.3	6.2	7.6	11.1	10.9	13.7	4.2	4.2	4.6*
Accidents	34.8	32.5	62.6	52.1	48.3	94.5	27.1	25.6	46.9
Motor vehicle accidents	12.2	12.1	14.7	16.2	15.9	19.8	10.5	10.4	12.1
Accident caused by fire and explosion of combustible material	4.1	3.3	13.6	8.0	6.5	24.7	2.4	1.9	8.1
Accidental drowning	7.2	6.9	11.8	12.5	12.3	14.8	4.9	4.5	10.3
All other accidents	11.2	10.3	22.6	15.3	13.6	35.2	9.4	8.8	16.5
Residual	8.1	7.4	16.3	12.5	10.5	35.2	6.1	6.0	7.0

Note: Sources and footnotes are the same as for the table on United States.

Table III.8   Childhood mortality rates per 100,000 population by age: Selected countries, 1950-63.

Age; Year	Canada	Belgium	Denmark[1]	England and Wales	Finland	France	Netherlands	Norway	Sweden	Switzerland	Australia[2]	United States
1-4 yrs.												
1963	—	111.1	91.6	90.5	104.0	108.5	97.1	98.1	67.2	—	95.8	99.5
1962	—	100.4	84.2	85.8	101.9	116.6	109.0	97.1	76.6	—	101.2	98.1
1961	—	101.5	87.6	92.7	109.4	114.3	101.5	96.7	79.9	—	109.3	101.7
1960	—	107.6	94.2	86.7	108.8	119.2	117.4	110.0	86.6	129.2	114.7	109.1
1959	—	130.6	94.3	90.6	137.5	139.6	132.7	96.5	84.9	130.2	118.4	107.0
1958	—	115.8	79.4	88.2	157.2	142.8	121.7	113.7	91.5	125.6	119.1	111.8
1957	—	130.0	112.6	97.0	213.7	165.8	127.0	108.1	94.9	158.6	135.8	112.0
1956	—	135.2	92.9	90.9	149.6	155.9	119.8	118.6	97.2	141.7	134.7	110.4
1955	—	160.1	100.4	100.3	169.6	181.3	124.6	132.3	100.6	161.8	149.4	113.6
1954	—	151.4	122.6	94.2	163.9	184.9	132.6	112.3	98.8	158.2	153.8	118.4
1953	—	152.5	118.4	117.8	189.5	194.1	164.6	130.7	105.1	154.6	159.4	130.3
1952	—	169.2	148.7	117.7	191.4	234.7	—	145.5	114.4	170.8	161.8	141.2
1951	—	193.9	121.3	135.1	195.1	243.6	165.1	159.1	122.8	198.0	173.5	137.1
1950	—	192.4	135.4	135.0	240.4	234.4	165.0	158.3	130.4	186.5	161.7	139.4
5-14 yrs.												
1963	48.9	41.8	35.5	36.0	44.9	36.7	42.7	42.3	37.0	47.2	40.9	43.5
1962	47.2	44.1	38.9	36.0	44.0	35.9	41.7	41.5	38.9	49.0	40.6	43.9
1961	47.8	42.5	36.4	36.1	45.7	34.9	41.5	39.4	38.0	46.0	42.3	43.9
1960	52.2	44.7	33.3	37.8	47.7	36.9	39.7	42.7	36.8	42.6	44.8	46.6

1959	56.4	48.2	38.2	37.3	48.8	40.3	48.4	46.8	38.3	45.5	45.0	46.8
1958	52.9	46.1	35.6	35.9	46.1	36.2	42.1	40.8	39.9	50.1	45.1	45.8
1957	56.6	51.2	36.7	39.4	61.2	44.0	48.0	47.8	46.5	53.8	47.5	48.2
1956	56.4	47.7	33.0	37.0	59.7	41.3	45.8	46.1	41.5	53.2	46.0	46.9
1955	60.0	52.5	31.9	40.8	60.7	41.6	49.4	47.1	46.0	51.8	50.8	48.4
1954	60.6	54.1	34.5	39.4	61.9	41.3	47.1	52.3	43.3	53.4	54.4	50.1
1953	69.9	49.0	43.4	45.0	70.4	50.1	67.9	52.4	51.8	61.7	60.0	54.6
1952	76.3	51.9	49.6	46.3	65.0	52.5	53.3	58.3	47.6	58.6	60.0	59.2
1951	76.0	61.0	41.8	51.9	80.0	59.6	57.4	65.2	53.9	66.6	66.5	59.3
1950	80.0	59.4	45.8	56.6	88.7	64.9	54.0	68.1	54.7	59.3	70.3	60.1

Source: Files of the Statistical Office of the United Nations and annual volumes Vital Statistics of the United States, National Center for Health Statistics, Public Health Service, Washington.

Note: For the 1-4 year age group, data not available for Netherlands for 1952 and for Switzerland for 1961, 1962 and 1963.

[1] Excluding Faeroe Islands and Greenland.

[2] Excludes full-blooded aborigines.

REFERENCES / INDEX

REFERENCES

Preface

1. S. Shapiro and I. M. Moriyama, "International Trends in Infant Mortality and Their Implication for the United States," *Am. J. Pub. Health*, 53:747-760 (May 1963).

2. E. P. Hunt and A. D. Chenoweth, "Recent Trends in Infant Mortality in the United States," *Am. J. Pub. Health*, 51:190-207 (February 1961).

3. I. M. Moriyama, "Recent Change in Infant Mortality Trend," *Pub. Health Rep.*, 75:391-405 (May 1960).

4. E. Oppenheimer, "Population Changes and Perinatal Mortality," *Am. J. Pub. Health*, 51:208-216 (February 1961).

5. K. C. Buetow, "An Epidemiological Approach to the Problem of Rising Neonatal Mortality in Baltimore," *Am. J. Pub. Health*, 51:217-227 (February 1961).

6. E. P. Hunt and S. M. Goldstein, *Trends in Infant and Childhood Mortality, 1961*, Children's Bureau Statistical Ser. No. 76 (1964).

7. *Infant Mortality Trends, United States and Each State, 1930-1964*, Pub. Health Service Publ. No. 1000, Ser. 20, No. 1 (November 1965).

8. E. P. Hunt and E. D. Huyck, "Mortality of White and Nonwhite Infants in Major U.S. Cities," *H. E. W. Indicators* (January 1966).

9. E. W. Curran, *International Conference on the Perinatal and Infant Mortality Problem of the United States*, Pub. Health Service Publ. No. 1000, Ser. 4, No. 3 (June 1966).

10. I. M. Moriyama, "Present Status of Infant Mortality Problem in the United States," *Am. J. Pub. Health*, 56:623-625 (April 1966).

11. S. Shapiro, E. R. Schlesinger, and R. E. L. Nesbitt, *Infant and Perinatal Mortality in the United States*, Pub. Health Service Publ. No. 1000, Ser. 3, No. 4 (October 1965).

12. *Infant and Perinatal Mortality Rates by Age and Color, United States, Each State and County, 1951-1955 and 1956-1960*, Children's Bureau, D. H. E. W., and Maternal and Infant Health Computer Project (Washington, D.C.: George Washington University, January 1967).

13. *Monthly Vital Statistics Report, Annual Summary for the United States, 1966* (Washington, D. C.: National Center for Health Statistics, July 1967) 15, 1-18.

14. *Monthly Vital Statistics Report, Births, Marriages, Divorces, and Deaths for 1967*, (Washington, D. C.: National Center for Health Statistics, February 26, 1968) 16, 1-8.

15. Report of the Program Area Committee on Child Health, A. P. H. A., "Requirements for Data on Infant and Perinatal Mortality," *Am. J. Pub. Health*, 57:1848-1861, (October 1967).

16. E. R. Schlesinger, "Infant and Perinatal Mortality," *Am. J. Pub. Health*, 57:1715-1716 (October 1967).

Part I. Infant and Perinatal Mortality

Chapter 1. Trends and Recent Status

1. *Vital Statistics of the United States, 1950* (Washington, D.C.: National Center for Health Statistics, 1954), I, 2–19.

2. *Ibid.*, pp. 12–14, 108–127.

3. United Nations Department of Economic and Social Affairs, *Population Bulletin of the United Nations*, No. 3 (1953).

4. L. Guralnick and E. D. Winter, "A Note on Cohort Infant Mortality Rates," *Pub. Health Rep.*, 80:692-694 (August 1965).

5. "The Effect of the Sixth Revision of the International List of Diseases and Causes of Death upon Comparability of Mortality Trends," *Vital Statistics-Special Rep.* (National Center for Health Statistics), Vol. 36, No. 10 (reprinted March 1960).

6. "Comparability of Mortality Statistics for the Fifth and Sixth Revisions: United States, 1950," *Vital Statistics-Special Rep.*, Vol. 51, No. 2 (December 1963).

7. H. N. Bundesen, E. L. Potter, W. I. Fishbein, F. C. Bauer, and G. V. Plotzke, "Progress in the Prevention of Needless Neonatal Deaths," *Annual Report of the Chicago Health Department, 1951*.

8. W. A. Silverman, *Dunham's Premature Infants* (New York: Paul C. Hoeber, 1961), pp. 224–250.

9. E. L. Potter, *Pathology of the Fetus and the Newborn* (Chicago: Year Book Publishers, 1952).

10. M. A. Valdes-Dapena, "Sudden and Unexpected Death in Infancy: A Review of the World Literature, 1954–1966," *Pediatrics*, 39:123-138 (January 1967).

11. J. Unger, "Weight at Birth and its Effect on Survival of the Newborn: United States by Geographic Divisions and by Urban and Rural Areas, Early 1950," *Vital Statistics-Special Rep.*, Vol. 45, No. 10 (April 1957).

12. F. Rosa and L. Resnick, "Birth Weight and Perinatal Mortality in the American Indian," *Am. J. Obs. & Gyn.*, 55:972-976 (April 1965).

13. *Report of the Study Group on Improving Registration of Fetal Deaths*, Public Health Conference on Records and Statistics, Doc. No. 601.12 (May 1966).

14. "Committee on Maternal and Child Care of the Council on Medical Services: A Guide for the Study of Perinatal Mortality and Morbidity," *J.A.M.A.*, 169:715 (February 1959).

Chapter 2. Other Parameters of Pregnancy Loss

1. M. Taback, "Birth Weight and Length of Gestation with Relation to Prematurity," *J.A.M.A.*, 146:897-901 (July 7, 1951).

2. S. Shapiro, "Influence of Birth Weight, Sex, and Plurality on Neonatal Loss in the United States," *Am. J. Pub. Health*, 44:1142-1153 (September 1954).

3. F. C. Battaglia, T. M. Frazier, and A. E. Hellegers, "Birth Weight, Gestational Age, and Pregnancy Outcome, with Special Reference to High Birth Weight-Low Gestational Age Infant," *Pediatrics*, 37:417-422 (March 1966).

4. S. Shapiro and J. Unger, "Weight at Birth and its Effect on Survival of the Newborn in the United States, Early 1950," *Vital Statistics-Special Rep.*, Vol. 39, No. 1 (July 1954).

5. E. R. Schlesinger and N. C. Allaway, "The Combined Effect of Birth Weight and Length of Gestation on Neonatal Mortality among Single Premature Births," *Pediatrics*, 15:698-704 (June 1955).

6. C. L. Erhardt, G. B. Joshi, F. G. Nelson, B. H. Kroll, and L. Weiner, "Influence of Weight and Gestation on Perinatal and Neonatal Mortality by Ethnic Group," *Am. J. Publ. Health*, 54:1841-1855 (November 1964).

7. J. Yerushalmy, B. J. van den Berg, C. L. Erhardt, and H. Jacobziner, "Birth Weight and Gestation as Indices of 'Immaturity'," *Am. J. Dis. Children*, 109:43-57 (January 1965).

8. J. Loeb, "Weight at Birth and Survival of Newborn, by Age of Mother and Total-Birth Order: United States, Early 1950," *Vital Statistics-Special Rep.*, Vol. 47, No. 2 (August 1958).

9. J. Pakter, H. J. Rosner, H. Jacobziner, and F. Greenstein, "Out-of-Wedlock Births in New York City: II. Medical Aspects," *Am. J. Pub. Health*, 51:846-865 (June 1961).

10. A. Gittelsohn, unpublished data for 1959-60 (Albany: New York State Dept. of Health).

11. E. R. Schlesinger and N. C. Allaway, "Trends in Familial Susceptibility to Perinatal Loss," *Am. J. Pub. Health*, 45:174-183 (February 1955).

12. E. R. Schlesinger and N. C. Allaway, "Use of Child-Loss Data in Evolving Priorities in Maternal Health Services," *Am. J. Pub. Health*, 47:570-577 (May 1957).

13. H. Chase, "Father's Occupation, Parental Age, and Infant's Birth Rank," *The Relationship of Certain Biologic and Socioeconomic Factors to Fetal, Infant, and Early Childhood Mortality*, Part I (Washington, D.C.: Children's Bureau, 1964).

14. P. M. Densen, unpublished data for 1961-63 (New York City Department of Health).

15. S. Shapiro, H. Jacobziner, P. M. Densen, and L. Weiner, "Further

Observations on Prematurity and Perinatal Mortality in a General Population and in the Population of a Prepaid Group Practice Medical Care Plan," *Am. J. Pub. Health*, 50:1304-1317 (September 1960).

16. A. Donabedian, L. Rosenfeld, and E. M. Southern, "Infant Mortality and Socioeconomic Status in a Metropolitan Community," *Pub. Health Rep.*, 80:1083-1094 (December 1965).

17. E. P. Hunt and E. E. Huyck, "Mortality of White and Nonwhite Infants in Major U.S. Cities," *H.E.W. Indicators* (January 1966).

18. L. Guralnick and E. D. Winter, "A Note on Cohort Infant Mortality Rates," *Pub. Health Rep.*, 80:692-694 (August 1965).

19. C. L. Erhardt, J. Pakter, and F. G. Nelson, "Season of Conception and its Relationship to Outcome of Pregnancy." Paper presented at Annual Meeting, Am. Pub. Health Assn., October 1965.

20. A. M. Lilienfeld and E. Parkhurst, "A Study of the Association of Factors of Pregnancy and Parturition with the Development of Cerebral Palsy," *Am. J. Hyg.*, 53:262-282 (May 1951).

21. B. Pasamanick and A. M. Lilienfeld, "Association of Maternal and Fetal Factors with Development of Mental Deficiency," *J.A.M.A.*, 159:155-160 (September 1955).

22. *Research Methodology and Needs in Perinatal Studies*, Proceedings of the Conference on Research Methodology and Needs in Perinatal Studies Held in Chapel Hill, N.C. (Springfield, Ill.: Charles C. Thomas, 1966). J. F. Donnelly, B. G. Greenberg, and H. B. Wells, "A Review of Methodology in the North Carolina Study of Fetal and Neonatal Deaths" (Chap. 1); S. Shapiro, "Methodology in the Study of Pregnancy Outcome and Childhood Disorders Being Conducted by the Health Insurance Plan" (Chap. 2); G. W. Mellin, "The Fetal Life Study of the Columbia-Presbyterian Medical Center: A Prospective Epidemiological Study of Prenatal Influences on Fetal Development and Survival" (Chap. 4); H. W. Berendes, "The Structure and Scope of the Collaborative Project on Cerebral Palsy, Mental Retardation, and other Neurological and Sensory Disorders of Infancy and Childhood" (Chap. 5).

23. C. L. Erhardt, "Pregnancy Losses in New York City, 1960" *Am. J. Pub. Health*, 53:1337-1352 (September 1963).

24. F. E. French and J. M. Bierman, "Probabilities of Fetal Mortality," *Pub. Health Rep.*, 77:835-847 (October, 1962).

25. S. Shapiro, E. W. Jones, and P. M. Densen, "A Life Table of Pregnancy Terminations and Correlates of Fetal Loss," *Milbank Memorial Fund Quarterly*, 40:7-45 (January 1962).

26. G. W. Mellin, "Fetal Life Tables—A Means of Establishing Perinatal Rates of Risk" *J.A.M.A.*, 180:11-14 (April 1962).

27. E. L. Potter, "The Abortion Problem," *GP*, 19:105-113 (April 1959).

28. R. McIntosh, K. K. Merritt, M. R. Richards, M. H. Samuels, and M. R. Bellows, "Incidence of Congenital Malformations—A Study of 5,964 Pregnancies," *Pediatrics*, 14:505-520 (November 1954).

29. S. Shapiro, L. Ross, and H. S. Levine, "Relationship of Selected Prenatal Factors to Pregnancy Outcome and Congenital Anomalies," *Am. J. Pub. Health*, 55:268-282 (February 1965).

30. J. M. Bierman, E. Siegal, F. E. French, and K. Simonian, "Analysis of the Outcome of All Pregnancies in a Community," *Am. J. Obs. & Gyn.*, 91:37-45 (January 1965).

31. J. Yerushalmy, J. M. Bierman, D. H. Kemp, A. Connor, and F. E. French, "Longitudinal Studies of Pregnancy of the Island of Kauai, Territory of Hawaii: Part I. Analysis of Previous Reproductive History," *Am. J. Obs. & Gyn.*, 71:80-96 (January 1956).

Chapter 3. Factors Influencing Trend

1. For detailed analysis of fertility rates see monograph: C. V. Kiser, W. H. Grabill, and A. A. Campbell, *Trends and Variations in Fertility in the United States* (Cambridge, Mass.: Harvard University Press, 1968).

2. *Vital Statistics of the United States, 1964*, Vol. I (Washington, D. C.: National Center for Health Statistics, 1966).

3. "Advance Report, Final Natality Statistics, 1965," *Monthly Vital Statistics Rep.*, Vol. 15, No. 11 (February 1967).

4. U. S. Bureau of the Census, *Current Population Rep.*, Ser. P-60, No. 47 (September 1965).

5. H. E. Martz, "Illegitimacy and Dependency," *H. E. W. Indicators* (September 1963).

6. U. S. Bureau of the Census, *U. S. Census of Population, 1950*, Vol. IV, Part 5; *U. S. Census of Population, 1960, Subject Reports, Women by Number of Children Ever Born*, PC (2)-3A (1964); and *Current Population Rep.*, Ser. P-20, No. 46 (December 1953).

7. U. S. Bureau of the Census, *U. S. Census of Population, 1960*, Vol. II, Part 2B.

8. J. D. Cowhig and L. Beale, "Levels of Living among Whites and Nonwhites," *H. E. W. Indicators* (October 1965).

9. "Neonatal, Stillbirth, and Perinatal Mortality and Operative Procedures for Delivery by Hospitals and Regions, New York State, Exclusive of New York City, 1950-1954" (Albany: New York State Department of Health).

10. "Neonatal, Stillbirth, and Perinatal Mortality and Operative Procedures for Delivery by Hospitals and Regions, New York State, Exclusive of New York City, 1955-1959" (Albany: New York State Department of Health, 1964).

11. J. Yerushalmy, unpublished data for 1950–52 (School of Public Health, University of California, Berkeley).

12. A. Gittelsohn, unpublished data for 1959–60 (Albany: New York State Department of Health).

Chapter 4. *Pregnancy Outcome and Maternal Conditions and Complications*

1. W. A. Silverman, *Dunham's Premature Infants* (New York: Paul C. Hoeber, 1961).

2. R. E. L. Nesbitt, Jr., E. R. Schlesinger, and S. Shapiro, "Role of Preventive Medicine in Reduction of Infant and Perinatal Mortality," *Pub. Health Rep.*, 81:691-702 (August 1966).

3. E. L. Potter, *Pathology of the Fetus and Infant* (Chicago: Year Book Publishers, 1961).

4. R. E. L. Nesbitt, Jr., *Perinatal Loss in Modern Obstetrics* (Philadelphia: F. A. Davis Co., 1957), p. 22.

5. D. E. Reid, *A Textbook of Obstetrics* (Philadelphia: W. B. Saunders Co., 1962), p. 990.

6. B. M. Hibbard and T. N. A. Jeffcoate, "Abruptio Placentae," *Obs. & Gyn.*, 27:155–167 (February 1966).

7. E. S. Haller, R. E. L. Nesbitt, Jr., and G. W. Anderson, "Clinical and Pathologic Concepts of Gross Intracranial Hemorrhage in Perinatal Mortality," *Obs. & Gyn. Survey*, 11:179–204 (April 1956).

8. M. Siegal and M. Greenberg, "Fetal Death, Malformation and Prematurity after Maternal Rubella," *New England J. Med.*, 262:389–393 (February 25, 1960).

9. J. L. Sever, K. B. Nelson, and M. R. Gilkeson, "Rubella Epidemic, 1964: Effect on 6000 Pregnancies," *Am. J. Dis. Children*, 110:395–407 (October 1965).

10. V. Apgar, "Drugs in Pregnancy," *J.A.M.A.*, 190:840–841 (November 30, 1964).

11. G. Thomascheck, L. Schmidtke, and H. Genz, "Studies of Toxoplasma Infection in Pregnant Subjects and Morbidity of Their Progeny," *Ztschr. Geburtsh. u. Gynak.*, 156:182 (1961).

12. J. Warkany and H. Kalter, "Congenital Malformations," *New England J. Med.*, 265:993–1001, 1046–1052 (November 16 and 23, 1961).

13. L. Z. Cooper, R. H. Green, S. Krugman, J. P. Giles, and G. S. Mirick, "Neonatal Thrombocytopenic Purpura and Other Manifestations of Rubella Contracted in Utero," *Am. J. Dis. Children*, 110:416–427 (October 1965).

14. R. H. Green, M. R. Balsamo, J. P. Giles, S. Krugman, and G. S. Mirick, "Studies of the Natural History and Prevention of Rubella," *Am. J. Dis. Children*, 110:348–365 (October 1965).

15. M. M. Cohen, D. H. Weintraub, and A. M. Lilienfeld, "The Relationship of Pulmonary Hyaline Membrane to Certain Factors in Pregnancy and Delivery," *Pediatrics*, 26:42–50 (July 1960).

16. K. Benirschke, "Routes and Types of Infection in the Fetus and Newborn," *Am. J. Dis. Children*, 99:714–721 (June 1960).

17. V. J. Freda, J. G. Gorman, and W. Pollack, "Successful Prevention of Experimental RH Sensitization in Man with an Anti-RH Gamma$_2$ Globulin Antibody Preparation," *Transfusion*, 4:26–32 (January–February 1964).

18. R. J. McKay, Jr. and J. F. Lucey, "Neonatology," *New England J. Med.*, 270:1231–1235, 1292–1299 (June 4 and 11, 1964).

19. J. Warkany, B. B. Monroe, and B. S. Sutherland, "Intrauterine Growth Retardation," *Am. J. Dis. Children*, 102:249–279 (August 1961).

20. M. Terris, "The Epidemiology of Prematurity: Studies of Specific Etiologic Factors," in *Research Methodology and Needs in Perinatal Studies*, ed. S. S. Chipman et al. (Springfield, Ill.: Charles C. Thomas, 1966), pp. 207–242.

21. E. H. Kass, "Bacteriuria and Pyelonephritis of Pregnancy," *Arch. Internal Med.*, 105:194–198 (February 1960).

22. S. Shapiro, L. J. Ross, and H. S. Levine, "Relationship of Selected Prenatal Factors to Pregnancy Outcome and Congenital Anomalies," *Am. J. Pub. Health*, 55:268–282 (February 1965).

23. C. R. Lowe, "Effect of Mothers' Smoking Habits on Birth Weights of Their Children," *Brit. Med. J.*, 2:673–676 (October 10, 1959).

24. H. Goldstein, I. D. Goldberg, T. M. Frazier, and G. E. Davis, "Cigarette Smoking and Prematurity," *Pub. Health Rep.*, 79:553–560 (July 1964).

25. T. M. Frazier, "Cigarette Smoking and Birth Weight—A Review of the Baltimore City Study," in *Research Methodology and Needs in Perinatal Studies*, ed. S. S. Chipman et al. (Springfield, Ill.: Charles C. Thomas, 1966), pp. 70–87.

26. B. MacMahon, M. Alpert, and E. J. Salber, "Infant Weight and Parental Smoking Habits," *Am. J. of Epidemiology*, 82:247–261 (November 1965).

27. J. Yerushalmy, "Mother's Cigarette Smoking and Survival of Infant," *Am. J. Obs. & Gyn.*, 88:505–518 (February 15, 1964).

28. J. Yerushalmy, "Statistical Considerations and Evaluation of Epidemiological Evidence," in *Tobacco and Health*, ed. G. James and T. Rosenthal (Springfield, Ill.: Charles C. Thomas, 1962), pp. 208–229.

29. A. M. Lilienfeld, E. Parkhurst, R. Patton, and E. R. Schlesinger, "Accuracy of Supplemental Medical Information on Birth Certificates," *Pub. Health Rep.*, 66:191–198 (February 16, 1951).

30. "Evaluation of Obstetric and Related Data Recorded on Vital

Records and Hospital Records: District of Columbia, 1952," *Vital Statistics—Special Rep.*, Vol. 45, No. 13 (November 1957).

31. W. Haenszel, "The Incidence of Premature Births, Complications of Pregnancy and Labor, and Delivery Procedures and Their Relationship to Fetal Mortality," *Conn. State Med. J.*, 15:148 (February 1951).

32. C. L. Erhardt and E. M. Gold, "Cesarean Section in New York City—Incidence and Mortality During 1954–55," *Obs. & Gyn.*, 11:241–260 (March 1958).

33. A. M. Lilienfeld, B. Pasamanick, and M. Rogers, "Relationship Between Pregnancy Experience and the Development of Certain Neuropsychiatric Disorders in Childhood," *Am. J. Pub. Health*, 45:637–643 (May 1955).

34. "Community Obstetrical Study—A Project to Develop and Demonstrate Methods for an Evaluation of Obstetrical and Newborn Services of Hospitals in Hartford County, Conn.," Progress Report (Brooklyn, State University of New York, Downstate Medical Center, December 1960).

35. J. E. Hall, S. G. Kohl, and H. R. Schechter, "Current Aspects of Cesarean Section and Perinatal Mortality," *Am. J. Obs. & Gyn.*, 75:387–395 (February 1958).

36. Special tabulations through cooperation of New York State Department of Health, Albany, N.Y.

Chapter 5. International Comparisons

1. S. Shapiro and I. M. Moriyama, "International Trends in Infant Mortality and Their Implications for the United States," *Am. J. Pub. Health*, 53:747–760 (May 1963).

2. E. W. Curran, *International Conference on the Perinatal and Infant Mortality Problem of the United States*, Pub. Health Service Publ. No. 1000, Ser. 4. No. 3 (June 1966).

3. The reader is also referred to the following comprehensive review of international data on infant and perinatal mortality: H. C. Chase, *International Comparison of Perinatal and Infant Mortality: The United States and Six West European Countries*, Pub. Health Service Publ. No. 1000, Ser. 3, No. 6 (March 1967).

4. Unpublished background documents for the International Conference on the Perinatal and Infant Mortality Problem of the United States made available by the National Center for Health Statistics.

5. All comparisons in this section are based on unpublished data, reference 4.

6. Eric Soop, "Sweden's Infant Mortality and the Definition of Live Birth," *Svenska Lakartidningen*, 55:1148 (1958).

7. Unpublished figures from the collaborative project on cerebral palsy, mental retardation, and other sensory and nervous system disorders of infancy and childhood, sponsored by the National Institute of Neurological Diseases and Blindness.

8. B. G. Greenberg, "Differential Factors in Infant Mortality," in reference 2, pp. 10–15.

Part II. Maternal Mortality

Chapter 7. Trends and Recent Status

1. J. L. McKelvey, "Factors Contributing to the Decline of Maternal and Infant Mortality," *Bull. Maternal and Infant Health,* 7:5–11 (1960).

2. *Maternal Mortality in New York City: A Study of All Puerperal Deaths* (Cambridge, Mass.: Harvard University Press, 1933).

3. C. L. Mendelson, "Heart Disease and Pregnancy," *Clin. Obs. & Gyn.,* 4:603–629 (September 1961).

4. C. S. Burwell and J. Metcalfe, *Heart Disease and Pregnancy: Physiology and Management* (Boston: Little, Brown, 1958).

5. B. Buemann and E. Kragelunc, "Clinical Assessment of Heart Disease during Pregnancy," *Acta Obs. et Gyn. Scandinav.,* 41:56–79 (1962).

6. D. E. Cannell and C. P. Vernon, "Congenital Heart Disease and Pregnancy," *Am. J. Obs. & Gyn.,* 85:744–753 (March 15, 1963).

7. C. J. Lund, "Pregnancy and Heart Disease," *Clin. Obs. & Gyn.,* 1:41–52 (March 1958).

8. F. E. Bryans, "Vascular Accidents in Maternal Mortality," *Clin. Obs. & Gyn.,* 6:861–873 (December 1963).

9. H. L. Sheehan, "Causes of Maternal Death in Toxemia," *Clin. Obs. & Gyn.,* 1:397–403 (June 1958).

10. J. N. Walton, "Subarachnoid Hemorrhage in Pregnancy," *Brit. Med. J.,* 1:869–871 (April 18, 1953).

11. J. L. Barnes and K. H. Abbott, "Cerebral Complications Incurred during Pregnancy and the Puerperium," *California Med.,* 91:237–244 (November 1959).

12. B. Gomberg, "Spontaneous Subarachnoid Hemorrhage in Pregnancy Not Complicated by Toxemia," *Am. J. Obs. & Gyn.,* 77:430–437 (February 1959).

13. R. A. Hingson and L. M. Hellman, *Anaesthesia for Obstetrics* (Philadelphia: J. B. Lippincott Co., 1956).

14. C. Baechler and H. de Watteville, "Role of Peridural Anesthesia in Obstetrics at the Maternity Hospital in Geneva," *Gynaecologia,* 160:1–10 (1965).

15. E. D. Brown, T. Engel, and R. G. Doublas, "Paracervical Block Analgesia in Labor," *Obs. & Gyn.*, 26:195–200 (August 1965).

16. L. G. Roth, "Pregnancy and Viral Hepatitis," *Clin. Obs. & Gyn.*, 1:87–96 (March 1958).

17. A. Peretz, E. Paldi, S. Brandstaedter, and D. Barzilai, "Infectious Hepatitis in Pregnancy," *Obs. & Gyn.*, 14:435–441 (October 1959).

Chapter 8. Review and Perspectives

1. N. J. Eastman and L. M. Hellman, *Williams' Obstetrics*, 13th ed. (New York: Appleton-Century-Crofts, 1966), p. 8.

2. D. E. Reid, *A Textbook of Obstetrics* (Philadelphia: W. B. Saunders Co., 1962), p. 1009.

3. M. M. Donnelly, "Hemorrhage as a Cause of Maternal Death in Iowa," *J. Iowa State Med. Soc.*, 45:62–65 (February 1955).

4. J. C. Moir, "The Obstetrician Bids, and the Uterus Contracts," *Brit. Med. J.*, 2:1025–1029 (October 24, 1964).

5. J. F. Jewett, "Changing Maternal Mortality in Massachusetts," *New England J. Med.*, 256:395–400 (February 28, 1957).

6. E. J. DeCosta, "Cesarean Section and Other Obstetric Operations," in *Textbook of Obstetrics and Gynecology*, ed. D. N. Danforth (New York: Paul C. Hoeber, 1966), p. 672.

7. C. D. Rodgers, C. P. Wickard, and M. R. McCaskill, "Labor and Delivery without Terminal Anesthesia," *Obs. & Gyn.*, 17:92–98 (January 1961).

8. H. B. Monahan and E. C. Spencer, "Deterrents to Prenatal Care," *Children*, 9:114–119 (May–June 1962).

Part III. Childhood Mortality

Chapter 9. Trends and Recent Status

1. J. A. James, "The Later Health of Premature Infants: A Field for Further Study," *Pediatrics*, 22:154–160 (June 1958).

2. I. M. Moriyama, "The Change in Mortality Trend in the United States," *Vital and Health Statistics Analytical Studies*, Pub. Health Service Publ. No. 1000, Ser. 3, No. 1 (March 1964).

3. G. M. Wheatley, "Childhood Accidents," in *Accident Prevention: The Role of Physicians and Public Health Workers* (New York: Blakiston, 1961), pp. 69–79.

4. A. M. Gittelsohn and S. Milham, "Declining Incidence of Central Nervous System Anomalies in New York State," *Brit. J. Preventive and Social Med.*, 16:153–158 (July 1962).

Chapter 10. International Comparisons

1. M. Spiegelman, "Recent Mortality in Countries of Traditionally Low Mortality," *Proceedings of World Population Conference, 1965* (New York: United Nations, 1967), II, 375.

2. H. Campbell, *Changes in Mortality Trends: England and Wales*, Pub. Health Service Publ. No. 1000, Ser. 3, No. 3 (November 1965).

Part IV. Health Services and Resources

Chapter 12. Health Services

1. Quoted from W. G. Smillie, *Public Health: Its Promise for the Future* (New York: Macmillan, 1955), p. 252.

2. E. R. Schlesinger, *Health Services for the Child* (New York: McGraw-Hill, 1953).

3. M. McMahon and C. L. Erhardt, "New York City Department of Health: Highlights of the First 100 Years," *Pub. Health Rep.*, 81:87–107 (January 1966).

4. E. R. Schlesinger, "The Sheppard-Towner Era: A Prototype Case Study in Federal-State Relationships," *Am. J. Pub. Health*, 57:1034 (June 1967).

5. M. Tayback and H. Wallace, "Maternal and Child Health Services and Urban Economics," *Pub. Health Rep.*, 77:827–833 (October 1962).

6. Report to the President: *A Proposed Program for National Action to Combat Mental Retardation* (Washington, D.C.: The President's Panel on Mental Retardation, October 1962).

7. *Projects Funded under the Maternal and Child Health and Crippled Children's Services Research Grants Program* (Washington, D.C.: Children's Bureau 1966).

8. E. Davens, "A View of Health Services for Mothers and Children," *Children*, 12:47–54 (March–April 1965).

9. J. B. Richmond, "Communities in Action: A Report on Project Head Start," *Pediatrics*, 37:905–912 (June 1966).

10. *Grants for Comprehensive Health Services for Children and Youth: Policies and Procedures* (Washington, D.C.: Children's Bureau, 1965).

11. J. W. B. Douglas and R. E. Waller, "Air Pollution and Respiratory Infection in Children," *Brit. J. Prev. and Soc. Med.*, 20:1–8 (January 1966).

12. "Public Health Nutrition Services for Children in the United States: A Resource for the Pediatrician," Report of Committee on Nutrition, American Academy of Pediatrics, *Pediatrics*, 36:789–803 (November 1965).

13. C. Stockburger, "The Migrant Child—Where is He?" *National Committee for the Day Care of Children Newsletter*, Vol. 6, No. 3 (January 1966).

14. *Manual of Standards in Obstetric-Gynecologic Practice*, 2d ed. (Chicago: American College of Obstetricians and Gynecologists, April 1965).

15. E. R. Schlesinger, "The Role of Community Health Services in Meeting the Needs of Mothers and Children," *Am. J. Pub. Health*, 49: 585–589 (May 1959).

16. Personal communication from Arthur J. Lesser, Children's Bureau, Washington, D.C. (February 21, 1967).

17. J. W. Eliot, C. Houser, and R. White, "The Development of Family Planning Services by State and Local Health Departments in the United States," *Am. J. Pub. Health*, 56:6–16, Part II (January 1966).

18. H. Abramson, "Comments from the Pediatric Point of View," in *Symposium on the Placenta*, Birth Defects Original Article Ser., The National Foundation, 1:92–95 (April 1965).

19. *Standards and Recommendations for Hospital Care of Newborn Infants* (Evanston, Ill.: American Academy of Pediatrics, 1964).

20. R. Guthrie and A. Susi, "A Simple Phenylalanine Method for Detecting Phenylketonuria in Large Populations of Newborn Infants," *Pediatrics*, 32:338–343 (September 1963).

21. K. Patau, "The Chromosomes," in *New Directions in Human Genetics*, Birth Defects Original Article Ser., The National Foundation, 1,2:71–74 (December 1965).

22. E. Jolly and H. L. Blum, "The Role of Public Health in Genetic Counseling," *Am. J. Pub. Health*, 56:186–190 (February 1966).

23. W. A. Silverman, *Dunham's Premature Infants* (New York: Paul C. Hoeber, 1961).

24. S. Milham, "Congenital Malformations Surveillance System Based on Vital Records," *Pub. Health Rep.*, 78:448–452 (May 1963).

25. H. H. Mitchell, "School Medical Service in Perspective," *Pediatrics*, 35:1011–1020 (June 1965).

26. G. James and H. Jacobziner, "A Pediatric Health Service—An Extension of the Child Health Conference," *Am. J. Pub. Health*, 55:982–993 (July 1965).

27. *Comprehensive Health Care: A Challenge to American Communities*, Report of the Task Force on Comprehensive Personal Health Services, National Commission on Community Health Services (Washington, D.C.: Public Affairs Press, 1967).

28. S. D. Pomrinse and M. S. Goldstein, "The 1959 Survey of Group Practice," *Am. J. Pub. Health*, 51:671–682 (May 1961).

29. E. M. Burns, "Social Policy and the Health Services: The Choices Ahead," *Am. J. Pub. Health*, 57:199–212 (February 1967).

Chapter 13. Facilities, Personnel, and Economics

1. *Hospitals* (Guide Issues), *J. Am. Hosp. Assoc.* (August 1949 and August 1963).
2. *Hill-Burton State Plan Data—A National Summary as of January 1, 1962*, Pub. Health Service Publ. No. 930-F2 (1962).
3. A. J. Lesser, "Accent on Prevention through Improved Service," *Children*, 11:13–18 (January–February 1964).
4. P. Q. Peterson and M. Y. Pennell, "Medical Specialists," Sec. 14 in *Health Manpower Source Book*, Pub. Health Service Publ. No. 263 (1962).
5. M. Y. Pennell and K. I. Baker, "Location of Manpower in 8 Health Occupations, 1962," Sec. 19 in *Health Manpower Source Book*, Pub. Health Service Publ. No. 263 (1965).
6. E. F. Daily, "Maternity Care in the United States—Planning for the Future," *Am. J. Obs. & Gyn.*, 49:128–143 (January 1945).
7. L. M. Hellman, "Nurse-Midwifery—An Experiment in Maternity Care." Paper presented at meeting of American College of Obstetricians and Gynecologists, May 1964.
8. Personal communication from O. W. Anderson. Data derived from household survey (1963) conducted by National Opinion Research Center for Health Information Foundation, University of Chicago.
9. "Statement of the Executive Board of the American Academy of Pediatrics," *Pediatrics*, 37:2–3 (January 1966).
10. H. M. Wallace, "Physician Manpower for Mothers and Children," *Am. J. Dis. Children*, 106:11–18 (July 1963).
11. "Manpower in the 1960's" Sec. 18 in *Health Manpower Source Book*, Pub. Health Service Publ. No. 263 (1964).
12. W. H. Stewart and V. V. Vahey, "Nursing Services to the Sick at Home in Selected Communities," *Am. J. Pub. Health*, 54:407–416 (March 1964).
13. M. W. Thomas, *The Practice of Nurse-Midwifery in the United States* (Washington, D.C.: Children's Bureau, 1965).
14. *Standards of Child Health Care* (Evanston, Ill.: Council on Pediatric Practice, American Academy of Pediatrics, 1967).
15. *Health Manpower: Action to Meet Community Needs*, report of the Task Force on Health Manpower, National Commission on Community Health Services (Washington, D.C.: Public Affairs Press, 1967).
16. H. R. Domke and G. Coffey, "The Neighborhood-Based Public Health Worker: Additional Manpower for Public Health Services," *Am. J. Pub. Health*, 56:603–608 (April 1966).

17. L. S. Reed and R. S. Hanft, "National Health Expenditures, 1950–64," *Social Security Bull.* (January 1966).

18. O. W. Anderson, P. Collette, and J. J. Feldman, *Family Expenditure Patterns for Personal Health Service, 1953 and 1958: Nationwide Surveys*, HIF Research Series No. 14 (New York: Health Information Foundation, 1960); and personal communication from O. W. Anderson.

19. O. W. Anderson, P. Collette, and J. J. Feldman, "Trends in Personal Health Spending," *Progress in Health Services* (Health Information Foundation, University of Chicago), Vol. 14, No. 5 (November–December 1965).

20. R. Andersen and O. W. Anderson, "Maternity Care and Costs: A Ten-Year Trend," *Progress in Health Services* (Health Information Foundation, University of Chicago), Vol. 15, No. 2 (March–April 1966), pp. 1–6.

21. C. W. Wilder, *Hospital Discharges and Length of Stay*, Pub. Health Service Publ. No. 1000, Ser. 10, No. 30 (June 1966).

22. R. Andersen and O. W. Anderson, *A Decade of Health Services* (Chicago, Ill.: University of Chicago Press, 1967).

INDEX

ABO incompatibility, 91. *See also* Hemolytic disease

Abnormal pulmonary ventilation: infant deaths from, 16; diagnosis, 26; classification, 26

Abortions: maternal mortality rates and rank order, 148, 149–150, 162; self-induced, 150; color, 150, 151; geographic areas, 154

Accidents: role in infant deaths, 27, 138; color and geographic areas, 40–41, 204–205, 215; sudden deaths attributed to, 27 125n; international comparisons, 125, 211, 212; childhood mortality rates and rank order, 176, 178, 182–183, 214; color, 178, 179, 183–184, 205, 214; sex, 180, 181, 184, 214; factors affecting, 184–185; types of, 185–188, 204–205, 216–217

Adolescents, health programs for, 139, 235, 243

Age differentials: infant mortality rate, 6–14, 20–25, 29–30, 133 (*see also* Neonatal, Perinatal, Post-neonatal mortality rates); maternal, relation to birth weight and neonatal mortality rates, 56–62, 128–129, 134, 135, 138, in fetal deaths, 74, 135, 156, in birth rates and birth-order rates, 78–79, 81–82, 134, 135, in obstetrical complication rates, 94–97, 101, 135, 154, in Caesarean section rates, 101–102, 105, 135, in maternal mortality rate, 146–147, 151, 156, 157, 162; childhood mortality rates, 167–171, 175–178, 189–190, 192, 197, 213 (*see also* Preschool children; School-age children); in personal health costs, 264–266

Air pollution, relation to childhood respiratory infections, 233

American Academy of Pediatrics: standards and recommendations, 240, 254, 259

American Association for Study and Prevention of Infant Mortality, 224

American Board of Obstetrics and Gynecology: efforts to improve obstetrical care, 159; diplomates, 253, 255, 256

American Board of Pediatrics, diplomates, 256

American Board of Preventive Medicine, 256

American Child Health Association, 224

American College of Obstetricians and Gynecologists: efforts to improve obstetrical care, 159–160; standards, 235

American Medical Association, 224

Anesthesia: maternal deaths from, 155–156; advances in, 155–156, 161–162

Anoxia, fetal, causes of, 89–90

Antibiotics, influence on mortality rates: infant, 15; maternal, 146; contagious diseases of childhood, 190; childhood, 190, 194–199; rheumatic fever and rheumatic heart disease, 194–196, 197; nephritis and nephrosis, 197; appendicitis, 198; nutritional deficiencies, 199; puerperal sepsis, 237

Appalachian Regional Development Act, 230

Appendicitis: childhood mortality rate and rank order, 177, 198, 215, factors in reduction, 198, color and sex, 198–199, in U.S. and England, 212

Arteriosclerotic heart disease, 154

Asphyxia: postnatal mortality rate, 17, 25, 26; role in infant deaths, 27; geographic area and color, 40, 41; intrauterine, relation to hyaline membrane deaths, 90

Asymptomatic bacteriuria, relation to pregnancy loss and damage, 92

Atelectasis: infant mortality rate, 17, 25-26; role in infant deaths, 27; geographic area and color, 41

Australia, mortality rates: infant, 114, 117; neonatal, 119; maternal, 158; childhood, 206, 207, 208

Babies Hospital (New York City) Fetal Life Study, 69

Belgium, mortality rates: infant, 117, 207; childhood, 207, 208

Birth injuries, infant mortality rates and rank order, 17, 25–27; sex, color, and age, 29–30; geographic area and color, 40; international comparisons, 124

Birth order: relation to low birth weight, 56–59; neonatal mortality rates, 59–60, 81, 128–129, 134, 135, 138; fetal deaths, 60–61, 74, 135; distributions, 78–79, 81, 134; obstetrical complications rate, 96–97, 135; Caesarean section rate, 101–102, 104–105, 135; international comparisons, 128–129

Birth rate: effect of changes on infant mortality rate, 5–6; relation to birth order and maternal age, 78–79; color, 81; effect on